Sleep in Critical Illness

Gerald L. Weinhouse • John W. Devlin
Editors

Sleep in Critical Illness

Physiology, Assessment, and Its Importance to ICU Care

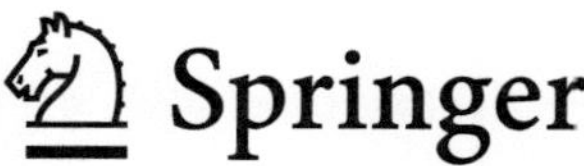 Springer

Editors
Gerald L. Weinhouse
Division of Pulmonary and Critical
Care Medicine
Brigham and Women's Hospital
Boston, MA, USA

John W. Devlin
Bouve College of Health Sciences
Northeastern University and Division of
Pulmonary and Critical Care Medicine
Brigham and Women's Hospital
Boston, MA, USA

ISBN 978-3-031-06446-3   ISBN 978-3-031-06447-0   (eBook)
https://doi.org/10.1007/978-3-031-06447-0

This Springer imprint is published by the registered company Springer Nature Switzerland AG
The registered company address is: Gewerbestrasse 11, 6330 Cham, Switzerland

Preface

The fields of critical care medicine and sleep medicine were both born in the early 1950s but have very different origins. Building on lessons learned from earlier decades of trauma care during global warfare, the world's first intensive care unit opened in 1953 in Copenhagen as hospital clinicians and administrators sought the most efficient setting to manage several hundred polio patients, many of whom needed artificial respiration and specialized care. This geographic cohorting of acutely ill patients helped launch the field of critical care medicine. While interest in sleep and dreams can be traced back thousands of years, it is through the development of electroencephalography in the late 1920s, and a number of brilliant scientific observations in subsequent decades, that sleep would transcend its image as a passive state pondered by philosophers and written about by poets to become recognized as an essential physiologic state to be studied by scientists. The discovery of rapid eye movement sleep in the early 1950's and the first publication with the terms REM and NREM sleep in 1957 by Dement and Kleitman were foundational to the field [1].

It wasn't until the turn of this century, however, that the growing fields of sleep and critical care medicine would meet. While observational studies at the end of the last century suggested patients slept poorly during critical illness, the significance of these findings was not yet realized. Moreover, prior to the 2000s, the more severely ill patients admitted to the ICU were deeply sedated in an effort, viewed at the time as being compassionate, to relieve stress and pain and facilitate the safe delivery of interventions. While deep sedation may have created an illusion of restful sleep to ICU clinicians and patients' families, it was masking the physiologic and clinical signs of disrupted sleep and potentially contributing to increased delirium, reduced ICU survival, prolonged ICU stays and worse post-ICU cognitive, psychologic, and functional outcomes.

Seminal studies by Cooper [2], Freedman [3], and Gabor [4] would serve as an epiphany for clinicians and investigators. These researchers discovered patients in the ICU had severely fragmented sleep with a relative lack of deep sleep stages. The importance of this finding has been bolstered over the past 20 years. Patients able to self-report sleep quality frequently complain of poor sleep throughout their ICU stay. The ICU factors that disrupt sleep and alter circadian rhythmicity are now well-established and ICU practice guidelines recommend the use of non-pharmacologic sleep improvement efforts [5]. However, evidence gaps regarding our understanding of the ICU and post-ICU outcomes of disrupted sleep, how to evaluate sleep in critically ill patients, the inter-relationship between disrupted sleep and delirium, and the interventions that have the greatest impact to improve sleep in critically ill adults continue to inspire translational and clinical research efforts.

Over the past 10 years, the number of papers cited in PubMed pertaining to sleep in the ICU has increased nearly ten-fold. To paraphrase a quote from the brilliant and visionary J. Allan Hobson, 'we have learned more in the past six years about sleep during critical illness then in the preceding six thousand years'.

This book is an homage to the pioneers who laid the foundations for the present generation of ICU sleep scientific inquiry. This book also honors those who carry the torch, many of whom kindly offered their time and expertise to author chapters and who continue to advance the science of sleep and circadian biology as it pertains to critical illness recovery. But most of all, this book is dedicated to our ICU patients who have suffered and continue to suffer the effects of acute critical illness and its aftermath which can have such a profound impact on their quality of life. It is also dedicated with gratitude to all those selfless patients and their surrogate decision makers who consented to their participation in the studies that have helped move the field forward.

"The best bridge between despair and hope is a good night's sleep."

E. Joseph Cossman, American inventor, businessman, entrepreneur and author

References

1. Dement W, Kleitman N. The relation of eye movements during sleep to dream activity: An objective method for the study of dreaming. Journal of Experimental Psychology 1957; 53:339–346.

2. Cooper AB, Thornley KS, Young GB, et al. Sleep in critically ill patients requiring mechanical ventilation. Chest 2000;117:809–18.

3. Freedman NS, Gazendam J, Levan L, et al. Abnormal sleep/wake cycles and the effect of environmental noise on sleep disruption in the intensive care unit. Am J Respir Crit Care Med 2001;163:451–7.

4. Gabor J, Cooper A, Crombach S, et al. Contribution of the intensive care unit environment to sleep disruption in mechanically ventilated patients and healthy subjects. Am J Crit Care Med 2003;167:708–15.

5. Devlin JW, Skrobik Y, Gelinas C, et al. Clinical Practice Guidelines for the Prevention and Management of Pain, Agitation/Sedation, Delirium, Immobility, and Sleep Disruption in Adult Patients in the ICU. Crit Care Med 2018;46(9):e825–e73.

Boston, MA, USA

Gerald L. Weinhouse
John W. Devlin

Contents

List of Contributors

Patricia S. Andrews Department of Psychiatry and Behavioral Sciences, Critical Illness, Brain dysfunction and Survivorship (CIBS) Center, Vanderbilt University Medical Center, Nashville, TN, USA

Florian Beck Department of Anesthesia and Intensive Care Medicine, Liege University Hospital, Liege, Belgium

Vincent Bonhomme Departments of Anesthesia and Intensive Care Medicine and Anesthesia, Liege University Hospital and Anesthesia and Perioperative Neuroscience Laboratory, GIGA-Consciousness Thematic Unit, GIGA-Research, Liege University, Liege, Belgium

Karen J. Bosma Department of Medicine, Division of Critical Care Medicine, Schulich School of Medicine and Dentistry, University of Western Ontario, London, ON, Canada

Caitlin S. Brown Department of Pharmacy, Mayo Clinic, Rochester, MN, USA

Patricia J. Checinski Department of Medicine, Vanderbilt University Medical Center, Nashville, TN, USA

Makayla Cordoza, PhD, RN School of Nursing, University of Pennsylvania, Philadelphia, PA, USA

Carolyn D'Ambrosio Section of Pulmonary, Critical Care and Sleep Medicine, Yale University School of Medicine, New Haven, CT, USA

John W. Devlin Bouve College of Health Sciences, Northeastern University and Division of Pulmonary and Critical Care Medicine, Brigham and Women's Hospital, Boston, MA, USA

David F. Dinges, PhD Division of Sleep and Chronobiology, Department of Psychiatry, University of Pennsylvania, Philadelphia, PA, USA

Xavier Drouot Centre d'Investigation Clinique INSERM 1402, Team Acute Lung Injury, VEntilatory support and Sleep, Centre Hospitalier Universitaire de Poitiers, and Université de Poitiers, Poitiers, France

Rosalind Elliott Malcolm Fisher Intensive Care Unit, Royal North Shore Hospital, Northern Sydney Local Health District and Faculty of Health, University of Technology Sydney, Sydney, Australia

E. Wesley Ely Critical Illness, Brain dysfunction and Survivorship (CIBS) Center, Division of Allergy, Pulmonary, and Critical Care Medicine, Vanderbilt University Medical Center, and Geriatric Research Education and Clinical Center (GRECC), VA Tennessee Valley Healthcare System, Nashville, TN, USA

Lauren E. Estep Division of Pulmonary, Allergy, Critical Care and Sleep Medicine, University of Arizona, Tucson, AZ, USA

Erica B. Feldman Division of Pulmonary, Critical Care, Sleep Medicine and Physiology, UC San Diego School of Medicine, La Jolla, CA, USA

Gilles L. Fraser (Ret.) Professor of Medicine, Tufts University, Boston, MA, USA

Brian K. Gehlbach Departments of Internal Medicine and Neurology, University of Iowa, Iowa City, IA, USA

Olivia Gosseries Coma Science Group, GIGA-Consciousness Thematic Unit, GIGA-Research, Liege University, Liege, Belgium

Mojdeh S. Heavner Department of Pharmacy Practice and Science, School of Pharmacy, University of Maryland, Baltimore, MD, USA

Kimia Honarmand Department of Medicine, Division of Critical Care Medicine, Schulich School of Medicine and Dentistry, University of Western Ontario, London, ON, Canada

Christopher W. Jones, PhD Division of Sleep and Chronobiology, Department of Psychiatry, University of Pennsylvania, Philadelphia, PA, USA

Biren B. Kamdar Division of Pulmonary, Critical Care, Sleep Medicine and Physiology, UC San Diego School of Medicine, La Jolla, CA, USA

Melissa P. Knauert Department of Internal Medicine, Section of Pulmonary, Critical Care and Sleep Medicine, Yale School of Medicine, New Haven, CT, USA

Amy S. Korwin Department of Internal Medicine, Section of Pulmonary, Critical Care and Sleep Medicine, Yale School of Medicine, New Haven, CT, USA

Sapna R. Kudchadkar Departments of Anesthesiology & Critical Care Medicine, Pediatrics, and Physical Medicine and Rehabilitation, Johns Hopkins University School of Medicine, Baltimore, MD, USA

Patricia R. Louzon Department of Pharmacy, AdventHealth Orlando, Orlando, FL, USA

Jennifer L. Martin VA Greater Los Angeles Healthcare System, Geriatric Research, Education and Clinical Center and David Geffen School of Medicine at the University of California, Los Angeles, CA, USA

Sharon McKinley University of Technology Sydney, Sydney, Australia

Marie-Anne Melone Department of Internal Medicine, University of Iowa, Iowa City, IA, USA

Department of Pulmonary, Thoracic Oncology and Respiratory Intensive Care, Rouen University Hospital, Rouen, France

Isabel Okinedo Department of Neuroscience, Vanderbilt University, Nashville, TN, USA

Sairam Parthasarathy Division of Pulmonary, Allergy, Critical Care & Sleep Medicine, University of Arizona College of Medicine, Tucson, AZ, USA

Mallory A. Perry Children's Hospital of Philadelphia Research Institute, Philadelphia, PA, USA

Alexander O. Pile Department of Biological Sciences, University of California San Diego, La Jolla, CA, USA

Julia Pilowsky Malcolm Fisher Intensive Care Unit, Royal North Shore Hospital, Northern Sydney Local Health District and Faculty of Health, University of Technology Sydney, Sydney, Australia

Margaret Pisani Section of Pulmonary, Critical Care and Sleep Medicine, Yale University School of Medicine, New Haven, CT, USA

Alejandro A. Rabinstein Division of Neurology, Mayo Clinic, Rochester, MN, USA

Shawniqua Williams Roberson Critical Illness, Brain dysfunction and Survivorship (CIBS) Center, Departments of Neurology and Biomedical Engineering, Vanderbilt University, Nashville, TN, USA

Yoanna Skrobik Department of Medicine, McGill University, Quebec, Canada

Wade Stedman Faculty of Medicine, University of Sydney, Sydney, Australia

Lauren Tobias Veterans Affairs Connecticut Healthcare System, West Haven, CT, USA

Section of Pulmonary, Critical Care and Sleep Medicine, Yale University School of Medicine, New Haven, CT, USA

Paula L. Watson Department of Medicine, Division of Allergy, Pulmonary, and Critical Care, Division of Sleep Disorders, Vanderbilt University Medical Center, Nashville, TN, USA

Gerald L. Weinhouse Division of Pulmonary and Critical Care, Brigham and Women's Hospital and School of Medicine, Harvard University, Boston, MA, USA

Characteristics of Sleep in Critically Ill Patients: Part I: Sleep Fragmentation and Sleep Stage Disruption

Patricia J. Checinski and Paula L. Watson

1 Introduction

Sleep is an essential physiologic function that is severely altered in critically ill adults. Poor sleep quality is one of the most common complaints of patients who survive their critical illness [1]. Patients' complaints include trouble initiating and maintaining sleep and frequent awakenings with difficulty returning to sleep. These sleep disruptions not only lead to emotional distress but may also contribute to cognitive dysfunction, intensive care unit (ICU) delirium, impaired immune function, prolonged mechanical ventilation, and cardiac disorders (see chapters "Biologic Effects of Disrupted Sleep", "Sleep Disruption and Its Relationship with Delirium: Electroencephalographic Perspectives", "Sleep Disruption and Its Relationship with Delirium: Clinical Perspectives", "ICU Sleep Disruption and Its Relationship to ICU Outcomes" and "Long-Term Outcomes: Sleep in Survivors of Critical Illness"). Sleep is regarded as a potentially modifiable risk factor influencing these clinical outcomes and sleep promotion is now recognized as an important factor in improving the care of critically ill adults [2]. Both subjective measurements, such as nurse and patient questionnaires, and objective measurements, such as polysomnography (PSG) and actigraphy, have been used to assess sleep quantity and characteristics in critically ill adults and to determine how sleep in the ICU differs from the normal sleep of healthy individuals (see chapter "Methods for Routine Sleep Assessment and Monitoring").

P. J. Checinski
Department of Medicine, Vanderbilt University Medical Center, Nashville, TN, USA
e-mail: patricia.checinski@vumc.org

P. L. Watson (✉)
Department of Medicine, Division of Allergy, Pulmonary, and Critical Care, Division of Sleep Disorders, Vanderbilt University Medical Center, Nashville, TN, USA
e-mail: paula.l.watson@vumc.org

G. L. Weinhouse, J. W. Devlin (eds.), *Sleep in Critical Illness*,
https://doi.org/10.1007/978-3-031-06447-0_1

1

Sleep investigations of critically ill adults have evaluated heterogenous populations (e.g., medical vs. surgical, low vs. high severity of illness) and have been performed at various stages of hospitalization. While some ICU studies have evaluated patients while they were sedated and mechanically ventilated, others have assessed patients supported on non-invasive ventilation as well as those who transitioned through the ICU quickly. Studies which used subjective assessment tools have concluded that sleep quality in the ICU is significantly decreased compared with what patients consider to be their normal sleep. Patients have reported that noise, particularly alarms and staff conversations, are the most disruptive environmental factors (see chapter "Risk Factors for Disrupted Sleep in the ICU"). Studies which used objective assessment tools have demonstrated variable total sleep times, changes in sleep architecture, severe sleep fragmentation, as well as alterations in circadian rhythm (see chapter "Characteristics of Sleep in Critically Ill Patients. Part II: Circadian Rhythm Disruption").

2 Total Sleep Time

Most ICU sleep studies demonstrate patients have a relatively normal total sleep time (TST) over the entire 24-h day, but wide variations exist both within study populations and between studies [3–6]. Sleep for these patients is often severely fragmented and occurs in short episodes that are distributed throughout the night and day. Cooper et al. reported the sleep characteristics of 20 intubated, mechanically ventilated ICU patients and categorized them into three groups—those with disrupted sleep (EEG features of both NREM and REM sleep), those with atypical sleep (EEG features intermediate between sleep and coma), and those in a coma [3]. In both the disrupted sleep and atypical sleep groups, the average TSTs over a 24-h period was normal (7 and 10 h, respectively) but there was marked variability in the TST among individual patients (Fig. 1).

Across ICU studies evaluating patients with varying frequencies of mechanical ventilation (MV) use, there does not appear to be a strong correlation between TST and MV use. For example, two ICU PSG studies evaluating primary mechanically ventilated adults (91% and 100%, respectively) reported a normal TST, while another study evaluating only mechanically ventilated adults showed decreased TST [3, 4, 7]. In PSG studies with few mechanically ventilated patients, one study (31% MV rate) found patients had a normal TST while another (24% MV rate) reported decreased TST [6, 8]. Finally, one study (54% MV rate) failed to find a difference in TST based on MV use [5]. Following extubation, the TST also remains low and is most reduced in patients who had received continuous sedation during the period of intubation. One study found a median TST of only 2.4 (IQR 1.1–4.2) hours during 16.7 (IQR 14.9–17.4) hours of PSG assessment in the 24 h after extubation [9].

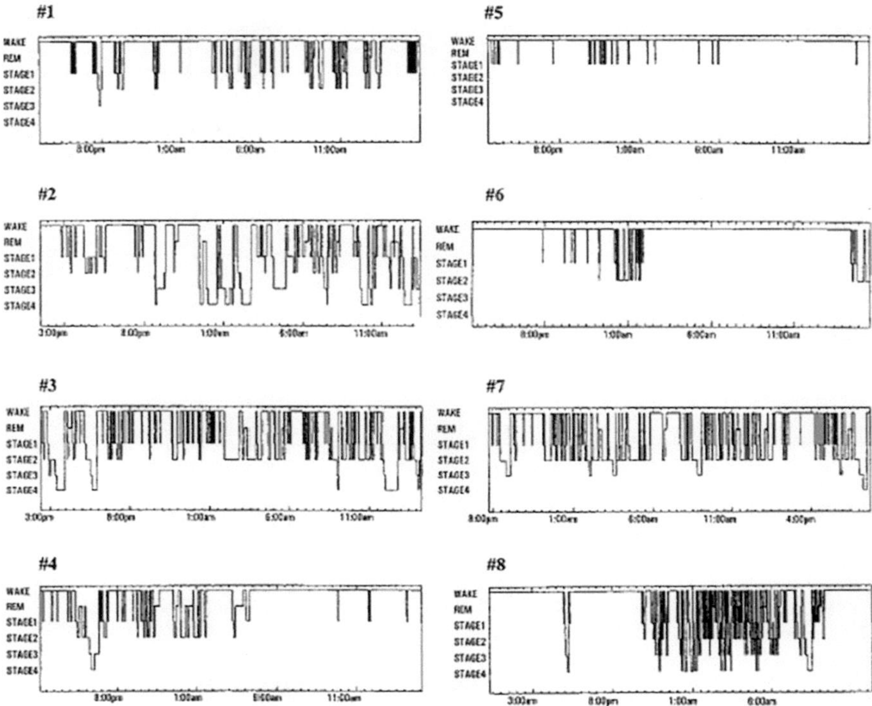

Fig. 1 24-h hypnograms of ICU patients. Sleep during critical care illness is severely fragmented and distributed evenly across 24 h. Oftentimes, a clear circadian rhythm is not seen in these patients (Adapted with permission from Cooper AB, Thornley KS, Young GB, Slutsky AS, Stewart TE, Hanly PJ. Sleep in critically ill patients requiring mechanical ventilation. Chest. 2000;117(3):809–818)

A systematic review of 13 ICU studies employing actigraphy rather than PSG reported a mean nocturnal recorded nighttime TST ranging from 4.4 to 7.8 h [10]. Over the entire 24-h period, the TST ranged from 7.1 to 12.1 h.

2.1 Challenges with TST Measurement

Important challenges exist with quantifying TST in critically ill adults: As discussed in chapter "Atypical Sleep and Pathologic Wakefulness", awake patients can have EEG features of sleep, a phenomenon termed pathologic wakefulness. Several studies have demonstrated the presence of EEG delta wave activity (characteristic of deep, slow wave NREM sleep) in patients who were awake and interactive, a finding which may lead to an erroneous TST measurement [3, 5, 11, 12]. Watson et al. studied 37 mechanically ventilated adults in an effort to describe atypical PSG findings and to assist in developing a pilot scoring scheme for sleep in the ICU [12]. Key

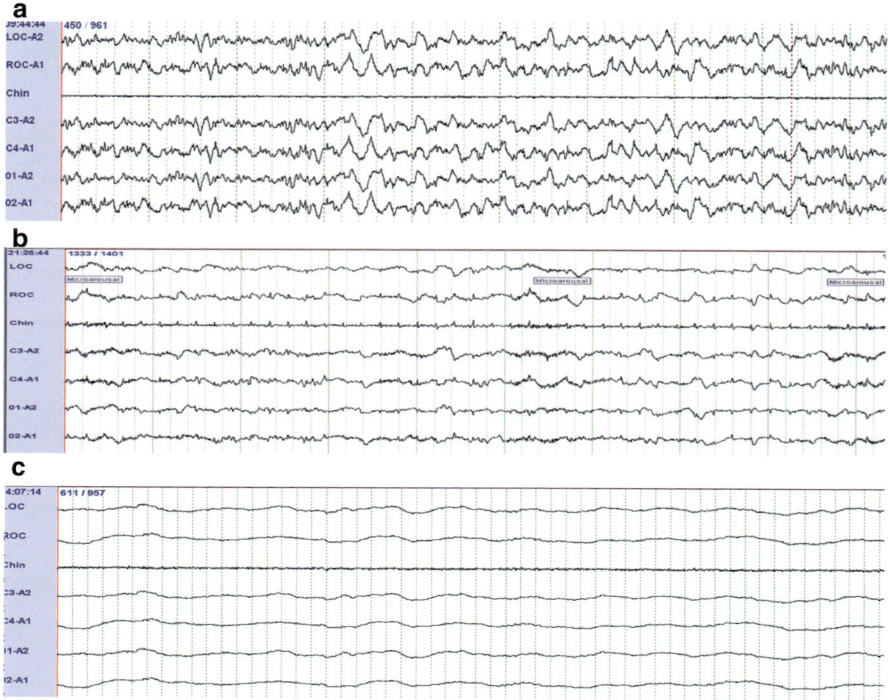

Fig. 2 (a) Example of pathologic wakefulness. Patient awake and following commands but EEG shows large percentage of delta waves consistent with N3 sleep. (b) Comatose patient with EEG pattern that would be labeled stage N1 sleep if standard AASM scoring criteria is used. (c) EEG from comatose patient showing complete lack of EEG/cortical activity (Adapted with permission from Watson PL, Pandharipande P, Gehlbach BK, et al. Atypical sleep in ventilated patients: empirical electroencephalography findings and the path toward revised ICU sleep scoring criteria. Crit Care Med. 2013;41(8):1958–1967)

findings include a predominance of theta activity (a frequency usually indicating sleep) in patients who were awake and interactive as well as greater than 20% delta activity [a frequency seen in SWS (slow wave sleep)] in one patient who was following simple instructions (Fig. 2a). In addition, comatose patients were found to have variable EEG patterns ranging from findings consistent with light sleep, stages N1 and N2 sleep, (Fig. 2b) to continuous isoelectric activity (Fig. 2c). The lack of correlation between EEG and physical exam findings can make the accurate assessment of sleep extremely difficult. A behavioral assessment of patients should therefore accompany all EEG recording when TST is being quantified. Continued work on developing a schema for scoring of sleep in the critically ill will help with future assessments of TST and quantification of time spent in the various sleep stages.

Actigraphy uses gross motor activity as an estimate of sleep and thus is unable to distinguish between physiologic sleep and motionless wakefulness. In critically ill patients, the use of physical restraints, sedating medications, and the more direct effects of their illness may cause a decrease in motor activity making this method of sleep measurement less reliable. Interestingly, even ICU patients who are young, non-mechanically ventilated, non-sedated, and non-restrained, have been found to have decreased activity compared to hospitalized patients not admitted to the ICU [13]. Studies comparing actigraphy to PSG, bispectral index (BIS), nurse assessment, and patient assessment have all found that actigraphy overestimates TST [14–19].

The variability in TST among adults admitted to the ICU is attributable to differences in admission diagnoses, severity of illness, use of mechanical ventilation, and medication exposure. Critically ill adults often receive sedating medications including benzodiazepines, dexmedetomidine, opioids, and propofol. As highlighted in chapters "Normal Sleep Compared to Altered Consciousness during Sedation" and "Effects of Common ICU Medications on Sleep", sedation is physiologically different from sleep and the use of sedating medications may result in decreased patient activity and altered EEG features of sleep that suggest TST is longer than it really is [20].

3   Sleep Fragmentation

3.1   Studies Employing Objective Assessment Methods

While the reported ICU TST in the literature varies, adults admitted to the ICU have consistently been found to experience significantly fragmented sleep, where sleep is distributed across the night and daytime periods, with a large proportion of sleep occurring during the day [3–9]. Arousals (an abrupt increase in EEG frequency lasting 3–15 s) and awakenings (EEG activation lasting >15 s) frequently occur in the ICU. Sleep fragmentation can be extreme; one ICU study found patients experienced 27 arousals per hour and an average duration of continuous sleep of only 3 min [5]. Patients in another study slept for just an average of 15 min at a time [4]. Arousals and awakenings also remain frequent following extubation; one study reported 25 events (arousals and awakenings) per hour [9]. Arousal frequency increases equally between the day and night [3]. Knauert et al. found similar results in patients with atypical sleep, with 32.3 NREM arousals per hour at night and 34.6 NREM arousals per hour in the daytime [8].

When patients with disrupted sleep were compared with those with atypical sleep in one ICU cohort study, both groups were found to have sleep distributed throughout the 24 h (disrupted group: 54% daytime and 46% nighttime; atypical group: 60% daytime and 40% nighttime) [3]. Figure 1 depicts hypnograms for the eight patients in the disrupted sleep group and illustrates the varying degrees of sleep fragmentation between individual patients. Freedman et al. reported similar findings with 57% of sleep occurring during the day and 43% at night [4]. Hypnograms illustrating the sleep distribution of these patients are shown in Fig. 3. The increase in daytime sleep has been further documented by several other studies

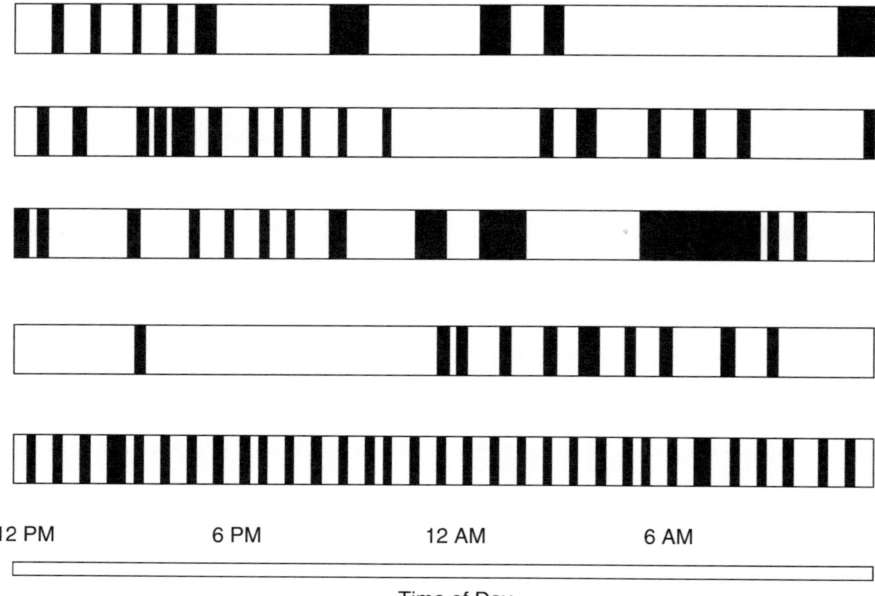

Fig. 3 Schematic representation of the redistribution of sleep and wake in five subjects over the 24-h period. Black areas represent episodes of sleep and white areas represent wakefulness. (Adapted with permission from Freedman NS, Gazendam J, Levan L, Pack AI, Schwab RJ. Abnormal sleep/wake cycles and the effect of environmental noise on sleep disruption in the intensive care unit. Am J Respir Crit Care Med. 2001;163(2):451–457)

[5–7]. The TST, day/night sleep distribution, sleep fragmentation, and sleep stage data from several PSG studies are summarized in Table 1.

Studies conducted in the ICU using actigraphy have also demonstrated marked sleep fragmentation. In one early study, patients monitored for 72 continuous hours were found to sleep for short periods during the day and night with sleep episodes lasting up to only 1 h [21]. The authors also reported abnormal melatonin secretion patterns (see chapter "Characteristics of Sleep in Critically Ill Patients. Part II: Circadian Rhythm Disruption"). A study of 16 non-ventilated burn patients demonstrated marked sleep fragmentation with sleep occurring in short episodes averaging only 15.6 min [19]. A systematic review of 13 ICU studies noted mean number of nocturnal awakenings ranged from 1.4 to 49 per night [10].

3.2 Studies Employing Subjective Assessment Methods

The Richards Campbell Sleep Questionnaire (RCSQ), specifically developed for use in critically ill adults, and shown to moderately correlate with PSG, asks patients to self-report their sleep across five domains (i.e., sleep latency, sleep efficiency, sleep depth, number of awakenings, and overall sleep quality) using visual analog

Table 1 Summary of sleep characteristics in critically ill adults [3–9]

Study type of sleep (N)	Proportion mechanically ventilated (%)	Total sleep time (hours) [mean (SD)]	Distribution of total sleep time between day (D) and night (N) periods (%)	Arousals (average number per/hour) [mean (SD)]	Awakenings (average number/hour) [mean (SD))	Slow wave sleep (as a % of total sleep time) [mean (SD)]	Rapid eye movement sleep REM (as a % of total sleep time) [mean (SD)]
Cooper et al.[a] (disrupted) N = 8	100%	D: 3.0 (1.9) N: 4.0 (2.9)	54 | 46	–	D: 17 (12) N: 22(25)	D: 15 (14) N: 10 (17)	D: 9 (6) N: 10 (14)
Cooper et al. (atypical) N = 5	100%	D: 6 (3) N: 4 (2)	60 | 40	D: 8 (5) N: 5 (3)	D: 6 (3) N: 7 (5)	D: 46 (47) N: 45 (51)	D: 4 (5) N: 4 (9)
Elliott et al.[b] N = 53	54%	5.0 (2.9–7.2)	41 | 59	27.0 (14.0–37.5)	–	0 (0–1)	0 (0–6)
Freedman et al. N = 17	91%[c]	8.8 (5.0)	57 | 43	11.6 + 5.0	–	9 (18)	6 (9)
Friese et al. N = 16	31%	8.3 (6.5)	–	–	6.2	0.3 (0.6)	3.3 (6.2)
Gabor et al. N = 7	100%	6.2 (2.5)	48 | 52	10.7 (5.9)	10.9 (7.6)	2.7 (3.3)	14.3 (9.8)
Knauert et al.[d] (typical) N = 14	24%[e]	6.2 (1.5)	32 | 68	NREM: 33.0 (13.3) REM: 18.7 (16.1)	–	3.9 (5.9)	12.9 (14.2)
Knauert et al. (atypical) N = 9	24%[e]	4.8 (3.4)	37 | 63	NREM: 26.5 (6.0) REM: 12.4 (4.9)	–	–	6.8 (6.0)
Thille et al.[b] N = 52	0%	2.4 (1.1–4.2)	–	25 (13–32)[f]	25 (13–32)[f]	17 (0–66)[g]	0 (0–8)[g]

D: daytime monitoring

N: nighttime monitoring

–: data not provided by study for specific outcome

[a] Study divided patients into two groups (disrupted sleep and atypical sleep) and provided data separately for daytime and nighttime monitoring

[b] Study expressed data values in median and interquartile range rather than mean and standard deviation

[c] Study initially recruited 22 patients but only 17 had scorable EEG data, this percentage reflects original 22 patients

[d] Study evaluated # of arousals between NREM and REM

[e] Study provided % ventilated for total study group and not for each group, typical and atypical

[f] Study grouped arousals and awakenings together to express value

[g] Study provided total amount of time spent in sleep stages rather than % of TST

scales ranging from 0 to 100 (higher score indicative of better sleep; score of <50 indicative of poor sleep) [22]. A number of studies have characterized ICU sleep using the RCSQ. In one mixed ICU cohort, the median (IQR) RCSQ was found to be moderately decreased at 58 (32–70) [5]. Among adults admitted to ICU for at least 2 nights, who were not sedated, the mean RCSQ was 45.5 [23]. In another ICU cohort, the mean RCSQ for awakenings was 46.4 and sleep quality 45.3; sleep depth had the lowest rating of 40.4 [24]. Although RCSQ assessment is both practical and inexpensive, a large proportion of ICU patients are unable to self-report their sleep quality due to delirium or sedation [22]. While the substitution of RCSQ assessments by nursing has been proposed, agreement between patients and nurses has been shown to be poor with nurses tending to overestimate sleep depth and return to sleep [25]. Sleep assessment methods are discussed in greater detail in chapter "Methods for Routine Sleep Assessment and Monitoring".

3.3 Causes of Sleep Fragmentation

Arousals and awakenings and sleep fragmentation resulting from it have been linked to frequent health care assessments, intensity of room lighting, noise levels, and ventilator mode, settings, and asynchrony [26]. A systemic review of 62 studies to evaluate risk factors for sleep disruption in critically ill individuals found most patients identify multiple variables affecting their sleep quality (see chapter "Risk Factors for Disrupted Sleep in the ICU" for a more detailed discussion of risk factors for sleep disruption) [27]. This review included an analysis of 17 studies that reported patient-identified factors and found that the most common causes of sleep disruption were anxiety/fear (42%), noise (42%), pain (39%), bed discomfort (38%), other discomfort (34%), attachment to a medical device (37%), care activities (33%), and light (33%). This review also highlighted significant interpatient variability in risk factors reported that is likely attributable to the variability in methods used between studies. For example, while six studies documented noise as an important ICU sleep disruptor, two other studies found no association [4, 5, 24, 28–31].

The Sleep in Intensive Care Questionnaire (SICQ) is a 7-question survey that allows patients to rate their sleep quality and perceived effect of the environment on sleep. Using this tool, patients identified noise as being most disturbing, followed by nursing interventions, light, diagnostic testing, vital signs, blood draws, and administration of medications [5]. However, when PSG was used to investigate causes of sleep fragmentation, it was found that only 11.5% of arousals and 17% of awakenings were related to environmental noise [4]. Gabor et al. further differentiated which sound level had the most frequent arousals/awakenings and found that 11.7% occurred at 10 dB while 30.8% occurred at 75 dB and greater [7]. In comparison, patient care interactions disturbed sleep an average of 7.8 times/hour of sleep with suctioning causing 62.8% of disruptions.

While it remains unclear if the use of mechanical ventilation itself disrupts sleep [27], several studies have evaluated the effect of ventilator modes on sleep quality. The use of pressure support (PS) mode is associated with more awakenings and arousals than assist-control (AC) mode [32]. However, Cabello et al. found no difference in fragmentation index or percentage of REM and SWS between patients on AC, clinically adjusted PS, and automatically adjusted PS modes [25]. There is a strong association between patient-ventilator asynchrony and sleep disruption; accordingly, hourly sleep arousals were found to be more frequent with PS ventilation compared to proportional assist ventilation in one study [33].

See chapter "Mechanical Ventilation and Sleep" for an in-depth discussion of mechanical ventilation and sleep.

3.4 *Sleep and Clinical Outcomes*

Sleep deprivation and fragmentation are associated with altered respiratory function, immune dysfunction and delirium. Only a few studies have evaluated the consequences of sleep on respiratory function. In healthy adults, a single night of sleep deprivation reduced respiratory endurance by reducing respiratory motor cortex output from the brain [34]. Among patients admitted to the ICU with acute respiratory failure and managed with non-invasive ventilation (NIV), the night to day TST ratio was significantly lower in those patients failing NIV compared to those who had NIV treatment success [35]. NIV failure was also associated with only 25% of the time spent in REM compared to the NIV success patients (6 vs. 26 min).

Sleep disruption may increase ICU delirium [36–38]. One early ICU study found patients with fewer uninterrupted 75 min sleep cycles, and thus more sleep fragmentation, had greater mental status alteration [37].

Sleep deprivation in healthy individuals has also been shown to adversely affect immune function [39]. Even one night of sleep deprivation negatively impacts vaccination response [40, 41]. Sleep deprivation has been linked to autonomic nervous system dysfunction which may lead to increased cardiac arrythmias [42]. Sleep arousals cause transient surges in sympathetic activity, blood pressure, and heart rate [43, 44]; sleep deprivation may adversely affect cardiovascular health due to increased pro-inflammatory cytokines (e.g., IL-6, TNF-α, CRP) [45].

For a detailed discussion of the myriad consequences of sleep deprivation, see chapters "Biologic Effects of Disrupted Sleep", "Sleep Disruption and Its Relationship with Delirium: Electroencephalographic Perspectives", "Sleep Disruption and Its Relationship with Delirium: Clinical Perspectives", "ICU Sleep Disruption and Its Relationship with ICU Outcomes", and "Long-Term Outcomes: Sleep in Survivors of Critical Illness".

4   Sleep Stage Disruption

4.1   Summary of PSG Studies

Sleep is divided into three non-rapid eye movement (NREM) stages (N1, N2, and N3) and rapid eye movement (REM). Normal sleep is characterized by an orderly transition through these stages [i.e., from the lightest (stage N1) to stages N2 and N3 (also known as SWS)], and REM. Healthy individuals typically cycle through these stages 4–5 times a night during sleep. Compared to healthy adults, critically ill patients experience frequent sleep disruption, often from fragmentation (see above) and thus spend greater time in light sleep (N1 and N2), less time (or no time) in deeper, restorative sleep (N3) and REM (Fig. 4) [46].

While N1 sleep accounts for only 5–10% of the TST in healthy adults, it is often the predominant sleep stage in critically ill adults [3–5] (Table 1). For example, in one ICU PSG study, N1 sleep accounted for 59% of TST; N2, N3 and REM accounted for 26%, 9%, and 6%, respectively [4]. Another PSG ICU study that dichotomized typical and atypical TST, found that N1 accounted for 22.7% of TST, N2 60.4%, N3 3.9%, and REM 12.9% of the TST spent with typical sleep [8]. Among TST spent with atypical sleep, REM accounted for only 6.8%. One other ICU study found the median time with SWS or REM sleep to both be zero [5]. Cooper et al. evaluated the percentages of SWS and REM during daytime and night-time and found no significant differences [3]. For example, in the disturbed sleep

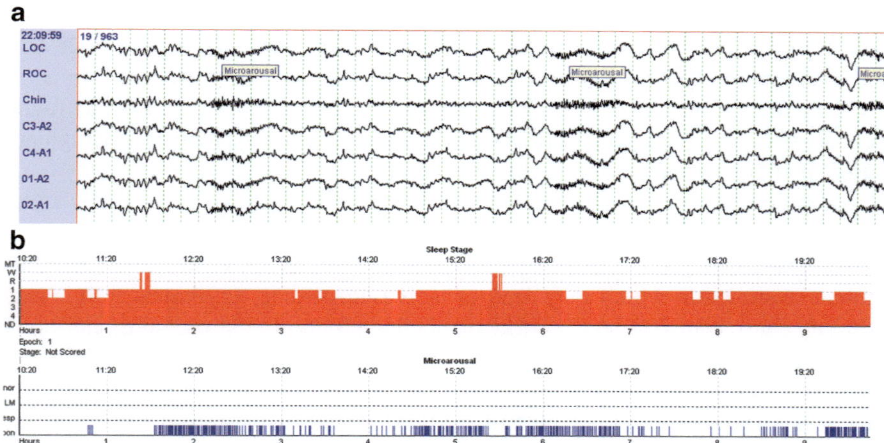

Fig. 4 Sleep in ICU patients is often severely fragmented and characterized by an increase in light sleep and a paucity of slow wave and REM sleep. (**a**) Polysomnography tracing from a critically ill, sedated patient demonstrating sleep fragmentation with microarousals noted approximately every 10 s. (**b**) Sleep histogram from the same patient showing a predominance of stage one sleep with frequent microarousals. (Adapted with permission from Weinhouse GL and Watson PL. Sedation and sleep disturbances in the ICU. Crit Care Clin 2009 Jul;25(3):539–49)

group, SWS and REM made up about 15% and 9% TST during the day and 10% and 10% TST during the night.

4.2   Causes of Sleep Stage Deprivation

The specific reasons for the reduced time spent in deep sleep in the ICU still remain unclear; it is likely to be multifactorial but medications may be a contributing factor. As reviewed in chapter "Effects of Common ICU Medications on Sleep", many common ICU medications are associated with reduced SWS and REM sleep. Vasopressors, sedatives, and analgesics in particular have this effect [20]. However, one ICU study of intubated patients found TST spent in REM was similarly low between ICU periods when patients were free of sedatives and opioids compared with when they were not [25]. In addition, a study of recently extubated patients free of sedatives found TST spent in REM or SWS to be very low [9].

The frequent interruption of the natural progression of sleep leading to sleep fragmentation in the ICU patients is an important contributor to the greatly reduced time spent in SWS and the sometimes-nonexistent time spent in REM sleep. Variability of TST in SWS and REM sleep may depend on when during the nocturnal period it is evaluated. One ICU PSG study that divided the nocturnal recording into early and late periods found SWS was more likely to occur during the earlier nocturnal period and REM sleep in the later nocturnal period [25].

4.3   Consequences of Sleep Stage Deprivation

Among ICU patients who failed a spontaneous breathing trial (SBT), patients with no REM sleep (compared with those who had REM) were found to require mechanical ventilation for an additional 2 days [47]. Among recently extubated patients, the presence of REM sleep was associated with re-intubation rates significantly lower than those without REM sleep [9].

Severe REM reduction (<6% of TST) is also associated with greater incidence of ICU delirium [48]. Atypical sleep, marked by loss of K-complexes and sleep spindles (hence loss of N2 sleep), is associated with a greater risk for severe encephalopathy and death [49].

SWS is associated with regulation of inflammation; reductions in SWS may therefore reduce the body's response to sepsis [28].

The impact of sleep deprivation on ICU and post-ICU outcomes are discussed in greater detail in chapters "ICU Sleep Disruption and Its Relationship to ICU Outcomes" and "Long-Term Outcomes: Sleep in Survivors of Critical Illness".

5 Conclusion

In summary, critically ill adults suffer from significant sleep fragmentation and sleep stage disruption, marked by frequent arousals and awakenings across both day and nighttime periods, that reduce the TST spent in restorative stages SWS and REM sleep. In addition to emotional distress, sleep disruption may contribute to delirium, prolonged mechanical ventilation, and immune dysfunction. Understanding the modifiable risk factors of sleep disruption and promoting sleep improvement strategies are crucial to improving ICU care. However, understanding the effects of sleep disruption on clinical outcomes is complicated in the ICU by multiple challenges, particularly in the face of sedative use that affects EEG findings and patient movement. Larger controlled studies dedicated to better understanding the effects of sleep fragmentation and sleep stage disruption on clinical outcomes of the critically ill are needed.

Funding/Support Dr. Watson received support from the National Institutes of Health (MO1 RR-00095) and the Vanderbilt CTSA grant UL1 RR024975–01 from NCRR/NIH.

References

1. Simini B. Patients' perceptions of intensive care. Lancet. 1999;354:571–2.
2. Devlin JW, Skrobik Y, Gelinas C, et al. Clinical practice guidelines for the prevention and management of pain, agitation/sedation, delirium, immobility, and sleep disruption in adult patients in the ICU. Crit Care Med. 2018;46(9):e825–73.
3. Cooper AB, Thornley KS, Young GB, Slutsky AS, Stewart TE, Hanly PJ. Sleep in critically ill patients requiring mechanical ventilation. Chest. 2000;117(3):809–18.
4. Freedman NS, Gazendam J, Levan L, Pack AI, Schwab RJ. Abnormal sleep/wake cycles and the effect of environmental noise on sleep disruption in the intensive care unit. Am J Respir Crit Care Med. 2001;163(2):451–7.
5. Elliott R, McKinley S, Cistulli P, Fien M. Characterisation of sleep in intensive care using 24-hour polysomnography: an observational study. Crit Care. 2013;17(2):R46.
6. Friese RS, Diaz-Arrastia R, McBride D, Frankel H, Gentilello LM. Quantity and quality of sleep in the surgical intensive care unit: are our patients sleeping? J Trauma. 2007;63(6):1210–4.
7. Gabor JY, Cooper AB, Crombach SA, et al. Contribution of the intensive care unit environment to sleep disruption in mechanically ventilated patients and healthy subjects. Am J Respir Crit Care Med. 2003;167(5):708–15.
8. Knauert MP, Yaggi HK, Redeker NS, Murphy TE, Araujo KL, Pisani MA. Feasibility study of unattended polysomnography in medical intensive care unit patients. Heart Lung. 2014;43(5):445–52.
9. Thille AW, Barrau S, Beuvon C, et al. Role of sleep on respiratory failure after extubation in the ICU. Ann Intensive Care. 2021;11(1):71.
10. Schwab KE, Ronish B, Needham DM, To AQ, Martin JL, Kamdar BB. Actigraphy to evaluate sleep in the intensive care unit. A systematic review. Ann Am Thorac Soc. 2018;15(9):1075–82.
11. Drouot X, Roche-Campo F, Thille AW, et al. A new classification for sleep analysis in critically ill patients. Sleep Med. 2012;13(1):7–14.

12. Watson PL, Pandharipande P, Gehlbach BK, et al. Atypical sleep in ventilated patients: empirical electroencephalography findings and the path toward revised ICU sleep scoring criteria. Crit Care Med. 2013;41(8):1958–67.
13. Gupta P, Martin JL, Needham DM, Vangala S, Colantuoni E, Kamdar BB. Use of actigraphy to characterize inactivity and activity in patients in a medical ICU. Heart Lung. 2020;49(4):398–406.
14. Beecroft JM, Ward M, Younes M, Crombach S, Smith O, Hanly PJ. Sleep monitoring in the intensive care unit: comparison of nurse assessment, actigraphy, and polysomnography. Intensive Care Med. 2008;34:2076–83.
15. van der Kooi AW, Tulen JH, van Eijk MM, et al. Sleep monitoring by actigraphy in short-stay ICU patients. Crit Care Nurs Q. 2013;36(2):169–73.
16. Bourne RS, Mills GH, Minelli C. Melatonin therapy to improve nocturnal sleep in critically ill patients: encouraging results from a small randomised controlled trial. Crit Care. 2008;12(2):R52.
17. Mistraletti G, Taverna M, Sabbatini G, et al. Actigraphic monitoring in critically ill patients: preliminary results toward an "observation-guided sedation". J Crit Care. 2009;24(4):563–7.
18. Kroon K, West S. 'Appears to have slept well': assessing sleep in an acute care setting. Contemp Nurse. 2000;9(3–4):284–94.
19. Raymond I, Ancoli-Israel S, Choiniere M. Sleep disturbances, pain and analgesia in adults hospitalized for burn injuries. Sleep Med. 2004;5(6):551–9.
20. Weinhouse GL. Pharmacology I: effects on sleep of commonly used ICU medications. Crit Care Clin. 2008;24(3):477–91, vi.
21. Shilo L, Dagan Y, Smorjik Y, et al. Patients in the intensive care unit suffer from severe lack of sleep associated with loss of normal melatonin secretion pattern. Am J Med Sci. 1999;317(5):278–81.
22. Richards KC, O'Sullivan PS, Phillips RL. Measurement of sleep in critically ill patients. J Nurs Meas. 2000;8(2):131–44.
23. Frisk U, Nordstrom G. Patients' sleep in an intensive care unit—patients' and nurses' perception. Intensive Crit Care Nurs. 2003;19(6):342–9.
24. Chen LX, Ji DH, Zhang F, et al. Richards-Campbell sleep questionnaire: psychometric properties of Chinese critically ill patients. Nurs Crit Care. 2019;24(6):362–8.
25. Cabello B, Thille AW, Drouot X, et al. Sleep quality in mechanically ventilated patients: comparison of three ventilatory modes. Crit Care Med. 2008;36(6):1749–55.
26. Pulak LM, Jensen L. Sleep in the intensive care unit: a review. J Intensive Care Med. 2016;31(1):14–23.
27. Honarmand K, Rafay H, Le J, et al. A systematic review of risk factors for sleep disruption in critically ill adults. Crit Care Med. 2020;48(7):1066–74.
28. Richards KC, Wang YY, Jun J, Ye L. A systematic review of sleep measurement in critically ill patients. Front Neurol. 2020;11:542529.
29. Fanfulla F, Ceriana P, D'Artavilla Lupo N, Trentin R, Frigerio F, Nava S. Sleep disturbances in patients admitted to a step-down unit after ICU discharge: the role of mechanical ventilation. Sleep. 2011;34(3):355–62.
30. Elbaz M, Leger D, Sauvet F, et al. Sound level intensity severely disrupts sleep in ventilated ICU patients throughout a 24-h period: a preliminary 24-h study of sleep stages and associated sound levels. Ann Intensive Care. 2017;7(1):25.
31. Roche-Campo F, Thille AW, Drouot X, et al. Comparison of sleep quality with mechanical versus spontaneous ventilation during weaning of critically III tracheostomized patients. Crit Care Med. 2013;41(7):1637–44.
32. Parthasarathy S, Tobin MJ. Effect of ventilator mode on sleep quality in critically ill patients. Am J Respir Crit Care Med. 2002;166(11):1423–9.
33. Bosma K, Ferreyra G, Ambrogio C, et al. Patient-ventilator interaction and sleep in mechanically ventilated patients: pressure support versus proportional assist ventilation. Crit Care Med. 2007;35(4):1048–54.

34. Rault C, Sangare A, Diaz V, et al. Impact of sleep deprivation on respiratory motor output and endurance. A physiological study. Am J Respir Crit Care Med. 2020;201(8):976–83.
35. Roche CF, Drouot X, Thille AW, et al. Poor sleep quality is associated with late noninvasive ventilation failure in patients with acute hypercapnic respiratory failure. Crit Care Med. 2010;38(2):477–85.
36. Weinhouse GL, Schwab RJ, Watson PL, et al. Bench-to-bedside review: delirium in ICU patients - importance of sleep deprivation. Crit Care. 2009;13(6):234.
37. Helton MC, Gordon SH, Nunnery SL. The correlation between sleep-deprivation and the intensive-care unit syndrome. Heart Lung. 1980;9(3):464–8.
38. Ely EW, Shintani A, Truman B, et al. Delirium as a predictor of mortality in mechanically ventilated patients in the intensive care unit. JAMA. 2004;291(14):1753–62.
39. Besedovsky L, Lange T, Born J. Sleep and immune function. Pflugers Arch. 2012;463(1):121–37.
40. Lange T, Perras B, Fehm HL, Born J. Sleep enhances the human antibody response to hepatitis A vaccination. Psychosom Med. 2003;65(5):831–5.
41. Spiegel K, Sheridan JF, Van Cauter E. Effect of sleep deprivation on response to immunization. JAMA. 2002;288(12):1471–2.
42. Tobaldini E, Costantino G, Solbiati M, et al. Sleep, sleep deprivation, autonomic nervous system and cardiovascular diseases. Neurosci Biobehav Rev. 2017;74(Pt B):321–9.
43. Sforza E, Chapotot F, Lavoie S, Roche F, Pigeau R, Buguet A. Heart rate activation during spontaneous arousals from sleep: effect of sleep deprivation. Clin Neurophysiol. 2004;115(11):2442–51.
44. Kondo H, Ozone M, Ohki N, et al. Association between heart rate variability, blood pressure and autonomic activity in cyclic alternating pattern during sleep. Sleep. 2014;37(1):187–94.
45. Faraut B, Boudjeltia KZ, Vanhamme L, Kerkhofs M. Immune, inflammatory and cardiovascular consequences of sleep restriction and recovery. Sleep Med Rev. 2012;16(2):137–49.
46. Weinhouse GL, Watson PL. Sedation and sleep disturbances in the ICU. Anesthesiol Clin. 2011;29(4):675–85.
47. Thille AW, Reynaud F, Marie D, et al. Impact of sleep alterations on weaning duration in mechanically ventilated patients: a prospective study. Eur Respir J. 2018;51(4)
48. Trompeo AC, Vidi Y, Locane MD, et al. Sleep disturbances in the critically ill patients: role of delirium and sedative agents. Minerva Anestesiol. 2011;77(6):604–12.
49. Knauert MP, Gilmore EJ, Murphy TE, et al. Association between death and loss of stage N2 sleep features among critically ill patients with delirium. J Crit Care. 2018;48:124–9.

Characteristics of Sleep in Critically Ill Patients: Part II: Circadian Rhythm Disruption

Marie-Anne Melone and Brian K. Gehlbach

1 Introduction

Circadian clocks provide temporal organization to an organism and are ubiquitous in nature. The ~24-h rotation of the Earth has been a major evolutionary force on the development of intrinsic circadian clocks [1]. Each cell has an endogenous clock, or oscillator, with a free-running period of approximately 24 h. To synchronize the oscillator with the 24-h rotation of the Earth it is necessary to reset or *entrain* its rhythm using extremal cues. These cues are named zeitgebers ("time-givers") and the most powerful cue for humans is the light/dark cycle.

Primitive non-transcriptional circadian rhythms may have first evolved 2.5 billion years ago at the time of the Great Oxidation Event to protect the organism from reactive oxygen species [2, 3]. Whatever their origin, circadian rhythms have conferred to species the ability to anticipate daily changes. Clock genes are numerous; approximately 40% of human genes are under circadian control [4]. Thus, there are many 24-h physiological rhythms, including sleep/activity cycles, core body temperature fluctuations, heart rate, hormone levels and metabolism [5, 6]. These circadian rhythms allow organisms to anticipate daily changes and align their activities to these changes to confer advantage. Environmental cycles have therefore driven the evolution of endogenous clock genes that tune internal physiology to external conditions. This chapter, a companion to the chapter "Characteristics of Sleep in

M.-A. Melone
Department of Internal Medicine, University of Iowa, Iowa City, IA, USA

Department of Pulmonary, Thoracic Oncology and Respiratory Intensive Care, Rouen University Hospital, Rouen, France
e-mail: marieanne.melone@chu-rouen.fr

B. K. Gehlbach (✉)
Departments of Internal Medicine and Neurology, University of Iowa, Iowa City, IA, USA
e-mail: brian-gehlbach@uiowa.edu

© The Author(s), under exclusive license to Springer Nature Switzerland AG 2022
G. L. Weinhouse, J. W. Devlin (eds.), *Sleep in Critical Illness*,
https://doi.org/10.1007/978-3-031-06447-0_2

Critically Ill Patients. Part I: Sleep Fragmentation and Sleep Stage Disruption"
(characteristics of sleep fragmentation and disruption) will introduce basic principles of circadian biology, describe potential circadian disrupters in intensive care
units, and characterize circadian profiles in critically ill patients.

2   Circadian Timing System Physiology

The basis of the circadian timing system is a molecular mechanism known as the
transcription-translation feedback loop. Suprachiasmatic nucleus (SCN) neurons
serve as a master clock to coordinate rhythms at an organismal level. This clock
interacts in a bidirectional manner with tissue-specific rhythms whose activity can
be shifted by specific time givers (Fig. 1).

2.1   *Molecular Basis*

A variety of clock genes maintain circadian rhythms in a constant environment (for
instance, stable darkness without other zeitgebers). A rhythm represents the ability to
oscillate. The nature of an oscillation describes a system that tends, in a regular manner,

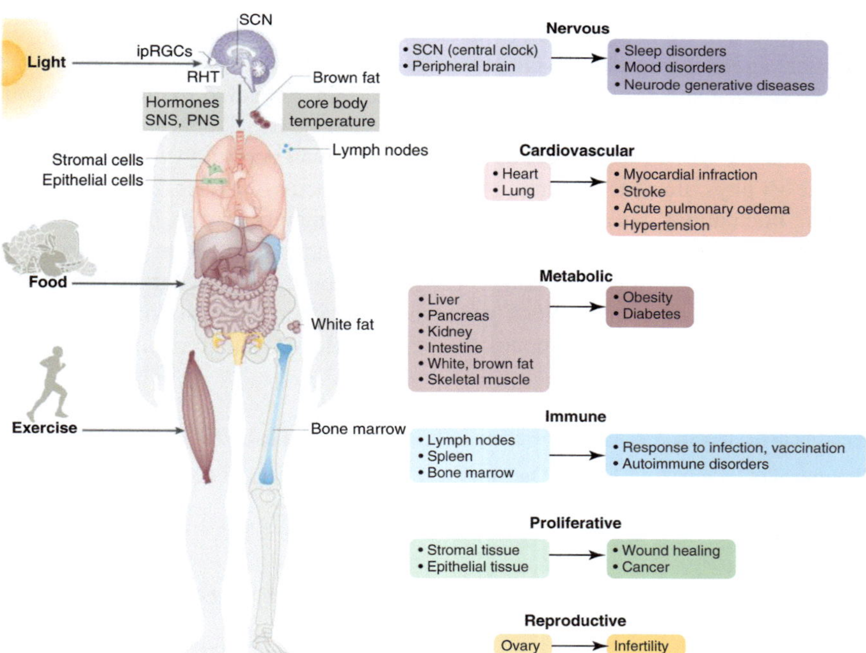

Fig. 1 The central clock and selected peripheral clocks in humans [106]

to move away from equilibrium before returning. To achieve this, a process whose product feeds back to slow the rate of the process itself is needed. This oscillator mechanism is under control of the Transcription-Translation Feedback Loop (TTFL) [7]. The TTFL involves clock genes working as activators of transcription then releasing proteins from the nucleus to the cytoplasm that negatively regulate their own transcription, leading to a negative feedback loop. To date, 6 interlocking TTFLs have been described. During the first step, CLOCK–BMAL1 heterodimers induce the expression of PER and CRY which inhibit the transcriptional activity of CLOCK–BMAL1 and represses their own expression. CLOCK–BMAL1 similarly induces the expression of other clock genes that regulate BMAL1 expression. This web of interconnected feedback loops constitutes the genetic network and allows a robust and precise circadian rhythm to be expressed.

2.2   Central Clock

The master, or central, clock has been localized to the SCN in the hypothalamus [8, 9]. The SCN is comprised of neuronal structures located in the anteroventral hypothalamus and subdivided in two anatomical parts: the ventral core region above the optic chiasm, and the dorsal shell region, which receives input from the core. The SCN receives direct input from melanopsin-containing retinal ganglion cells via the retinohypothalamic tract. The SCN projects in turn to the brain and hormonal systems thereby enabling the synchronization of other oscillators throughout the brain and body.

The SCN regulates sleep timing via its regulation of melatonin secretion (discussed below) and via direct projections to sleep regulatory systems such as the dorsomedial hypothalamic nucleus [10]. Indeed, Nauta et al. described syndromes of prolonged wakefulness with anterior hypothalamic lesions and prolonged sleep with posterior hypothalamic lesions [11]. Sleep/wake regulation results from the interaction of a circadian alerting process and a homeostatic process that relates increasing sleep pressure to increased duration of wakefulness. The nighttime reduction in the circadian alerting signal promotes consolidation of sleep. Additional evidence of interaction between sleep and circadian rhythms is demonstrated by the effect of sleep loss on clock gene expression [12]. SCN fibers also project to the pineal gland, where melatonin is synthesized, and to other hypothalamus areas regulating core body temperature, cortisol, and the autonomic system [8].

To conclude, SCN neuronal activity coordinates the timing of sleep and wake rhythms and plays a major role in the regulation and coordination of multiple biological, immunological, and metabolic functions.

2.3   Entrainment

SCN neurons possess endogenous rhythmicity meaning they oscillate over a period of time even in the absence of external influences. In addition, the transplantation of these neurons into animals with their own SCN removed restores their circadian rhythms [13]. The master clock has a free-running period in humans of ~24.2 h [14]. The central clock therefore needs to be *entrained*, or synchronized, by external cues to fit the 24-h rotation of the Earth. Light is the most powerful cue to entrain the SCN, although constant light exposure results in desynchronization of SCN activity [15]. The SCN receives photic time of day information from these photoreceptors, which express the photopigment melanopsin [16, 17]. Intrinsically photosensitive retinal ganglion cell (iPRGC) activity depends on five different influencing factors:

1. **Timing**. Exposure to light during the early biological night causes a phase delay, thereby preparing the body for a later day. Exposure to light during the late biological night causes a phase advance, thereby preparing the body for an earlier day. In clinical practice light therapy can advance the timing of the sleep/wake cycle in patients with Delayed Sleep Phase Syndrome [18].
2. **Dose (intensity)**. Approximately 7000–13,000 lux is a highly effective circadian zeitgeber. For comparison, spring day light levels may range from 32,000 to 60,000 lux. But even 80 lux can significantly phase-shift circadian clocks [19].
3. **Exposure duration**. In drosophila, constant light perturbs degradation of PERIOD/TIMELESS (PER/TIM) heterodimeric complexes [20].
4. **Wavelength**. Intrinsically photosensitive retinal ganglion cells exhibit maximal sensitivity in the blue spectrum, while low-intensity red light does not appear to suppress melatonin production [21].
5. **Prior light history**. Overall, non-circadian light exposures have the potential to modify gene expression patterns, alter melatonin secretion, and disrupt the duration and timing of sleep [22].

2.4   *Peripheral Clocks*

Peripheral oscillators are distributed throughout the body in a variety of tissues and organs. For instance, hepatocytes have clock genes that continue to oscillate in the absence of zeitgebers [23]. Similarly, other parts of the brain sustain circadian rhythms independently of the SCN [24]. In SCN-ablated mice, peripheral tissues are still rhythmic, but they do not work in a coordinated way, suggesting the SCN is a synchronizer [25].

Previously considered to be less important in humans, the timing of food intake has, in more recent studies, been found to be a zeitgeber for various peripheral tissues in humans and may play an important role in regulating metabolism. Mistimed glucose, corticoids, and insulin may alter *Per* gene expression in the liver in vivo potentially leading to alterations in the immune response, corticosteroid production, and metabolism [26, 27]. In addition, peripheral clocks outside of the liver may be shifted by restricted feeding [26]. For instance, there is an increase in locomotion, corticosterone secretion, body temperature, and several metabolic parameters, in anticipation of mealtime in mice models [27].

Ambient temperature sensation also serves as a cue to coordinate the timing of sleep and activity [28]. Even organ-specific microenvironments can have different effects on the respective peripheral organ. For instance, hypoxia recently was found to shift clock genes expression differently in the liver, lung, and kidney suggesting a specific synchronizing effect of exercise on the molecular clockwork of peripheral tissues [29]. Moreover, timed exercise can reset the circadian clock in skeletal muscles [30, 31]. Social activity is probably the least powerful zeitgeber. Most nonsighted individuals exhibit free-running circadian rhythms despite the presence of numerous social cues (employment, family, alarm clocks, guide dogs, etc.).

To summarize, the body is designed to align feeding/fasting, sleep/wake, and activity/inactivity cycles to survive in a specific environment. Failure to do so leads to adverse health consequences [32, 33] (Fig. 1). Nowadays, light widely used throughout 24 h via indoor lights and electronic devices can alter clock gene expression and melatonin secretion with potential harmful effects on external and internal synchronization. Jet lag and shift work are known to desynchronize internal oscillations and environmental cues leading to metabolic, cardiovascular, neoplastic, and mental health disorders [34, 35].

3   Measurement of Circadian Rhythms

Circadian rhythmicity can be evaluated by different biomarkers representing the output of the biological clock. The most widely biomarkers used are melatonin, core body temperature, and cortisol (Fig. 2).

3.1   *Melatonin, 6-Sulfatoxymelatonin Levels*

Melatonin is synthesized in the pineal gland in response to regulation by the SCN and is primarily secreted at night [36, 37]. Melatonin is primarily metabolized by the liver and excreted in urine as 6-sulfatoxymelatonin (6-SMT). Melatonin levels can be measured in blood, saliva, and urine. In ICU studies, the urinary metabolite of melatonin, 6-SMT, has typically been measured [38], although renal and hepatic dysfunction must be considered as potential masking factors in this population. Moreover, alterations in the serum melatonin concentration may result from decreased melatonin metabolism in the liver from direct suppression of hepatic cytochrome activity by proinflammatory cytokines [39]. Alterations in the urinary excretion of 6-SMT have been reported in septic intensive care unit patients [40].

The frequency of sampling differs between studies ranging from every 6 h to hourly. Some authors have highlighted discrepancies between urine and serum melatonin samples [41, 42] but the effect may have been exaggerated by infrequent sampling of urine specimens. Indeed, hourly sampling routines, while labor-intensive, are likely to increase the precision of circadian assessments in this patient

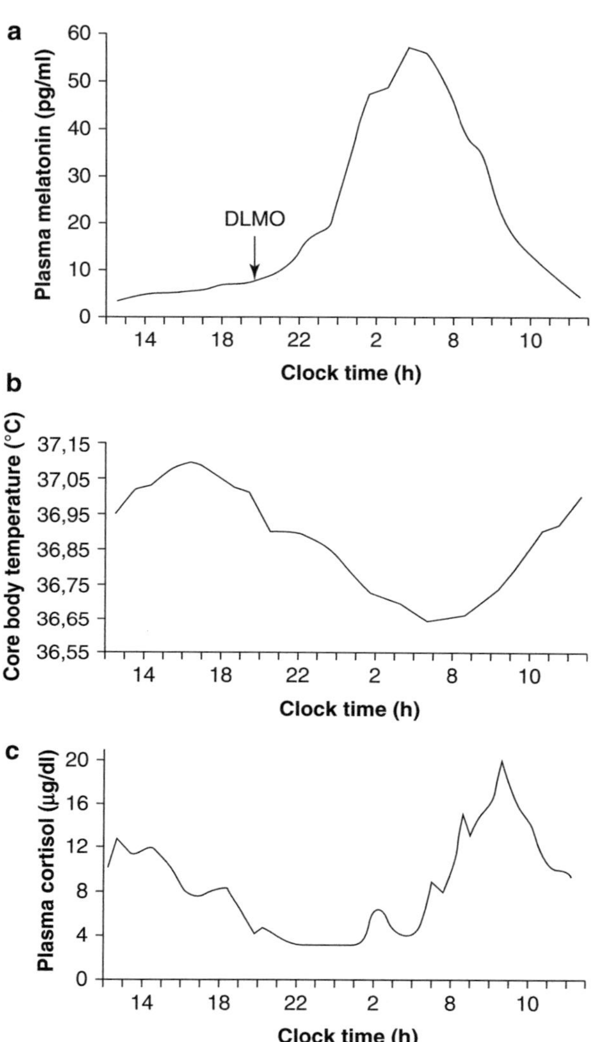

Fig. 2 Human circadian rhythms of the plasma melatonin level, core body temperature and plasma cortisol level [107]

population. Overall, serum samples are likely to be more accurate phase markers than urinary 6-SMT but require indwelling catheters for frequent assessment.

In normal subjects, peak serum melatonin levels occur between 1:00 and 3:00 a.m., with very low levels during the daytime between 10:00 a.m. and 6:00 p.m. Overall melatonin secretion gradually declines with age and also varies between individuals [43]. Potential melatonin-based analyses include: (1) Total 24-h melatonin or 6-SMT excretion. (2) Analysis of individual 24-h temporal profiles. (3) Determination of the acrophase (peak value) and nadir of each 24-h profile, along with the rhythm amplitude, defined as 50% of the difference between the values of the acrophase and nadir. (4) Determination of DLMO (dim light melatonin onset), characterizes the time of the onset of melatonin rise.

3.2 Cortisol Levels

Cortisol is a corticosteroid hormone, synthesized in the zona fasciculata of the adrenal cortex in the adrenal gland in response to regulation by the hypothalamic-pituitary-adrenal axis with input from the SCN [44]. The secretion of cortisol decreases throughout the day, with its nadir occurring approximately 2 h after sleep onset and with a sharp increase at the end of the biological night to reach a peak in the early morning [45]. Free plasma cortisol levels are the most accurate reflection of cortisol activity, but the technique is complex and expensive. Salivary cortisol can be assessed as a surrogate of serum free cortisol [46].

Several factors influence the secretion of cortisol, including stress and light, both of which stimulate secretion [47]. Sleep onset and deep sleep reduce cortisol whereas sleep deprivation increases it [48, 49]. Potential measures include: (1) Determination of the nadir and the acrophase. (2) The time of the onset of the rise and the timing of the quiescent period. (3) The amplitude of the 24-h rhythm.

3.3 Core Body Temperature

Core body temperature (CBT) displays a circadian rhythm under control of the SCN which regulates the hypothalamic preoptic thermoregulatory control center [50]. Average CBT is approximately 37.0 °C in healthy subjects, with a nearly 1 °C sinusoidal circadian fluctuation and a period of 24 h. CBT nadir typically occurs at approximately 4:00 a.m., while peak CBT occurs at the end of the day. Body temperature can be monitored at different sites, either peripherally (oral, axillary, thoracic skin surface) or centrally (rectal, esophageal, or intestinal). Central monitoring methods are the most accurate to assess the CBT rhythm [51]. CBT oscillations generated by the SCN modulate peripheral clock gene expression and act as a cue for the entrainment of cell-specific oscillators throughout the body [52]. Conversely, the molecular clock is needed for generating CBT rhythms [53]. Additionally, CBT oscillations result from multiple processes (metabolism, muscular contraction, dissipation of heat via sweating, blood flow changes in the skin, respiration). As a result, CBT dysrhythmias are common in critically ill patients and may reflect not only the effect of acute illness, therapeutic interventions, and the ICU environment on the central clock, but also masking effects (see below).

3.4   Actigraphy

Actigraphy uses a 3-axis accelerometer with an algorithm to determine sleep/wake state and is validated by the American Academy of Sleep Medicine to diagnosis circadian rhythm and sleep-wake disorders [54]. Recently, this technology has been studied in the ICU in a prospective observational study of 80 patients that compared actigraphy with polysomnography (PSG). The authors reported that actigraphy and PSG showed good agreement in determining both total sleep, time ($r = 0.873$) and wakefulness ($r = 0.769$), though with actigraphy over-reporting total sleep time. Actigraphy demonstrated a moderate level of agreement in identifying awakening ($r = 0.227$) in ventilated patients (specificity 83.7%) [55] (see chapter "Methods for Routine Sleep Assessment and Monitoring").

3.5   Circadian Gene Expression

Accumulating evidence suggests that nearly half of the genome oscillates with a circadian rhythm [4]. In human studies, quantitative real-time PCR is frequently used to analyze the gene expression of several core "clock genes"—*BMAL1, CLOCK, PER,* and *CRY*—through the collection of whole blood samples at regular intervals.

3.6   Challenges to Assessing CR in Critically Ill Adults

As discussed above, numerous zeitgebers exist not only in the external environment but also in the microenvironment of each organ. Light/dark cycles, food availability (via food-entrainable oscillators in the gut), physical activity, social interaction, and sleep/wake cycles can all be perturbed in the ICU (Fig. 3).

Accurately assaying an individual's biological clock requires scrupulous management or accounting of potential masking factors (hepatic or renal dysfunction, administration of norepinephrine or other drugs that stimulate melatonin secretion, and environmental influences). The results of these studies may also vary because of differences in the choice of phase marker or its sampling frequency or differences in the ICU environment and illness. Which factors disrupt circadian rhythms in ICU? Are some forms of circadian disruption adaptive to the illness? We will review in the next section ICU and medical conditions that may affect circadian rhythms (Table 1).

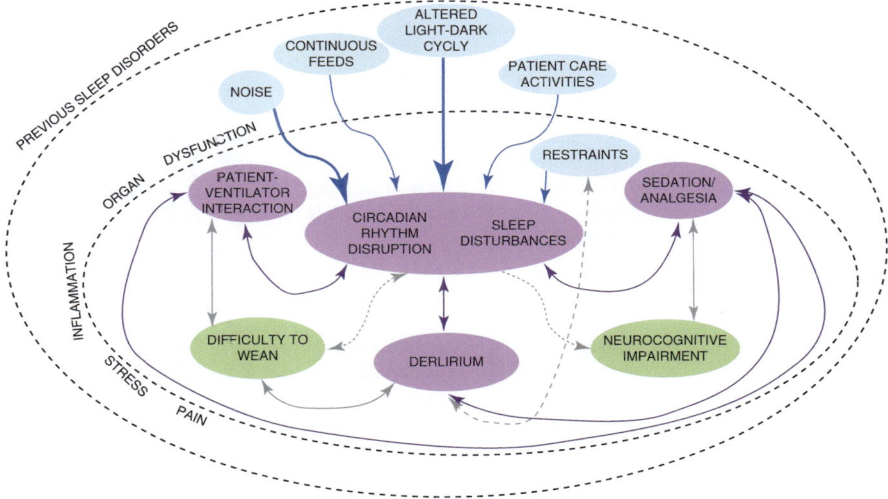

Fig. 3 Determinants and physiological consequences of sleep and circadian rhythm disruption in the intensive care unit (ICU) [108]

Table 1 Effects of various ICU and medical conditions on clock gene expression and melatonin circadian rhythmicity

Circadian disrupters	Changes	Consequences	Chronobiologic interventions
Light–dark cycle	– Dim light levels [61] – Daytime light levels range from 30 to 165 lux – Nocturnal light levels vary from 2.4 to 145 lux [89, 90] – Up to 10,000 lux during procedures (e.g., central line insertion) [91]	– Dim light levels were not able to entrain the melatonin-based rhythm [40] – 6-SMT acrophase occurs at 8:30 a.m. (phase delay) as compared with between midnight and 5:00 a.m. in healthy adults [57, 58]	– Exposure of 400 to 5000 lux from 9 a.m. to noon reduces phase delay in the melatonin secretion rhythm [58]
Fasting/feeding cycle	– Continuous feeding for 24 h in intubated and sedated patients – Prolonged fasting due to different interventions (surgery, exams, extubating…)	– Altered gene expression in the liver and melatonin secretion potentially leading to alterations in the immune response, corticosteroid production, and metabolism [62, 63]	– Reprogramming clocks through appropriately timed feeding routines may positively impact immunity

(continued)

Table 1 (continued)

Circadian disrupters	Changes	Consequences	Chronobiologic interventions
Medications			
Catecholamines	– Directly stimulate melatonin secretion which is under sympathetic regulation [92]	– Higher levels of melatonin secretion were observed in patients receiving catecholamines [41]	– Melatonin supplementation *chapter "*Best Practices for Improving Sleep in the ICU. Part II: Pharmacologic*"*
Propofol	– Suppresses slow wave sleep (SWS) [93]	– Negatively influences clock gene expression in the SCN master clock [94]	– Daily sedative interruption
Selective α-2-adrenergic agonists (e.g. clonidine, dexmedetomidine)	– Improve sleep efficiency – Increase stage N2 sleep [95]	– Alter ACTH, cortisol, and melatonin secretion [96]	
Benzodiazepines	– Increase N2 sleep – Decrease SWS and REM sleep [97]	– In six healthy volunteers receiving a 2-mg of alprazolam at 21:00 h, suppressed melatonin concentrations were found throughout the night [98]	
Opioids	– Suppress both SWS and REM [99]	– In a recent study, 72 patients with sepsis or respiratory failure under MV received either non-sedation (but analgesia by morphine) or sedation (propofol, midazolam). Melatonin levels were suppressed in sedated patients when compared to non-sedated patients [100]	

Table 1 (continued)

Circadian disrupters	Changes	Consequences	Chronobiologic interventions
Sleep disrupters (see chapter "Risk Factors for Disrupted Sleep in the ICU")			
Mechanical ventilation	– see chapter "Mechanical Ventilation and Sleep"	– Frisk et al. reported markedly lower 6-SMT excretion with MV compared with periods without MV [56] – Gehlbach et al. found significant variability in the timing of 6SMTexcretion, suggesting that the circadian rhythms of critically ill patients were "free-running". The loss of normal sleep/wake cycles induced by either sedation or MV may have contributed to disruption of the melatonin-based rhythm [57]	
Physical activity	– Drastically reduced by physiologic stressors and the presence of indwelling devices [66] – Half of total sleep time occurs during the daytime [101] – Significant activity occurs at night [102]	– Modifies clock gene rhythmicity [30, 31, 103]	– Mobilization, although in some cases premature mobilization may be counterproductive [65, 66]

(continued)

Table 1 (continued)

Circadian disrupters	Changes	Consequences	Chronobiologic interventions
Acute and chronic disease			
Sepsis	– Acute inflammation with high levels of proinflammatory cytokines	– Urinary 6-SMT excretion exhibited loss of circadian rhythmicity with no daytime decline in septic patients compared to non-septic and control patients [104] – Lower expression of *Cry-1* and *Per-2*, are correlated with higher levels of TNF-α and IL-6, in patients during the acute phase of sepsis compared to non-septic patients [105] – Urinary 6-SMT was related to severity of illness and procalcitonin levels and low *Bmal1*, *per2*, and *cry1* expression in septic patients [83]	– To be determined
Severity of illness		– APACHE III score has been found to be significantly predictive of circadian displacement [74] – Acuna et al. also found a negative correlation between SOFA and melatonin levels in septic patients [83]	
Chronic diseases	– Neurodegenerative or psychiatric disorders, jet lag, shift work, aging…	– The presence of any of these predisposing factors have the potential to magnify the ICU environmental impact on sleep and circadian rhythmicity	

4 Circadian Disrupters

4.1 ICU Environment

In general, the light–dark cycle of a typical ICU is weak and phase-delayed when compared to the solar cycle. Many studies have reported a phase delay in the melatonin secretion rhythm although the direct relationship between dim ICU light environment and circadian "dysrhythms" is difficult to disentangle considering the numerous other circadian disrupters (noise, medication, disease) in this setting [56–60].

In one study that measured 24-h light and sound levels in patients' rooms, the authors reported frequent underutilization of available light sources [61]. Behavioral interventions using objective measurements to increase daytime light, reduce nighttime noise, and improve circadian alignment should be included in ICU sleep promotion strategies. The encouraging results of a small pilot trial of timed light therapy in critically ill patients suggests that at least a portion of the circadian dysrhythms is attributable to a nontherapeutic ICU environment where the light/dark cycle is concerned [58]. Confirmation of this result in a larger sample is required (see chapter "Best Practices for Improving Sleep in the ICU. Part I: Non-pharmacologic").

As, discussed above, food is an important zeitgeber and mistimed feeding may induce internal desynchrony [23, 26, 62, 63]. Optimizing the timing of feeding in relation to the day/night cycle for critically ill patients receiving enteral nutrition could potentially resynchronize rhythms. Currently, such evidence is lacking. But correction of nutritional dysrhythmias is a promising avenue for investigation that may positively impact immunity (see chapter "Best Practices for Improving Sleep in the ICU. Part I: Non-pharmacologic").

Sleep disrupters are numerous in the ICU and are reviewed in chapter "Risk Factors for Disrupted Sleep in the ICU" [64]. As discussed above, homeostatic and circadian processes work together to coordinate sleep/wake cycles. Therefore, sleep-wake disruption can negatively influence circadian rhythmicity. The effects of mechanical ventilation (MV) on sleep and circadian rhythmicity are reviewed in chapter "Mechanical Ventilation and Sleep". In general, MV requires high-level care, prolonged treatment in a medical facility, and the frequent administration of sedation, all with the potential to negatively impact circadian rhythmicity. Indeed, numerous medications affect circadian rhythmicity (see chapter "Effects of Common ICU Medications on Sleep").

There is chronobiologic evidence from other populations to suggest that disruption in physical activity during critical illness may alter circadian rhythmicity [30, 31]. But it is noteworthy that early mobilization during critical illness, while promising, has not been definitively proven to improve clinical outcomes [65]. Moreover, quiescence during acute critical illness may be protective and attempting to counter this response too early could, in theory, be harmful [66].

4.2   Acute and Chronic Disease

In addition to the ICU environment, critical illness itself may lead to disruptions of circadian rhythmicity. For instance, the circadian regulation of the inflammatory response and immune system has been extensively studied [67]. A bidirectional relationship exists between the degree of clock gene expression alteration and the degree of inflammation [68–70]. Moreover, findings suggest that infection and pro-inflammatory cells induce the production of melatonin, perhaps for protective purposes, and that a failure to do so may be associated with a less effective immune response against infection. (Please see chapter "ICU Sleep Disruption and Its

Relationship with ICU Outcomes" for additional discussion on the outcomes of sleep during sepsis). Neurodegenerative or psychiatric disorders, jet lag, shift work, and aging are all associated with circadian disruption [33–35]. The presence of any of these predisposing factors have the potential to magnify the ICU environmental impact on sleep and circadian rhythmicity.

5 Circadian Rhythms in the Critically Ill

Circadian rhythms in critically ill patients are significantly disturbed due to the ICU environment, sleep disruption, and acute and chronic illness. The most frequently reported alterations in the biomarkers of circadian rhythmicity (melatonin, CBT, cortisol) are a decrease in the amplitude of the circadian rhythm and a phase shift in timing.

5.1 Core Body Temperature

Acute illness such as inflammation or brain injury can influence the activity of the SCN, which regulates the hypothalamic preoptic thermoregulatory control center, leading to CBT dysrhythmia [71–73]. Most studies have reported dispersion of the CBT minimum over the entire 24 h whereas in healthy subjects this would be expected to occur between 4:00 and 6:00 a.m. [74, 75]. Severity of illness and poor prognosis have been associated with temperature curve displacement [74–76]. Paul et al. prospectively measured tympanic temperature hourly in 13 sedated ICU patients. They did not find any normal circadian profiles of the temperature curve in the overall population, and reported more severe alterations in patients with brain injuries [72]. Pina et al. prospectively analyzed hourly CBT and 4-h interval urine cortisol and melatonin profiles in eight burn patients. When compared to healthy controls, patients demonstrated alterations in circadian rhythms that tended to improve with time [77].

5.2 Melatonin

The melatonin secretion pattern has been studied in different groups of critically ill patients. The results of these studies vary somewhat depending on the study population and the methodology. In general, a disturbed melatonin excretion pattern has been consistently reported, with either low levels at different times of day with an absence of nocturnal rise, a preserved but dampened rise and delayed phase, or high levels of melatonin at all times of the day (see details in Table 1). Collectively, these results suggest an influence on the melatonin-based rhythm by the many disrupters in the patient and the ICU itself (encephalopathy, use of mechanical ventilation, catecholamine administration, dim lighting, frequent nursing care arousal stimuli, nighttime noise pollution, etc.) [41]. In some cases, the utility of melatonin as a "hand of the clock" (e.g. phase marker) may be reduced, as with the use of 24-h urinary 6SMT profiles in patients with acute kidney injury. The clinical evidence regarding melatonin replacement in critically ill adults is reviewed in chapter "Best Practices for Improving Sleep in the ICU. Part II: Pharmacologic".

To conclude, the ICU light/dark cycle may fail to entrain the SCN if daytime light is too low, particularly in patients with sedative-induced eye closure. Patients may also be subjected to various mistimed zeitgebers that may influence melatonin circadian timing.

5.3   Cortisol

Many studies have shown loss of the 24-h circadian profile of cortisol in critically ill patients with respiratory failure, trauma, brain or burn injuries [59, 72, 77–79]. ACTH secretion also showed altered circadian rhythmicity during the night in a study of 40 critically ill patients, with a lower amplitude of rhythm in patients compared to controls [80].

5.4   Genetic Changes

To our knowledge, four studies have evaluated the molecular changes of gene clock expression in ICU patients. Coiffard et al. recently demonstrated that all trauma patients had disrupted circadian rhythms of cortisol, cytokines, leukocytes, and clock genes [81]. Maas et al. reported changes in clock gene expression in 15 critically ill patients, including 10 with sepsis and five with intracerebral hemorrhage, compared to 11 healthy controls [82]. Additionally, Acuna et al. enrolled 12 healthy volunteers, 24 ICU non septic control patients, and 20 septic ICU patients. Levels of *Bmal1*, *Clock*, and *Per2* expression were greater in the non-septic ICU patient and healthy volunteers than in septic ICU patients, suggesting that this reduction may favor the production of NF-kB dependent inflammatory response in septic patients [83]. Diaz et al. concluded that patients staying for a week in ICU exhibited altered expression of 4 clock genes (*Clock*, *Bmal1*, *Cry1*, and *Per2*) showing that the loss of circadian rhythmicity occurs at a molecular level [84].

To conclude, these preliminary studies have demonstrated the depth of clock gene alteration and their relationship to the inflammatory response in sepsis. Whether these alterations are adaptive to the host, and in which clinical contexts these alterations are maladaptive, is unclear.

6   Potential Clinical Consequences

Dysrhythmias that occur in specific populations such as shift workers or sleep deprived people are known to be associated with adverse outcomes (e.g., cardiovascular, metabolic, psychiatric, and oncologic diseases). Loss of rhythmicity may impair function: for example, the cardiomyocytes of *Bmal1* knockout mice exhibit impaired glucose utilization and contractility leading to reduced lifespan [85]. Animal models suggest that temporal organization of the immune system results in a more effective host response during the active phase when compared to the rest phase [86, 87].

As discussed above, in the population of ICU patients with sepsis, melatonin levels and the depth of clock gene alteration were correlated with severity of illness and the magnitude of inflammatory response. The highest levels of melatonin were seen in recovered septic patients [83]. Moreover, temperature curve displacement and cortisol circadian deregulation have been associated with the severity of illness and poor prognosis [59, 74]. Evidence of relationship between melatonin dysrhythmia and delirium have been suggested [88].

To summarize, circadian misalignment has the potential to impair recovery from critical illness. However, accurately assaying an individual's biological clock requires scrupulous consideration of potential masking factors (hepatic or renal dysfunction, medications that alter melatonin secretion, and environmental influences). Whether circadian dysrhythmias directly contribute to morbidity and mortality in critically ill patients remains unknown. The correction of iatrogenic circadian dysrthyhmias, at least, may be beneficial for patients' sleep and neurobehavioral performance and may improve clinical outcomes. Chapters "Best Practices for Improving Sleep in the ICU. Part I: Non-pharmacologic" and "Best Practices for Improving Sleep in the ICU. Part II: Pharmacologic" will discuss how interventions focused on improving circadian alignment can be employed in the ICU.

7   Conclusion

The circadian timing system regulates and coordinates countless physiological rhythms, including sleep/activity cycles, core body temperature fluctuations, endothelial function, hormone levels, and metabolism. The alignment of these internal activities with the external environment contributes to the fitness of the organism. In contrast, circadian misalignment between master and peripheral clocks and the environment leads to adverse health consequences. The ICU environment consists of weak and mistimed zeitgebers (light/dark cycles, food availability, physical activity, social interaction, and sleep/wake cycles) that may result in circadian dysrhythmias that inhibit recovery. Efforts to strengthen day/night routines and enhance circadian rhythmicity should be included in ICU sleep promotion strategies. Whether certain circadian dysrhythms observed in sepsis and other forms of critical illness should be modulated or are, in fact, adaptive, is not known.

References

1. Pittendrigh CS. Temporal organization: reflections of a Darwinian clock-watcher. Annu Rev Physiol. 1993;55:16–54.
2. Loudon AS. Circadian biology: a 2.5 billion year old clock. Curr Biol. 2012;22(14):R570–1.
3. O'Neill JS, van Ooijen G, Dixon LE, Troein C, Corellou F, Bouget FY, et al. Circadian rhythms persist without transcription in a eukaryote. Nature. 2011;469(7331):554–8.
4. Zhang R, Lahens NF, Ballance HI, Hughes ME, Hogenesch JB. A circadian gene expression atlas in mammals: implications for biology and medicine. Proc Natl Acad Sci U S A. 2014;111(45):16219–24.
5. Ceriani MF, Hogenesch JB, Yanovsky M, Panda S, Straume M, Kay SA. Genome-wide expression analysis in Drosophila reveals genes controlling circadian behavior. J Neurosci. 2002;22(21):9305–19.
6. Claridge-Chang A, Wijnen H, Naef F, Boothroyd C, Rajewsky N, Young MW. Circadian regulation of gene expression systems in the Drosophila head. Neuron. 2001;32(4):657–71.
7. Takahashi JS. Transcriptional architecture of the mammalian circadian clock. Nat Rev Genet. 2017;18(3):164–79.
8. Hastings MH, Maywood ES, Brancaccio M. Generation of circadian rhythms in the suprachiasmatic nucleus. Nat Rev Neurosci. 2018;19(8):453–69.
9. Welsh DK, Takahashi JS, Kay SA. Suprachiasmatic nucleus: cell autonomy and network properties. Annu Rev Physiol. 2010;72:551–77.
10. Saper CB, Scammell TE, Lu J. Hypothalamic regulation of sleep and circadian rhythms. Nature. 2005;437(7063):1257–63.
11. Nauta WJ. Hypothalamic regulation of sleep in rats; an experimental study. J Neurophysiol. 1946;9:285–316.
12. Franken P. A role for clock genes in sleep homeostasis. Curr Opin Neurobiol. 2013;23(5):864–72.
13. Ralph MR, Foster RG, Davis FC, Menaker M. Transplanted suprachiasmatic nucleus determines circadian period. Science. 1990;247(4945):975–8.
14. Czeisler CA, Duffy JF, Shanahan TL, Brown EN, Mitchell JF, Rimmer DW, et al. Stability, precision, and near-24-hour period of the human circadian pacemaker. Science. 1999;284(5423):2177–81.
15. Ohta H, Yamazaki S, McMahon DG. Constant light desynchronizes mammalian clock neurons. Nat Neurosci. 2005;8(3):267–9.
16. Duffy JF, Czeisler CA. Effect of light on human circadian physiology. Sleep Med Clin. 2009;4(2):165–77.
17. Provencio I, Jiang G, De Grip WJ, Hayes WP, Rollag MD. Melanopsin: an opsin in melanophores, brain, and eye. Proc Natl Acad Sci U S A. 1998;95(1):340–5.
18. Rosenthal NE, Joseph-Vanderpool JR, Levendosky AA, Johnston SH, Allen R, Kelly KA, et al. Phase-shifting effects of bright morning light as treatment for delayed sleep phase syndrome. Sleep. 1990;13(4):354–61.
19. Boivin DB, Duffy JF, Kronauer RE, Czeisler CA. Dose-response relationships for resetting of human circadian clock by light. Nature. 1996;379(6565):540–2.
20. Ceriani MF, Darlington TK, Staknis D, Mas P, Petti AA, Weitz CJ, et al. Light-dependent sequestration of timeless by cryptochrome. Science. 1999;285(5427):553–6.
21. Thapan K, Arendt J, Skene DJ. An action spectrum for melatonin suppression: evidence for a novel non-rod, non-cone photoreceptor system in humans. J Physiol. 2001;535(Pt 1):261–7.
22. Casiraghi L, Spiousas I, Dunster GP, McGlothlen K, Fernandez-Duque E, Valeggia C, et al. Moonstruck sleep: synchronization of human sleep with the moon cycle under field conditions. Sci Adv. 2021;7(5).
23. Sinturel F, Gos P, Petrenko V, Hagedorn C, Kreppel F, Storch KF, et al. Circadian hepatocyte clocks keep synchrony in the absence of a master pacemaker in the suprachiasmatic nucleus or other extrahepatic clocks. Genes Dev. 2021;35(5–6):329–34.

24. Paul JR, Davis JA, Goode LK, Becker BK, Fusilier A, Meador-Woodruff A, et al. Circadian regulation of membrane physiology in neural oscillators throughout the brain. Eur J Neurosci. 2020;51(1):109–38.

25. Yoo SH, Yamazaki S, Lowrey PL, Shimomura K, Ko CH, Buhr ED, et al. PERIOD2::LUCIFERASE real-time reporting of circadian dynamics reveals persistent circadian oscillations in mouse peripheral tissues. Proc Natl Acad Sci U S A. 2004;101(15):5339–46.

26. Asher G, Sassone-Corsi P. Time for food: the intimate interplay between nutrition, metabolism, and the circadian clock. Cell. 2015;161(1):84–92.

27. Patton DF, Mistlberger RE. Circadian adaptations to meal timing: neuroendocrine mechanisms. Front Neurosci. 2013;7:185.

28. Yadlapalli S, Jiang C, Bahle A, Reddy P, Meyhofer E, Shafer OT. Circadian clock neurons constantly monitor environmental temperature to set sleep timing. Nature. 2018;555(7694):98–102.

29. Manella G, Aviram R, Bolshette N, Muvkadi S, Golik M, Smith DF, et al. Hypoxia induces a time- and tissue-specific response that elicits intertissue circadian clock misalignment. Proc Natl Acad Sci U S A. 2020;117(1):779–86.

30. Harfmann BD, Schroder EA, Esser KA. Circadian rhythms, the molecular clock, and skeletal muscle. J Biol Rhythm. 2015;30(2):84–94.

31. Hower IM, Harper SA, Buford TW. Circadian rhythms, exercise, and cardiovascular health. J Circadian Rhythms. 2018;16:7.

32. Evans JA, Davidson AJ. Health consequences of circadian disruption in humans and animal models. Prog Mol Biol Transl Sci. 2013;119:283–323.

33. Musiek ES, Holtzman DM. Mechanisms linking circadian clocks, sleep, and neurodegeneration. Science. 2016;354(6315):1004–8.

34. Kecklund G, Axelsson J. Health consequences of shift work and insufficient sleep. BMJ. 2016;355:i5210.

35. Weingarten JA, Collop NA. Air travel: effects of sleep deprivation and jet lag. Chest. 2013;144(4):1394–401.

36. Claustrat B, Brun J, Chazot G. The basic physiology and pathophysiology of melatonin. Sleep Med Rev. 2005;9(1):11–24.

37. Lewy AJ, Tetsuo M, Markey SP, Goodwin FK, Kopin IJ. Pinealectomy abolishes plasma melatonin in the rat. J Clin Endocrinol Metab. 1980;50(1):204–5.

38. Bojkowski CJ, Arendt J, Shih MC, Markey SP. Melatonin secretion in humans assessed by measuring its metabolite, 6-sulfatoxymelatonin. Clin Chem. 1987;33(8):1343–8.

39. Crawford JH, Yang S, Zhou M, Simms HH, Wang P. Down-regulation of hepatic CYP1A2 plays an important role in inflammatory responses in sepsis. Crit Care Med. 2004;32(2):502–8.

40. Verceles AC, Silhan L, Terrin M, Netzer G, Shanholtz C, Scharf SM. Circadian rhythm disruption in severe sepsis: the effect of ambient light on urinary 6-sulfatoxymelatonin secretion. Intensive Care Med. 2012;38(5):804–10.

41. Maas MB, Lizza BD, Abbott SM, Liotta EM, Gendy M, Eed J, et al. Factors disrupting melatonin secretion rhythms during critical illness. Crit Care Med. 2020;48(6):854–61.

42. Mahlberg R, Tilmann A, Salewski L, Kunz D. Normative data on the daily profile of urinary 6-sulfatoxymelatonin in healthy subjects between the ages of 20 and 84. Psychoneuroendocrinology. 2006;31(5):634–41.

43. Brzezinski A. Melatonin in humans. N Engl J Med. 1997;336(3):186–95.

44. Buijs RM, Wortel J, Van Heerikhuize JJ, Feenstra MG, Ter Horst GJ, Romijn HJ, et al. Anatomical and functional demonstration of a multisynaptic suprachiasmatic nucleus adrenal (cortex) pathway. Eur J Neurosci. 1999;11(5):1535–44.

45. Veldhuis JD, Iranmanesh A, Johnson ML, Lizarralde G. Amplitude, but not frequency, modulation of adrenocorticotropin secretory bursts gives rise to the nyctohemeral rhythm of the corticotropic axis in man. J Clin Endocrinol Metab. 1990;71(2):452–63.

46. Umeda T, Hiramatsu R, Iwaoka T, Shimada T, Miura F, Sato T. Use of saliva for monitoring unbound free cortisol levels in serum. Clin Chim Acta. 1981;110(2–3):245–53.

47. Leproult R, Colecchia EF, L'Hermite-Baleriaux M, Van Cauter E. Transition from dim to bright light in the morning induces an immediate elevation of cortisol levels. J Clin Endocrinol Metab. 2001;86(1):151–7.
48. Chapotot F, Buguet A, Gronfier C, Brandenberger G. Hypothalamo-pituitary-adrenal axis activity is related to the level of central arousal: effect of sleep deprivation on the association of high-frequency waking electroencephalogram with cortisol release. Neuroendocrinology. 2001;73(5):312–21.
49. Chapotot F, Gronfier C, Jouny C, Muzet A, Brandenberger G. Cortisol secretion is related to electroencephalographic alertness in human subjects during daytime wakefulness. J Clin Endocrinol Metab. 1998;83(12):4263–8.
50. Morrison SF, Nakamura K. Central mechanisms for thermoregulation. Annu Rev Physiol. 2019;81:285–308.
51. Edwards B, Waterhouse J, Reilly T, Atkinson G. A comparison of the suitabilities of rectal, gut, and insulated axilla temperatures for measurement of the circadian rhythm of core temperature in field studies. Chronobiol Int. 2002;19(3):579–97.
52. Buhr ED, Yoo SH, Takahashi JS. Temperature as a universal resetting cue for mammalian circadian oscillators. Science. 2010;330(6002):379–85.
53. Doi M, Shimatani H, Atobe Y, Murai I, Hayashi H, Takahashi Y, et al. Non-coding cis-element of Period2 is essential for maintaining organismal circadian behaviour and body temperature rhythmicity. Nat Commun. 2019;10(1):2563.
54. Auger RR, Burgess HJ, Emens JS, Deriy LV, Thomas SM, Sharkey KM. Clinical practice guideline for the treatment of intrinsic circadian rhythm sleep-wake disorders: advanced sleep-wake phase disorder (ASWPD), delayed sleep-wake phase disorder (DSWPD), Non-24-hour sleep-wake rhythm disorder (N24SWD), and irregular sleep-wake rhythm disorder (ISWRD). An update for 2015: An American Academy of sleep medicine clinical practice guideline. J Clin Sleep Med. 2015;11(10):1199–236.
55. Delaney LJ, Litton E, Melehan KL, Huang HC, Lopez V, Van Haren F. The feasibility and reliability of actigraphy to monitor sleep in intensive care patients: an observational study. Crit Care. 2021;25(1):42.
56. Frisk U, Olsson J, Nylen P, Hahn RG. Low melatonin excretion during mechanical ventilation in the intensive care unit. Clin Sci (Lond). 2004;107(1):47–53.
57. Gehlbach BK, Chapotot F, Leproult R, Whitmore H, Poston J, Pohlman M, et al. Temporal disorganization of circadian rhythmicity and sleep-wake regulation in mechanically ventilated patients receiving continuous intravenous sedation. Sleep. 2012;35(8):1105–14.
58. Gehlbach BK, Patel SB, Van Cauter E, Pohlman AS, Hall JB, Zabner J. The effects of timed light exposure in critically ill patients: a randomized controlled pilot clinical trial. Am J Respir Crit Care Med. 2018;198(2):275–8.
59. Sertaridou EN, Chouvarda IG, Arvanitidis KI, Filidou EK, Kolios GC, Pnevmatikos IN, et al. Melatonin and cortisol exhibit different circadian rhythm profiles during septic shock depending on timing of onset: a prospective observational study. Ann Intensive Care. 2018;8(1):118.
60. Shilo L, Dagan Y, Smorjik Y, Weinberg U, Dolev S, Komptel B, et al. Patients in the intensive care unit suffer from severe lack of sleep associated with loss of normal melatonin secretion pattern. Am J Med Sci. 1999;317(5):278–81.
61. Danielson SJ, Rappaport CA, Loher MK, Gehlbach BK. Looking for light in the din: an examination of the circadian-disrupting properties of a medical intensive care unit. Intensive Crit Care Nurs. 2018;46:57–63.
62. Cisse YM, Borniger JC, Lemanski E, Walker WH 2nd, Nelson RJ. Time-restricted feeding alters the innate immune response to bacterial endotoxin. J Immunol. 2018;200(2):681–7.
63. Yasumoto Y, Hashimoto C, Nakao R, Yamazaki H, Hiroyama H, Nemoto T, et al. Short-term feeding at the wrong time is sufficient to desynchronize peripheral clocks and induce obesity with hyperphagia, physical inactivity and metabolic disorders in mice. Metabolism. 2016;65(5):714–27.

64. Honarmand K, Rafay H, Le J, Mohan S, Rochwerg B, Devlin JW, et al. A systematic review of risk factors for sleep disruption in critically ill adults. Crit Care Med. 2020;48(7):1066–74.
65. Doiron KA, Hoffmann TC, Beller EM. Early intervention (mobilization or active exercise) for critically ill adults in the intensive care unit. Cochrane Database Syst Rev. 2018;3:CD010754.
66. Maas MB, Lizza BD, Kim M, Abbott SM, Gendy M, Reid KJ, et al. Stress-induced behavioral quiescence and abnormal rest-activity rhythms during critical illness. Crit Care Med. 2020;48(6):862–71.
67. Keller M, Mazuch J, Abraham U, Eom GD, Herzog ED, Volk HD, et al. A circadian clock in macrophages controls inflammatory immune responses. Proc Natl Acad Sci U S A. 2009;106(50):21407–12.
68. Spengler ML, Kuropatwinski KK, Comas M, Gasparian AV, Fedtsova N, Gleiberman AS, et al. Core circadian protein CLOCK is a positive regulator of NF-kappaB-mediated transcription. Proc Natl Acad Sci U S A. 2012;109(37):E2457–65.
69. Narasimamurthy R, Hatori M, Nayak SK, Liu F, Panda S, Verma IM. Circadian clock protein cryptochrome regulates the expression of proinflammatory cytokines. Proc Natl Acad Sci U S A. 2012;109(31):12662–7.
70. Haimovich B, Calvano J, Haimovich AD, Calvano SE, Coyle SM, Lowry SF. In vivo endotoxin synchronizes and suppresses clock gene expression in human peripheral blood leukocytes. Crit Care Med. 2010;38(3):751–8.
71. Coiffard B, Diallo AB, Mezouar S, Leone M, Mege JL. A tangled threesome: circadian rhythm, body temperature variations, and the immune system. Biol-Basel. 2021;10(1).
72. Paul T, Lemmer B. Disturbance of circadian rhythms in analgosedated intensive care unit patients with and without craniocerebral injury. Chronobiol Int. 2007;24(1):45–61.
73. Kirkness CJ, Burr RL, Thompson HJ, Mitchell PH. Temperature rhythm in aneurysmal subarachnoid hemorrhage. Neurocrit Care. 2008;8(3):380–90.
74. Gazendam JAC, Van Dongen HPA, Grant DA, Freedman NS, Zwaveling JH, Schwab RJ. Altered circadian rhythmicity in patients in the ICU. Chest. 2013;144(2):483–9.
75. Papaioannou VE, Sertaridou EN, Chouvarda IG, Kolios GC, Pneumatikos IN. Determining rhythmicity and determinism of temperature curves in septic and non-septic critically ill patients through chronobiological and recurrence quantification analysis: a pilot study. Intensive Care Med Exp. 2019;7(1):53.
76. Varela M, Churruca J, Gonzalez A, Martin A, Ode J, Galdos P. Temperature curve complexity predicts survival in critically ill patients. Am J Respir Crit Care Med. 2006;174(3):290–8.
77. Pina G, Brun J, Tissot S, Claustrat B. Long-term alteration of daily melatonin, 6-sulfatoxymelatonin, cortisol, and temperature profiles in burn patients: a preliminary report. Chronobiol Int. 2010;27(2):378–92.
78. Bartanusz V, Corneille MG, Sordo S, Gildea M, Michalek JE, Nair PV, et al. Diurnal salivary cortisol measurement in the neurosurgical-surgical intensive care unit in critically ill acute trauma patients. J Clin Neurosci. 2014;21(12):2150–4.
79. Savaridas T, Andrews PJ, Harris B. Cortisol dynamics following acute severe brain injury. Intensive Care Med. 2004;30(7):1479–83.
80. Boonen E, Meersseman P, Vervenne H, Meyfroidt G, Guiza F, Wouters PJ, et al. Reduced nocturnal ACTH-driven cortisol secretion during critical illness. Am J Physiol Endocrinol Metab. 2014;306(8):E883–92.
81. Coiffard B, Diallo AB, Culver A, Mezouar S, Hammad E, Vigne C, et al. Circadian rhythm disruption and sepsis in severe trauma patients. Shock. 2019;52(1):29–36.
82. Maas MB, Iwanaszko M, Lizza BD, Reid KJ, Braun RI, Zee PC. Circadian gene expression rhythms during critical illness. Crit Care Med. 2020;48(12):e1294–e9.
83. Acuna-Fernandez C, Marin JS, Diaz-Casado ME, Rusanova I, Darias-Delbey B, Perez-Guillama L, et al. Daily changes in the expression of clock genes in sepsis and their relation with sepsis outcome and urinary excretion of 6-sulfatoximelatonin. Shock. 2020;53(5):550–9.
84. Diaz E, Diaz I, Del Busto C, Escudero D, Perez S. Clock genes disruption in the intensive care unit. J Intensive Care Med. 2020;35(12):1497–504.

85. Young ME, Brewer RA, Peliciari-Garcia RA, Collins HE, He L, Birky TL, et al. Cardiomyocyte-specific BMAL1 plays critical roles in metabolism, signaling, and maintenance of contractile function of the heart. J Biol Rhythm. 2014;29(4):257–76.
86. Edgar RS, Stangherlin A, Nagy AD, Nicoll MP, Efstathiou S, O'Neill JS, et al. Cell autonomous regulation of herpes and influenza virus infection by the circadian clock. Proc Natl Acad Sci U S A. 2016;113(36):10085–90.
87. Halberg F, Johnson EA, Brown BW, Bittner JJ. Susceptibility rhythm to *E. coli* endotoxin and bioassay. Proc Soc Exp Biol Med. 1960;103:142–4.
88. Dessap AM, Roche-Campo F, Launay JM, Charles-Nelson A, Katsahian S, Brun-Buisson C, et al. Delirium and circadian rhythm of melatonin during weaning from mechanical ventilation: an ancillary study of a weaning trial. Chest. 2015;148(5):1231–41.
89. Meyer TJ, Eveloff SE, Bauer MS, Schwartz WA, Hill NS, Millman RP. Adverse environmental conditions in the respiratory and medical ICU settings. Chest. 1994;105(4):1211–6.
90. Verceles AC, Liu X, Terrin ML, Scharf SM, Shanholtz C, Harris A, et al. Ambient light levels and critical care outcomes. J Crit Care. 2013;28(1):110 e1–8.
91. Dunn H, Anderson MA, Hill PD. Nighttime lighting in intensive care units. Crit Care Nurse. 2010;30(3):31–7.
92. Palazidou E, Franey C, Arendt J, Stahl S, Checkley S. Evidence for a functional role of alpha-1 adrenoceptors in the regulation of melatonin secretion in man. Psychoneuroendocrinology. 1989;14(1–2):131–5.
93. Murphy M, Bruno MA, Riedner BA, Boveroux P, Noirhomme Q, Landsness EC, et al. Propofol anesthesia and sleep: a high-density EEG study. Sleep. 2011;34(3):283–91A.
94. Ben-Hamouda N, Poirel VJ, Dispersyn G, Pevet P, Challet E, Pain L. Short-term propofol anaesthesia down-regulates clock genes expression in the master clock. Chronobiol Int. 2018;35(12):1735–41.
95. Alexopoulou C, Kondili E, Diamantaki E, Psarologakis C, Kokkini S, Bolaki M, et al. Effects of dexmedetomidine on sleep quality in critically ill patients a pilot study. Anesthesiology. 2014;121(4):801–7.
96. Munoz-Hoyos A, Fernandez-Garcia JM, Molina-Carballo A, Macias M, Escames G, Ruiz-Cosano C, et al. Effect of clonidine on plasma ACTH, cortisol and melatonin in children. J Pineal Res. 2000;29(1):48–53.
97. Golombek DA, Martini M, Cardinali DP. Melatonin as an anxiolytic in rats: time dependence and interaction with the central GABAergic system. Eur J Pharmacol. 1993;237(2–3):231–6.
98. McIntyre IM, Norman TR, Burrows GD, Armstrong SM. Alterations to plasma melatonin and cortisol after evening alprazolam administration in humans. Chronobiol Int. 1993;10(3):205–13.
99. Dimsdale JE, Norman D, DeJardin D, Wallace MS. The effect of opioids on sleep architecture. J Clin Sleep Med. 2007;3(1):33–6.
100. Oxlund J, Knudsen T, Strom T, Lauridsen JT, Jennum PJ, Toft P. Serum melatonin concentration in critically ill patients randomized to sedation or non-sedation. Ann Intensive Care. 2021;11(1):40.
101. Freedman NS, Gazendam J, Levan L, Pack AI, Schwab RJ. Abnormal sleep/wake cycles and the effect of environmental noise on sleep disruption in the intensive care unit. Am J Respir Crit Care Med. 2001;163(2):451–7.
102. Munro CL, Liang Z, Elias MN, Ji M, Chen X, Calero K. Sleep and activity patterns are altered during early critical illness in mechanically ventilated adults. Dimens Crit Care Nurs. 2021;40(1):29–35.
103. Hodge BA, Wen Y, Riley LA, Zhang X, England JH, Harfmann BD, et al. The endogenous molecular clock orchestrates the temporal separation of substrate metabolism in skeletal muscle. Skelet Muscle. 2015;5:17.
104. Mundigler G, Delle-Karth G, Koreny M, Zehetgruber M, Steindl-Munda P, Marktl W, et al. Impaired circadian rhythm of melatonin secretion in sedated critically ill patients with severe sepsis. Crit Care Med. 2002;30(3):536–40.

105. Li CX, Liang DD, Xie GH, Cheng BL, Chen QX, Wu SJ, et al. Altered melatonin secretion and circadian gene expression with increased proinflammatory cytokine expression in early-stage sepsis patients. Mol Med Rep. 2013;7(4):1117–22.
106. Patke A, Young MW, Axelrod S. Molecular mechanisms and physiological importance of circadian rhythms. Nat Rev Mol Cell Biol. 2020;21(2):67–84.
107. Hofstra WA, de Weerd AW. How to assess circadian rhythm in humans: a review of literature. Epilepsy Behav. 2008;13(3):438–44.
108. Telias I, Wilcox ME. Sleep and circadian rhythm in critical illness. Crit Care. 2019;23(1):82.

Atypical Sleep and Pathologic Wakefulness

Xavier Drouot

1 Introduction

Sleep in humans can be evaluated by analyzing the electrical activity generated by the brain as recorded by electroencephalography (EEG). (Please refer to chapters "Characteristics of Sleep in Critically Ill Patients. Part I: Sleep Fragmentation and Sleep Stage Disruption" and "Methods for Routine Sleep Assessment and Monitoring" for further background on sleep characterization and assessment). In their pioneering work, Allen Rechtschaffen and Antony Kales proposed polysomnographic criteria to classify different sleep stages [1]. For example, stage 2 sleep is defined by the presence of at least one K complex or one sleep spindle present in a 30-second epoch or in the 3 preceding or next minutes. Sleep in critically ill patients has been studied for decades [2–4]; its association with delirium has been an important research focus (chapters "Sleep Disruption and Its Relationship with Delirium: Electroencephalographic Perspectives" and "Sleep Disruption and Its Relationship with Delirium: Clinical Perspectives" review the relationship between sleep disruption and delirium).

Cooper et al. were the first to report ICU adults having sleep EEG patterns not corresponding with Rechtschaffen and Kales classification categories [5] (Table 1). For example, stage 2 sleep occurred in only 5 of 26 patients and transitions between stages 1, 3, 4 and REM sleep occurred without intervening stage 2 sleep. These authors used the term "atypical sleep" for the first time, noting ICU adults also displayed abnormal features on their awake EEG. They defined "pathological wakefulness" as EEG

X. Drouot (✉)
Centre d'Investigation Clinique INSERM 1402, Team Acute Lung Injury,
VEntilatory support and Sleep, Centre Hospitalier Universitaire de Poitiers,
and Université de Poitiers
Poitiers, France
e-mail: xavier.drouot@chu-poitiers.fr

G. L. Weinhouse, J. W. Devlin (eds.), *Sleep in Critical Illness*,
https://doi.org/10.1007/978-3-031-06447-0_3

Table 1 Comparison between conventional sleep and atypical sleep. Please refer to Drouot's criteria and Watson's criteria for detailed description [9, 10]

Domain	Normal sleep	Atypical sleep
Transitions sleep-wake	Present, clear	Present (Drouot), can be absent (Watson)
N2 figures	Present	Absent or strongly reduced density
N3 sleep: Delta waves	Present	Present and normal (Drouot), can be absent or abnormal (Watson)
Dynamic of sleep depth	Transition from light sleep to deep sleep	No transition from light to deep sleep
REM sleep	Present	Reduced or absent
Arousals	Present	Present or absent
Sleep cycles	Present	Absent

epochs where behavioral correlates of wakefulness [e.g., saccadic eye movements and sustained electromyography (EMG) activity] coincide with EEG features of slow wave sleep (i.e., high amplitude, low-frequency theta waves, 3–7 Hz) not seen in normal sustained wakefulness [5]. This pioneering work inspired other research teams, who also reported unusual EEG features in critically ill adults [6–8].

2 Defining Characteristics

Two different teams have proposed specific rules to identify and characterize atypical sleep and pathological wakefulness [9, 10].

2.1 Watson's Criteria

Paula Watson and collaborators examined polysomnographic recordings in 37 mechanically ventilated patients [9]. They noted frequent atypical polysomnographic findings such as absence of N2 sleep markers, presence of polymorphic delta, and burst suppression or isoelectric EEG. These investigators also reported a dissociation between the EEG signal and the behavioral state. Such dissociations consisted of: (a) abnormally slow EEG frequency in the theta or delta range (0.5–7 Hz) (normally generated during sleep) in awake patients and (b) low-amplitude, high-frequency beta EEG activity (typically indicative of wakefulness) present during coma. For example, awake patients able to interact with nurses were noted to predominantly exhibit theta (4–7 Hz) or delta activity (0.5–4 Hz). Conversely, alpha activity, an EEG frequency typically seen in the awake state, was observed in several unresponsive comatose patients.

These observations led investigators to recommend the abandonment of standard sleep scoring criteria in favor of the following proposed modified scoring system:

Step 1: Assess the patient for behavioral evidence of wakefulness or sleep. Step 2: For patients with behavioral evidence of wakefulness: (a) If the EEG is typical of wakefulness, the patient should be scored normal awake or (b) if the EEG is atypical, the patient should be scored pathological wakefulness. Step 3: For patients who are behaviorally sleeping or sedated, scoring is based on PSG features: wake, N1-N3, REM if conventional criteria are met, or atypical A1 to A6 if conventional features are absent (see [9] for tracing examples).

Interestingly, these authors reported that some patients could have normal sleep at any time during the study and a minority could have normal slow wave sleep and REM sleep. This underlines the possible co-existence of atypical sleep and normal sleep in a patient at different ICU time points [9].

2.2 Drouot's Criteria

These investigators acknowledged scoring sleep in sedated patients is challenging given the influence of sedating medications on the EEG. Several medications employed for sedation trigger delta slow waves that resemble spontaneous slow wave sleep [11] (see chapter "Effects of Common ICU Medications on Sleep"). Their classification has been built on PSG results from 57 non-sedated and responsive ICU adults.

Atypical sleep using this system is characterized by prolonged periods of continuous, high amplitude (50–100 µV), irregular delta activity; fast frequencies, rapid eye movements and low chin muscle tone are not superimposed and characteristics of N2 sleep (K complexes and sleep spindles) are absent. Except for the absence of K complex and sleep spindle, atypical sleep was visually identical to slow wave sleep. All patients with atypical sleep also exhibited periods highly suggestive of wakefulness, with rapid eye movements and sustained chin muscle activity (Fig. 1). This last criterion therefore implies some fluctuations between "atypical sleep" and "pathological wakefulness". These fluctuations could be spontaneous or provoked and evident at visual inspection. For the novice scorer, it is important to highlight that these fluctuations may often be subtle.

Pathological wakefulness was defined by the association of slowed EEG rhythms with an altered EEG reactivity to eyes opening. In their study, Drouot et al. found peak EEG frequency was significantly lower in pathological wakefulness than in normal awake patients (5.8 Hz [5.4–6.5] vs. 8.2 Hz [7.8–8.8], respectively, $p < 0.0001$) (Fig. 2). They evaluated EEG reactivity to eye opening as proxy for wakefulness as has previously been done during EEG classification efforts in patients with hepatic encephalopathy [12]. Normally, EEG background activity is present only with eyes closed and disappears with eye opening. Drouot and his collaborators proposed evaluating this EEG reactivity to eye opening and classify it into three grades (Fig. 3). They reported background frequency below 7 Hz associated with altered EEG reactivity (grade 1 or 2) had sensitivity of 100% and

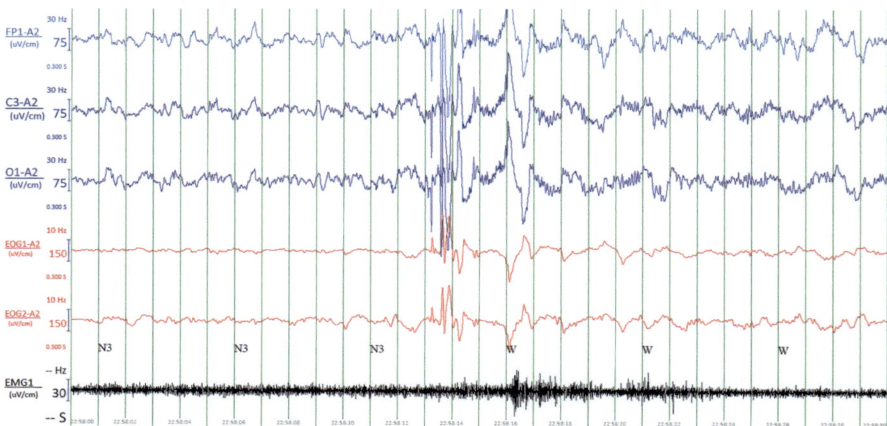

Fig. 1 Awakening during atypical sleep. One epoch (30s) of polysomnography recording showing atypical sleep (left half) and an awakening (right half) illustrating that transitions between "sleep state" and "wake state" are always present in patient with atypical EEG patterns in the Drouot classification. For all figures: Blue signals are EEG (FP1-A2, C3-A2, O1-A2); red signals are electro-oculograms and black signal is chin electromyogram

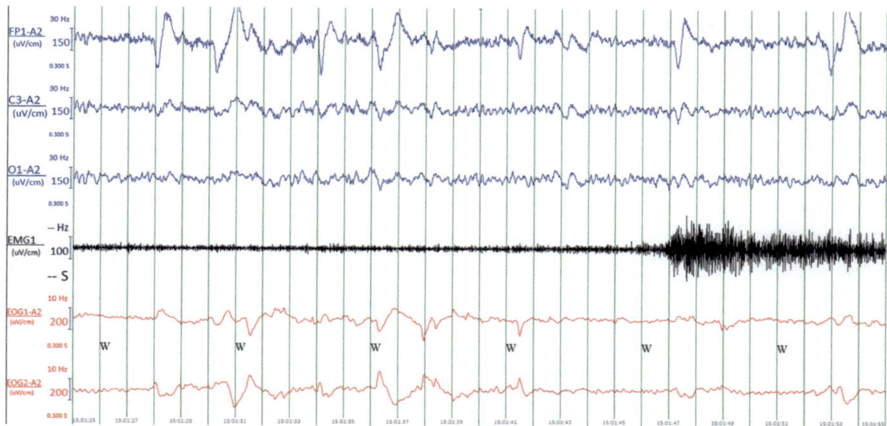

Fig. 2 Pathological wakefulness. One epoch (30s) of polysomnography recording showing pathological wakefulness. Note the numerous EEG theta waves (evocative of sleep) and the eye movements and the chin EMG amplitude fluctuations corresponding to movements

specificity of 97% in detecting pathological wakefulness [10]. Pathological wakefulness and atypical sleep were frequently found together in the same patient.

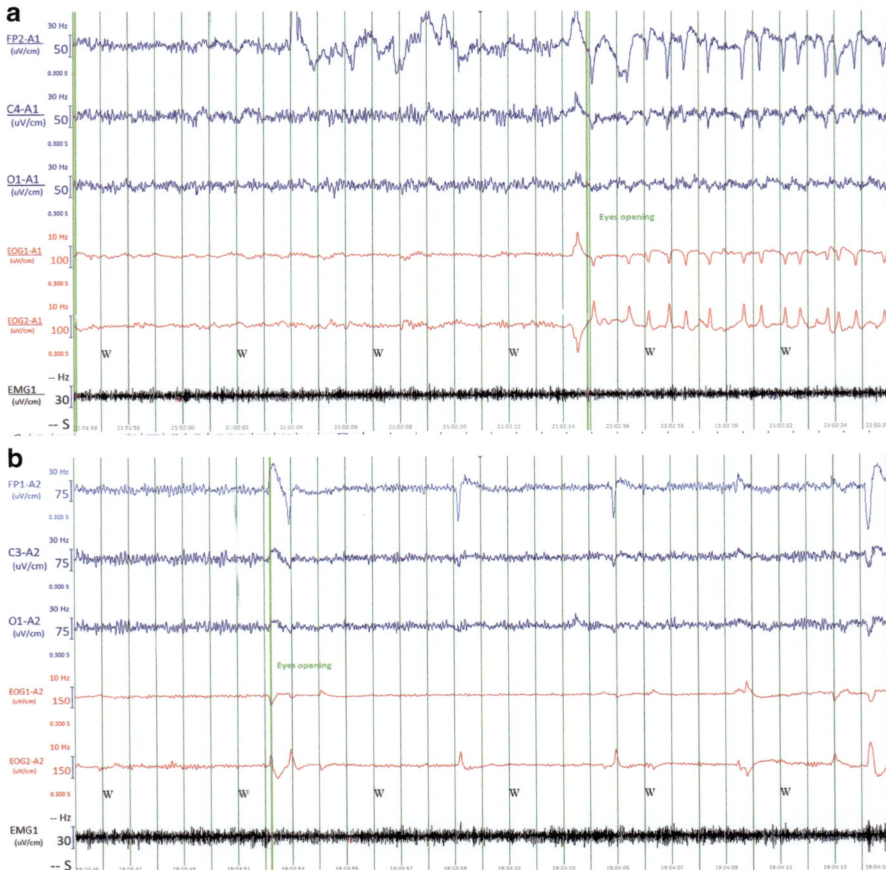

Fig. 3 Altered EEG reactivity to eye opening. (**a**) One epoch (30s) of polysomnography recording showing normal EEG reactivity. Note the disappearance of the alpha waves when eyes opened (green line). (**b**) One epoch (30s) of polysomnography recording showing altered EEG reactivity to eyes opening. Note that EEG signal change is perceptible at eyes opening, but background EEG activity is still visible with eye opened. When EEG reactivity is absent, no EEG changes are visible when patient open the eyes (not shown)

2.3 Comparisons Between the Watson and Drouot Criteria

The first difference between the two scoring systems is that for patients receiving sedation Watson's criteria can be used but Drouot's cannot (Table 2) [9, 10]. The second difference relates to fluctuation between the awake (i.e., normal or pathological) and sleep (i.e., normal or atypical) states. In Drouot's system, the EEG must fluctuate between the awake and sleep states given these transitions are a mandatory scoring component. In contrast, Watson's atypical sleep criteria does not require the

Table 2 Comparison between Drouot and Watson criteria [9, 10][a]

Domain	Watson criteria	Drouot criteria
Sedation	Can evaluate both sedated and non-sedated patients	Only can evaluate non-sedated patients
Pathological wakefulness criteria	Any EEG frequency other than alpha or beta with behavioral characteristics of wakefulness	Altered EEG reactivity to eyes opening (grade 1 or 2) and background EEG frequency <7 Hz
Atypical sleep criteria	Absence of K complex and spindle and presence[a] of polymorphic delta, FIRDA, triphasic activity, burst-suppression pattern, suppressed pattern or isoelectric activity	Absence of K complex and spindle with polymorphic delta activity with arousals
Transition between pathological wake and atypical sleep	No criteria Continuous EEG without transitions between two states can be scored atypical sleep	Presence of transitions ("arousals" and "awakenings") between pathological wake and atypical sleep are mandatory (continuous EEG without transition between to states cannot be scored atypical sleep)
Algorithm		
Step 1	Determine if awake or asleep/coma	Determine if awake or asleep/coma
Step 2	If awake: Assess EEG and search for normal (alpha/beta waves) or abnormal wake EEG activity (theta/delta waves)	When awake: Assess EEG reactivity to eyes opening
Step 3	Score using standard criteria or atypical sleep A_t1 to A_t6	Score atypical sleep or pathological wakefulness

[a] Please refer to Table 1 in Watson [9] for a detailed description. FIRDA: frontal intermittent rhythmic delta activity

occurrence of these transitions as these criteria considers monotonic and continuous EEG tracing with burst suppression patterns (A_t4), suppressed patterns (A_t5) and isoelectric activity (A_t6). However, whether atypical sleep stages (specifically A_t4, A_t5 and A_t6) could be considered as encephalopathy instead of sleep states have been debated [9, 13].

In summary, Drouot's criteria should be used in non-sedated patients given sedation may influence brain functioning during sleep, a condition propitious for pathophysiological studies or outcome studies. Although Watson's criteria can be used in sedated patients, it is important to keep in mind that sedation might mask or block natural sleep brain waves [14].

3 Monitoring Tools

Polysomnography associated with a behavioral assessment of patients' responsiveness is used to identify atypical sleep and pathological wakefulness (Please see chapters "Characteristics of Sleep in Critically Ill Patients. Part I: Sleep Fragmentation and Sleep Stage Disruption" and "Methods for Routine Sleep Assessment and Monitoring"). The EEG recording is probably the only reliable tool to assess and monitor atypical sleep and pathological wakefulness. Behavioral responsiveness is assessed by asking patients to sequentially open and close their eyes while visually evaluating EEG reactivity. Under normal conditions, there are clear EEG differences between periods when eyes are opened and when they are closed. When the EEG is similar between eyes open and closed periods, EEG reactivity is considered to be absent. When the difference is partial, EEG reactivity is considered to be altered (Fig. 3). Pathological wakefulness can also be detected with spectral EEG analysis given EEG recordings have been shown to be different between normal and pathological wakefulness periods [10]. The fact that spectral analysis was performed using a single EEG channel suggests single channel use may be sufficient to detect pathological wakefulness. Similar EEG analysis using more complex algorithms are under development to detect sleep and atypical sleep by automation in critically ill patients. Once technology is more refined, automated EEG analysis may represent a novel sleep evaluation approach in routine ICU practice.

4 Prevalence

The prevalence of atypical sleep and pathological wakefulness is highly variable and depends on patient risk factors (see below) and on the awareness of those who score the recordings to detect unusual sleep EEG patterns. In sedated or unconscious patients, the prevalence of at least one unusual electroencephalogram pattern (pathological wake or atypical sleep) ranges from 60% to 97% [5, 9, 15]. In conscious, non-sedated or lightly sedated ICU patients, the prevalence of abnormal sleep EEG patterns ranges from 23% to 31% [8, 10, 16–18]. When factors known to alter an electroencephalogram (sedation, coma or history of epilepsy, stroke) are used as exclusion criteria, the prevalence of atypical sleep is likely to be lower (0–19%) [19, 20].

5   Pathophysiology and Risk Factors

5.1   Pathophysiology

The pathophysiology of atypical sleep is largely unknown, and no studies have attempted to clarify its origin. Data can only be inferred from studies reporting atypical sleep prevalence in different ICU subpopulations exposed to different potential risk factors. Several investigators have reported patients with atypical sleep receive more sedation than patients with normal sleep [5, 21]. Thille et al. found patients with atypical sleep spent more days under sedation and received a higher cumulative dose of midazolam. In the study by Cooper et al., patients with atypical sleep were merged with patients in coma; therefore, similar conclusions could not be made [5]. In contrast, Knauert et al. found no significant differences in narcotics, benzodiazepine and propofol administration in patients with atypical sleep compared to patients with normal sleep EEG patterns [17, 20]. Thille et al. reported the number of days with sedation was not different in patients with and without atypical sleep (p = 0.08) in patients extubated the day before PSG, although the study was underpowered to show such a difference [21]. These discrepancies may be explained by the variability in the duration of delay between sedation discontinuation and PSG assessment. Therefore, it remains unclear if sedation is a strong pathophysiological risk factor for atypical sleep.

5.2   Risk Factors

Risk factors are attributes, characteristics or exposures that increase the likelihood of a person developing a disease. Several methodological criteria are required to make inferences between risk factors and a disease. The study question or hypothesis has to be formulated so that it can be tested using statistical analysis. Patient populations (i.e., exposed or control) need to be defined to characterize risk factors and indicators of exposure have to be appropriate [22]. There are many risk factors for sleep disruption in the ICU (see chapter "Risk Factors for Disrupted Sleep in the ICU"). However, only a minority of these have been associated with the presence of atypical sleep given the limited number of investigations in this area.

Severity of illness at admission [5, 15] and the increased use of invasive ventilation has been associated with atypical sleep and pathological wakefulness in the ICU [15]. Among adults admitted to the ICU with acute respiratory failure and treated for ≥ 2 or more days with non-invasive ventilation, hypercapnia was associated with atypical sleep [23]. The authors reported a negative correlation between spindle density and arterial PCO_2; patients with atypical sleep had a lower sleep spindle density. In 17 non-sedated, adults admitted to the ICU with a chronic obstructive pulmonary disease exacerbation, Boyko and al. reported that 59% of patients displayed atypical sleep [24].

An association between atypical sleep and sepsis has been reported by Freedman et al., [16]. Interestingly, in four patients, an EEG pattern evocative of atypical sleep and pathological wakefulness appeared in the 8 h prior to the presence of clinical signs of sepsis (e.g., fever, hypotension). These data have been replicated in a more recent study reporting atypical sleep in 49% of non-sedated patients and ventilated patients with severe sepsis [24]. However, further research is required given severe sepsis is known to alter brain function and modify the EEG and to trigger sepsis-associated encephalopathy [25], a condition sharing EEG features with atypical sleep and pathological wakefulness.

Sepsis-associated encephalopathy is associated with non-specific electroencephalographic patterns [25]. Some of these findings are not included in EEG descriptions of atypical sleep, such as seizures or periodic epileptiform discharges. However, some EEG patterns associated with sepsis (such as increased theta rhythms, predominant delta waves, triphasic waves and suppression of EEG activity) have been reported in atypical sleep, especially by Watson et al. [9]. In addition, sepsis can be associated with a significant drop in the relative peak frequency of the alpha band or an intermittent delta activity or an impaired EEG reactivity [26–28] which all are patterns included in Drouot's criteria. Confusion may arise because EEG changes in septic encephalopathy might appear before clinical symptoms of sepsis [29, 30] but also because alteration of sleep wake cycle are part of the clinical symptoms of severe sepsis [31].

Lastly, prolonged sleep deprivation, common in the ICU, by itself can slow down background EEG frequency and trigger the appearance of theta waves during wakefulness. Sleep loss can alter EEG reactivity to eye opening (with persistence of alpha waves in subjects with opened eyes) very similar to what has been noted in pathological wakefulness [32, 33]. Sleep after sleep deprivation or sleep occurring during prolonged sleep restriction is characterized by decreased spindle [34] and K complex densities [35]. The prolonged and severe sleep deprivation experienced by ICU patients might be an ingredient leading to atypical sleep and pathological wakefulness.

Studies investigating risk factors for atypical sleep are too rare to draw conclusions. Despite most critically ill adults experiencing many risk factors for sleep disruption during their ICU stay, a method to characterize these risk factors as they pertain to atypical sleep does not exist. Atypical sleep can be thought of as the most degraded form of human sleep, a sort of rudimentary sleep pattern where the brain is reduced to very basic functioning, devoid of its natural complexity. For instance, sleep spindles and K-complexes emerge from the complex interplay between thalamus and cortex during sleep [36]. A loss a functional connectivity could lead to atypical sleep. Atypical sleep and pathological wake might be a specific brain dysfunction, that could be a sort of "sleep deprivation related encephalopathy".

6   Clinical Consequences

It remains uncertain whether atypical sleep is associated with poor outcomes. Sedation and sepsis remain important confounding factors for atypical sleep but risk factor models incorporating these variables have not been published.

6.1   Respiratory Outcomes

Among ICU patients admitted with hypercapnic acute respiratory failure, the presence of atypical sleep on ICU day 3 was associated with a longer duration of non-invasive ventilation, a need for intubation, or death on ICU day 6 [8]. In this study, admission severity of illness and ICU daily severity of illness and respiratory parameters on each ICU day of PSG assessment were similar between patients with and without atypical sleep. Among patients meeting extubation criteria, the presence of atypical sleep was associated with a prolonged weaning period [21]. However, others have reported a lack of association between atypical sleep and prolonged weaning [37]. One recent study found atypical sleep not to be associated with respiratory failure after extubation [20]. However, compared to patients with normal sleep EEG patterns, patients with atypical sleep had lower negative airway pressure generated against occlusion during the first 0.1 s of spontaneous inspiration (P0.1), suggesting that atypical sleep could alter brain ventilatory drive [21]. Atypical sleep is more frequent in patients who are mechanically ventilated but severity of illness, an important risk for atypical sleep, is also greater among intubated patients [15].

6.2   Neurologic Outcomes

Delirium is a clinical manifestation of acute encephalopathy; abnormal sleep organization in this population is prevalent (see chapters "Sleep Disruption and Its Relationship with Delirium: Electroencephalographic Perspectives" and "Sleep Disruption and Its Relationship with Delirium: Clinical Perspectives"). In one cohort of cardiac surgery patients admitted to the ICU, atypical sleep was found to be more than four-times greater among those patients who developed postoperative delirium [38]. Among patients treated with NIV for hypercapnic respiratory failure, delirium occurrence is great among patients where a PSG assessment(s) revealed atypical sleep [10]. Other studies have reported an association between atypical sleep and neurological status at ICU discharge among patients with encephalopathy [39] or head injury [18]. Two studies have reported an association with atypical sleep and mortality [40, 41].

7 Treatment

It is not known if reducing the incidence of atypical sleep will improve ICU outcomes; no intervention studies designed to reduce atypical sleep have been published. Our lack of understanding of the pathophysiology of atypical sleep in the ICU currently precludes identifying potential treatment strategies. As knowledge of the risk factors for atypical sleep evolve, strategies focused on reducing modifiable risk factors should be investigated. For example, sedation reduction and early discontinuation, sleep promotion protocols, and early identification of patients at risk for atypical sleep may help reduce the occurrence of atypical sleep.

8 Conclusion

Atypical sleep and pathological wakefulness are abnormal forms of sleep and wakefulness very frequently observed in critically ill patients, that could be the most degraded form of human sleep. In the case of atypical sleep, patients display specific EEG patterns that can be identified on EEG signals. Specific rules have been proposed to score sleep in ICU patients. While the pathophysiology of atypical sleep and pathological wakefulness is complex, research efforts are important given atypical sleep seems to be associated with poor outcomes. Sleep-promoting strategies should be implemented as early as possible in the ICU stay to prevent the occurrence of atypical sleep.

References

1. Rechtschaffen A, Kales A. A manual for standardized terminology, techniques and scoring system for sleep stages of human subjects. Washington, DC: Public Health Service, US Government Printing Office; 1968. p. 1–12.
2. Helton MC, Gordon SH, Nunnery SL. The correlation between sleep deprivation and the intensive care unit syndrome. Heart Lung. 1980;9(3):464–8.
3. Johns MW, Large AA, Masterton JP, Dudley HA. Sleep and delirium after open heart surgery. Br J Surg. 1974;61(5):377–81.
4. Broughton R, Baron R. Sleep patterns in the intensive care unit and on the ward after acute myocardial infarction. Electroencephalogr Clin Neurophysiol. 1978;45(3):348–60.
5. Cooper AB, Thornley KS, Young GB, Slutsky AS, Stewart TE, Hanly PJ. Sleep in critically ill patients requiring mechanical ventilation. Chest. 2000;117(3):809–18.
6. Watson PL. Measuring sleep in critically ill patients: beware the pitfalls. Crit Care. 2007;11(4):159.
7. Elliott R, Nathaney A. Typical sleep patterns are absent in mechanically ventilated patients and their circadian melatonin rhythm is evident but the timing is altered by the ICU environment. Aust Crit Care. 2014;27(3):151–3.

8. Roche Campo F, Drouot X, Thille AW, et al. Poor sleep quality is associated with late noninvasive ventilation failure in patients with acute hypercapnic respiratory failure. Crit Care Med. 2010;38(2):477–85.

9. Watson PL, Pandharipande P, Gehlbach BK, et al. Atypical sleep in ventilated patients: empirical electroencephalography findings and the path toward revised ICU sleep scoring criteria. Crit Care Med. 2013;41(8):1958–67.

10. Drouot X, Roche-Campo F, Thille AW, et al. A new classification for sleep analysis in critically ill patients. Sleep Med. 2012;13(1):7–14.

11. Murphy M, Bruno MA, Riedner BA, et al. Propofol anesthesia and sleep: a high-density EEG study. Sleep. 2011;34(3):283–291A.

12. Amodio P, Marchetti P, Del Piccolo F, et al. Spectral versus visual EEG analysis in mild hepatic encephalopathy. Clin Neurophysiol. 1999;110(8):1334–44.

13. Bridoux A, Thille AW, Quentin S, et al. Sleep in ICU: atypical sleep or atypical electroencephalography? Crit Care Med. 2014;42(4):e312–3.

14. Gehlbach BK, Chapotot F, Leproult R, et al. Temporal disorganization of circadian rhythmicity and sleep-wake regulation in mechanically ventilated patients receiving continuous intravenous sedation. Sleep. 2014;35(8):1105–14.

15. Foreman B, Westwood AJ, Claassen J, Bazil CW. Sleep in the neurological intensive care unit: feasibility of quantifying sleep after melatonin supplementation with environmental light and noise reduction. J Clin Neurophysiol. 2015;32(1):66–74.

16. Freedman NS, Gazendam J, Levan L, Pack AI, Schwab RJ. Abnormal sleep/wake cycles and the effect of environmental noise on sleep disruption in the intensive care unit. Am J Respir Crit Care Med. 2001;163(2):451–7.

17. Knauert MP, Yaggi HK, Redeker NS, Murphy TE, Araujo KL, Pisani MA. Feasibility study of unattended polysomnography in medical intensive care unit patients. Heart Lung. 2014;43(5):445–52.

18. Valente M, Placidi F, Oliveira AJ, et al. Sleep organization pattern as a prognostic marker at the subacute stage of post-traumatic coma. Clin Neurophysiol. 2002;113(11):1798–805.

19. Kondili E, Alexopoulou C, Xirouchaki N, Georgopoulos D. Effects of propofol on sleep quality in mechanically ventilated critically ill patients: a physiological study. Intensive Care Med. 2012;38(10):1640–6.

20. Thille AW, Barrau S, Beuvon C, et al. Role of sleep on respiratory failure after extubation in the icu. Ann Intensive Care. 2021;11(1):71.

21. Thille AW, Reynaud F, Marie D, et al. Impact of sleep alterations on weaning duration in mechanically ventilated patients: a prospective study. Eur Respir J. 2018;51(4).

22. Blumenthal UJ, Fleisher JM, Esrey SA, Peasey A. Epidemiology: A tool for the assessment of risk. In: Organization WH, editor. Water quality: Guidelines, standards, and health: assessment of risk and risk management for water-related infectious disease. London: IWA Publishing; 2001. p. 135.

23. Quentin S, Thille AW, Roche-Campo F, et al. Atypical sleep in icu: role of hypercapnia and sleep deprivation. Paper presented at: ATS meeting; May 19, 2014; San Diego. https://www. atsjournals.org/doi/pdf/10.1164/ajrccm-conference.2014.189.1_MeetingAbstracts.A3615

24. Boyko Y, Jennum P, Oerding H, Lauridsen JT, Nikolic M, Toft P. Sleep in critically ill, mechanically ventilated patients with severe sepsis or copd. Acta Anaesthesiol Scand. 2018;62:1120–6.

25. Pantzaris ND, Platanaki C, Tsiotsios K, Koniari I, Velissaris D. The use of electroencephalography in patients with sepsis: a review of the literature. J Transl Int Med. 2021;9(1):12–6.

26. Berisavac II, Padjen VV, Ercegovac MD, et al. Focal epileptic seizures, electroencephalography and outcome of sepsis associated encephalopathy-a pilot study. Clin Neurol Neurosurg. 2016;148:60–6.

27. Rosengarten B, Krekel D, Kuhnert S, Schulz R. Early neurovascular uncoupling in the brain during community acquired pneumonia. Crit Care. 2012;16(2):R64.

28. Velissaris D, Pantzaris ND, Skroumpelou A, et al. Electroencephalographic abnormalities in sepsis patients in correlation to the calculated prognostic scores: a case series. J Transl Int Med. 2018;6(4):176–80.
29. Nielsen RM, Urdanibia-Centelles O, Vedel-Larsen E, et al. Continuous EEG monitoring in a consecutive patient cohort with sepsis and delirium. Neurocrit Care. 2020;32(1):121–30.
30. Young GB, Bolton CF, Archibald YM, Austin TW, Wells GA. The electroencephalogram in sepsis-associated encephalopathy. J Clin Neurophysiol. 1992;9(1):145–52.
31. Sonneville R, Verdonk F, Rauturier C, et al. Understanding brain dysfunction in sepsis. Ann Intensive Care. 2013;3(1):15.
32. Rodin EA, Luby ED, Gottlieb JS. The electroencephalogram during prolonged experimental sleep deprivation. Electroencephalogr Clin Neurophysiol. 1962;14:544–51.
33. Naitoh P, Kales A, Kollar EJ, Smith JC, Jacobson A. Electroencephalographic activity after prolonged sleep loss. Electroencephalogr Clin Neurophysiol. 1969;27(1):2–11.
34. De Gennaro L, Ferrara M, Bertini M. Effect of slow-wave sleep deprivation on topographical distribution of spindles. Behav Brain Res. 2000;116(1):55–9.
35. Sforza E, Chapotot F, Pigeau R, Paul PN, Buguet A. Effects of sleep deprivation on spontaneous arousals in humans. Sleep. 2004;27(6):1068–75.
36. Steriade M. The corticothalamic system in sleep. Front Biosci. 2003;8:d878–99.
37. Dres M, Younes M, Rittayamai N, et al. Sleep and pathological wakefulness at the time of liberation from mechanical ventilation (sleewe). A prospective multicenter physiological study. Am J Respir Crit Care Med. 2019;199(9):1106–15.
38. Chen Q, Peng Y, Lin Y, Li S, Huang X, Chen LW. Atypical sleep and postoperative delirium in the cardiothoracic surgical intensive care unit: a pilot prospective study. Nat Sci Sleep. 2020;12:1137–44.
39. Sutter R, Barnes B, Leyva A, Kaplan PW, Geocadin RG. Electroencephalographic sleep elements and outcome in acute encephalopathic patients: a 4-year cohort study. Eur J Neurol. 2014;21(10):1268–75.
40. Boyko Y, Toft P, Ording H, Lauridsen JT, Nikolic M, Jennum P. Atypical sleep in critically ill patients on mechanical ventilation is associated with increased mortality. Sleep Breath. 2019;23(1):379–88.
41. Knauert MP, Gilmore EJ, Murphy TE, et al. Association between death and loss of stage n2 sleep features among critically ill patients with delirium. J Crit Care. 2018;48:124–9.

Normal Sleep Compared to Altered Consciousness During Sedation

Florian Beck, Olivia Gosseries, Gerald L. Weinhouse, and Vincent Bonhomme

1 Introduction

Sedation is an integral part of intensive care management that is often necessary for restoring homeostasis, facilitating mechanical ventilation, protecting the brain, ensuring patient comfort, and reducing anxiety [1]. Sedated patients may, at times, appear to be asleep and this has led to the common misperception that sleep and sedation are equivalent. In fact, patients are often told they will "go to sleep" when they are about to be sedated. However, the relationship between sedation and sleep is complex.

While both sleep and sedation, when compared to the waking state, share behavioral and physiologic similarities they exhibit distinct electroencephalogram and

F. Beck
Department of Anesthesia and Intensive Care Medicine, Liege University Hospital, Liege, Belgium
e-mail: fbeck@chuliege.be

O. Gosseries
Coma Science Group, GIGA-Consciousness Thematic Unit, GIGA-Research, Liege University, Liege, Belgium
e-mail: ogosseries@uliege.be

G. L. Weinhouse (✉)
Division of Pulmonary and Critical Care, Brigham and Women's Hospital and School of Medicine, Harvard University, Boston, MA, USA
e-mail: gweinhouse@bwh.harvard.edu

V. Bonhomme
Departments of Anesthesia and Intensive Care Medicine and Anesthesia, Liege University Hospital and Anesthesia and Perioperative Neuroscience Laboratory, GIGA-Consciousness Thematic Unit, GIGA-Research, Liege University, Liege, Belgium
e-mail: vincent.bonhomme@chuliege.be

G. L. Weinhouse, J. W. Devlin (eds.), *Sleep in Critical Illness*, https://doi.org/10.1007/978-3-031-06447-0_4

brain activity changes. Moreover, a patient who is sedated rather than sleeping may have very different sleep-related outcomes including their subjective sense of restfulness, recovery of sleep debt, learning and memory, elimination of neuronal waste products, immune modulation, protein synthesis, emotional regulation, and endocrine regulation. In this chapter, we will review these similarities and differences between sleep and sedation in the context of the care of the critically ill (Fig. 1).

2 Phenomenological and Behavioral Changes

Sleep and sedation have distinct phenomenological and behavioral characteristics (Table 1); some of which may appear similar under certain conditions. These two conditions are best compared across four domains: (1) spontaneous, reflex, or purposeful movements, (2) responses to external stimuli, (3) perception of the external environment, and (4) richness of mental content.

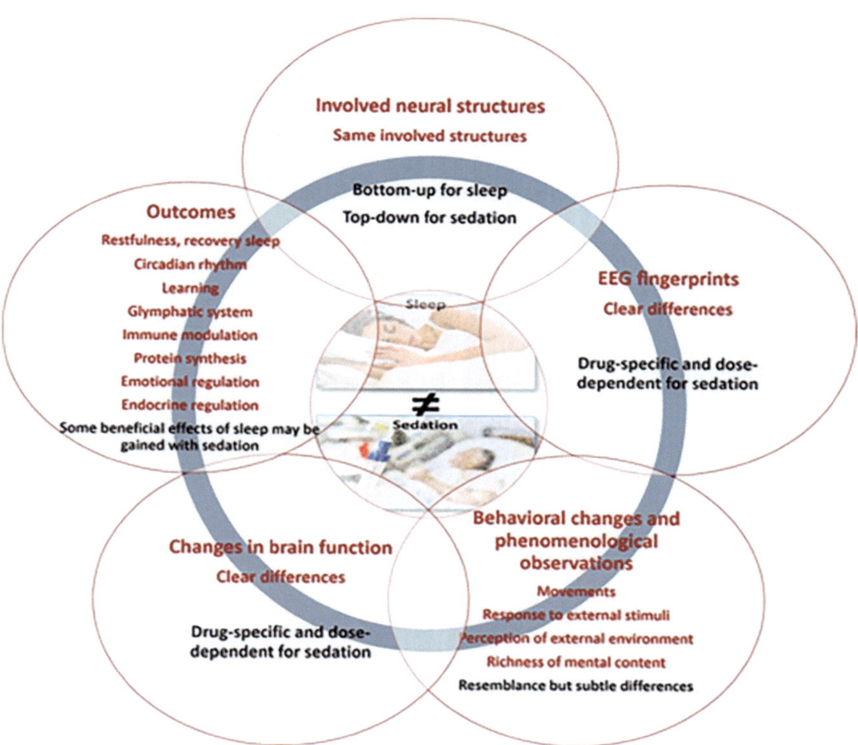

Fig. 1 Domains for comparison between sleep and sedation. EEG = electroencephalogram

Table 1 Comparison of behaviors and neural structures between sedation and sleep stages

Domain	Sedation	Sleep
Behavior—Movements	Dose-dependent reduction; not seen with KET (abnormal involuntary movements occur instead)	NREM: Reduced-none REM: Almost none
Behavior—Muscle tone	Dose-dependent reductions; not seen with KET or DEX	NREM: Decreased REM: Very decreased
Behavior—Response to stimuli	Dose-dependent reduction; with DEX preserved until high doses administered	Stage-dependent; lowest during N3 NREM REM: reduced
Behavior—Perception of environment	Dose-dependent reduction Possible episodes of connected consciousness (with or without recall)	Absent, except during lucid dreams
Behavior—Richness of mental content	Possible dreams (with or without recall); more frequent with DEX and KET (distorted) No memory consolidation with GABA agents	Dreaming possible Dreams most likely recalled if during REM Important role of sleep in memory consolidation (remembering and forgetting)
Involved neural structures	Same for sleep and sedation, including cortex and subcortical sleep-wake cycle regulating systems Most probably dominating bottom-up dynamic for sleep and top-down for sedation, (DEX is the exception)	

REM = rapid-eye movement sleep; NREM = non rapid-eye movement sleep; N3 NREM = stage 3 NREM sleep; GABA = mainly acting through a potentiation of γ-amino-butyric acid neurotransmission (propofol, benzodiazepines, barbiturates, and halogenated anesthetics); DEX = dexmedetomidine; KET = ketamine

Sleep is an actively generated brain function characterized by an organized cycling between rapid-eye-movement (REM) and non-REM sleep, as different from one another as they are from wakefulness, and governed by circadian and homeostatic influences. REM and the stages of non-REM sleep are defined according to their electroencephalographic (EEG) signature, eye movements (evaluated using electrooculogram), and muscle tone (as measured using electromyogram). NREM is further divided into three stages from lighter (N1 to N2) to deeper (N3) sleep. In contrast, phenomenological changes during sedation are dose-dependent and non-cyclic. Not all sedative agents produce the same behavioral and phenomenological characteristics. For example, the effects of agents acting mainly through the promotion of γ-amino-butyric-acid (GABA) neurotransmission, such as propofol, benzodiazepines, barbiturates, and halogenated anesthetics are distinct from agents acting on other neurotransmitter systems.

During sleep and sedation, spontaneous movements may be diminished or absent. Movement during sleep is stage-dependent; the least amount of movement and muscle tone is seen during REM sleep. As GABA-promoting sedative dosing increases, spontaneous movements and muscle tone are increasingly suppressed, reappearing when medication is decreased or discontinued. However, non-GABA sedative agents may preserve muscle tone, and even induce abnormal involuntary

non-purposeful movements. For example, dexmedetomidine, an α_2-adrenergic agonist, is characterized by preserved muscle tone and spontaneous ventilation.
Likewise, sedation with ketamine, a N-methyl-D-aspartate (NMDA) glutamate
receptor antagonist, is frequently associated with involuntary movements of the
limbs, also with preserved muscle tone and spontaneous ventilation [2].

During sleep, response to external stimuli such as verbal command or gentle
shaking is stage-dependent with patients in deep (N3) non-REM and REM stage
sleep being the least responsive. With the exception of dexmedetomidine, as the
dose of the sedative progressively increases, responsiveness progressively decreases.
In contrast, patients receiving dexmedetomidine, remain responsive until very high
doses are infused; this property is a potential advantage over other sedatives in the
ICU setting given it enables patients to communicate with their medical team and
families and participate in their own care [3].

A lack of response to external stimulation does not necessarily mean the absence
of a conscious experience [4]. Both sedation and sleep may be associated with
internally-generated mental imagery, or dreaming. When occurring in the absence
of any awareness of the external environment, dreaming is sometimes described as
disconnected consciousness [5]. During lucid dreaming (dreams where the dreamer
is aware they are dreaming), however, the ability to communicate with the external
environment persists [6, 7]. Whatever the conscious experience during sleep or
sedation, it is not necessarily followed by explicit recall. Internally-generated mental imagery may occur during all sleep stages, but is most likely recalled if occurring
during REM sleep. In this instance, the purpose of dreaming is thought to be related
to memory consolidation [8].

Mental imagery during sedation is more frequent with dexmedetomidine and ketamine, but may occur with all sedative agents, particularly during emergence from
sedation after it is weaned. Dreaming during ketamine is intense; hallucinations and
distorted self-perception are common [9]. Most likely, dreaming during GABAergic
sedation does not subserve the memory consolidation function of dreaming during
normal sleep. To the contrary, propofol and benzodiazepines produce anterograde
amnesia rather than the memory improvements known to occur with sleep.

3   Mechanistic Correlates and Targets

In the healthy awake individual, mental content, cognitive functions, and motor
behavior are generated by activity within the cerebral cortex. Within the cortex,
pyramidal neurons operate in a tight balance between excitatory projections from
subcortical structures and inhibitory projections from interneurons. Complex interactions between brain regions, organized in networks with constantly evolving
topological properties over space and time, are at the origin of these high-order
functions. However, this network connectivity is only possible when the cortex has
a sufficiently high degree of arousal.

Wakefulness and cortical arousal are promoted by excitatory projections from subcortical arousal centers located in the midbrain, pons and hypothalamus. The arousal-promoting projections are cholinergic, orexinergic and monoaminergic. Cholinergic nuclei are found in both the lateral-dorsal tegmental area (LDT) and the pedunculopontine tegmental area (PPT), located in the pons and basal forebrain. The orexinergic nuclei are found in the lateral hypothalamus (LH). The monoaminergic nuclei encompass several structures including the locus coeruleus (LC—norepinephrine) and dorsal raphe (DR—serotonin) located in the pons, the ventral periaqueductal grey area (vPAG—dopamine) and the tuberomamillary nucleus (TMN—histamine). Those arousal centers are restrained by inhibitory GABAergic and galaninergic projections from the preoptic area (POA) and emerge from the ventrolateral preoptic nucleus (VLPO) located in the anterior hypothalamus. Other inhibitory projections include the thalamic reticular nucleus (TRN), which regulates the output pathways of the thalamus, and the supraoptic nucleus of the hypothalamus (SON) [10–13].

The transition from wakefulness to sleep occurs via a "bottom-up" approach (i.e., from the subcortical to cortical region) through a series of neurophysiologic events influenced by both homeostatic mechanisms and circadian rhythms. The VLPO promotes and maintains sleep by sending GABA and galanin-mediated inhibitory projections to all major arousal centers. Decreased cortical activation is reflected by a reduction in excitatory projections to the cortex, which manifests as a lower frequency cortical neuron spontaneous firing. A presumed mechanism for the transition from wakefulness to NREM sleep is LC inhibition resulting in reduction of norepinephrine which in turn disinhibits the VLPO [14]. LC is extremely active during wakefulness and progressively less active during NREM, until REM is reached, where it becomes inactive. Other structures, such as the TRN, SON, and median preoptic nucleus, are also presumably involved in promoting NREM sleep. Deeper NREM stages are associated with higher neuronal hyperpolarization in the thalamus and cortex. REM sleep is promoted by different brainstem structures including the sublaterodorsal nucleus, ventrolateral periaqueductal grey, gigantocellular nucleus and the LH [10, 11, 13].

In contrast to sleep, drug-induced sedation appears to have a partial "top-down" (i.e., cortical to subcortical) mechanism of action. This is linked to the biochemical targets of the sedative and provides a unique EEG signature. GABA receptors are distributed throughout the brain and hence GABA agonist (e.g., barbiturates, benzodiazepines, and propofol) exposure results in central nervous system effects that are more global and result in multiple behavioral and phenomenological differences compared with physiological sleep. The enhanced inhibitory postsynaptic potentials (IPSP) of GABAergic sedatives diffusely reduce neurotransmission at the cortical level in both the thalamus and brainstem. The primary sites of action for these sedatives are the GABAergic postsynaptic connections between the inhibitory interneurons and pyramidal neurons in the cortex, the neurons in the TRN, and the GABAergic postsynaptic connections of the VLPO onto the arousal nuclei [10, 11, 15].

NMDA antagonists (e.g., ketamine) produce complex changes in neurotransmission [16]. Ketamine NMDA receptor antagonism indirectly excites neurons by suppressing their inhibition by GABAergic interneurons. This occurs at the level of the cortex, the limbic system, and the hippocampus [10, 15]. Through a similar disinhibition mechanism, it also increases release in the brain of dopamine, acetylcholine and other amines [17]. As a result, some cortical pyramidal cells are disinhibited, with an activation of specific brain regions including the anterior cingulate and medial prefrontal cortices while the insula, the hippocampus, and the precuneus, and other regions are inhibited [18, 19]. α_2-adrenergic agonists such as dexmedetomidine are exceptions to the "top-down" pattern of GABA agonists and NMDA antagonists. They primarily target the presynaptic α_2-receptors on neurons from the LC, which results in less norepinephrine release and reduced VLPO inhibition. Increased GABAergic and galaninergic VLPO activity consequently inhibits arousal centers [10, 14]. Hence, α_2-adrenergic agonists initiate sedation through mechanisms that are closely aligned to physiological sleep.

Modulation of neurotransmitters typically active during the waking state will impact sedation. For example, nicotinic acetylcholine receptor activation in the medial central nucleus of the thalamus weakens the hypnotic state induced by the inhaled anesthetic sevoflurane, a potent halogenated anesthetic with mainly GABAergic properties [20]. This has also been observed with propofol [21]. Likewise, the activation of histamine receptors in the basal forebrain is able to partially reverse a halogenated anesthetic-related hypnotic state [20]. Conversely, antihistamines, which are known to have a sedative effect, are sometimes given as a premedication before anesthesia.

4 Electroencephalogram Signatures

Sleep and sedation both induce specific neural oscillations that translate into specific EEG patterns (Table 2). A standard EEG approach or a perturbational transcranial magnetic stimulation with high-density EEG (TMS-EEG) can be used to characterize the electrophysiological changes associated with either sleep or sedation. During physiological sleep, the EEG evolves through different phases. The EEG pattern of N1 sleep is characterized by decreased β oscillations (13–25 Hz) and loss of occipital α oscillations (9–12 Hz) that are associated with relaxed wakefulness. During N2, slow δ oscillations (slow <1 Hz, δ: 1–4 Hz), K-complexes and sleep spindles (12–16 Hz) appear. K-complexes occur spontaneously as transient low frequency oscillations but they can also be evoked by sensory (auditory, somatosensory) stimulation. Sleep spindles are transient, present as single events, and are often, but not exclusively, associated with the "up" state of a slow wave. They reflect rebound bursting in thalamocortical neurons, and are generated in part by the TRN. N3 sleep is characterized by even larger slow wave oscillations than in N2. These slow waves reflect a toggling state of membrane potentials in cortical and thalamic neurons. These neurons switch between an "up" or depolarized state,

Table 2 Comparison of electroencephalogram signature and transcranial magnetic stimulation changes between sedation and sleep stages

Domain	Sedation	Sleep
EEG	Drug-class specific, dose-dependent, and often different from sleep K-complexes never found GABA: prevalent β (excitation) at low doses; evolution from regular β-γ to slow-δ and continuous α, burst-suppression at high doses DEX: resembles NREM sleep KET fast and irregular slow oscillations, high β-low γ	No burst-suppression pattern and γ oscillations N1 NREM: decreased β and loss of occipital α N2 NREM: slow δ, K-complexes, spindles N3 NREM: largest slow waves REM: activity approaching the waking state, mixed frequencies (propensity for θ or γ), PGO waves, no K-complexes or sleep spindles
TMS	GABA: breakdown of cortical response complexity DEX: increased cortical excitability KET: preserved cortical response complexity	NREM: slow and stereotyped cortical response REM: preserved cortical response complexity

REM = rapid-eye movement sleep; NREM = non rapid-eye movement sleep; N1, N2 and N3 = NREM sleep stages; GABA = mainly acting through a potentiation of γ-amino-butyric acid neurotransmission (propofol, benzodiazepines, barbiturates, and halogenated anesthetics); EEG = electroencephalogram; TMS = Transcranial Magnetic Stimulation; PGO = ponto-geniculate occipital; dex = dexmedetomidine; ket = ketamine

interpreted as intense synaptic activity and "down" or hyperpolarized state, reflecting the inactivated period. The alternation between the up and down states generates the slow oscillations, for which an unaltered thalamocortical network is required [11, 13, 22]. The complexity of the cortical response to TMS, which corresponds with the functional differentiation and integration of information by the brain, collapses during NREM sleep [23].

In contrast, REM sleep is characterized by cortical activity that approaches the waking state. In this case, the EEG pattern is made of mixed frequencies with a propensity for θ (5–8 Hz) or γ (26–80 Hz) oscillations, ponto-geniculate-occipital waves (PGO waves or P-waves) and the absence of K-complexes or sleep spindles [11, 13, 22]. During REM sleep, the complexity of the cortical response to TMS persists [23].

During sedation, EEG changes are drug-class specific, dose-dependent, and often different from sleep. Light propofol sedation evolves on the EEG from regular β-γ oscillations, larger than during the awake state, to slow-δ oscillations. Typically, at a low dose, a paradoxical propofol-induced excitation occurs, where β-oscillations are prevalent. As the dose increases, the higher frequency oscillations disappear and slow-δ oscillations of greater amplitude in the foreground appear accompanied by continuous α oscillations in the frontal region. The presence of such a frontal α pattern does not preclude volitional response to external stimulation [24]. At even higher doses, however, a burst suppression pattern (intermittent EEG bursts separated by electrical silence and associated with deep coma) appears [15, 25]. Similar to deep NREM sleep, propofol administration produces a breakdown of the complexity of the cortical response to TMS [26]. EEG changes associated with the administration of halogenated anesthetics, benzodiazepines, and barbiturates closely resemble those induced by propofol [27].

Ketamine is associated with an active EEG signature, composed of fast and irregular slow oscillations. The fast oscillations are located in the high β-low γ frequency range [15]. The complexity of the cortical response to TMS is preserved during ketamine administration [26]. Dexmedetomidine has also an EEG signature that is dose-dependent; however, unlike other sedatives it more closely resembles NREM sleep. At low doses, dexmedetomidine induces a combination of slow-δ oscillations with spindles in the high α-low β spectrum, lasting 1 or 2 s and closely resembling N2 sleep spindles. At higher doses, spindles disappear and the amplitude of the slow-δ oscillations strengthen to approximate N3 sleep patterns [15].

In summary, although sleep and sedation may sometimes share similarities in the observed EEG changes (such as slow-δ, and α oscillations of high amplitude) during their use, none are exactly the same, with the exception of dexmedetomidine and N2 sleep. In contrast to sleep, medications used to sedate critically ill patients may produce burst suppression and γ oscillations and K-complexes are not observed.

5   Changes in Brain Function

Sleep and sedation are associated with characteristic changes in brain function (Table 3). These changes can be assessed non-invasively in humans using several functional brain imaging techniques such as positron emission tomography (PET), functional magnetic resonance imaging (fMRI), high-density EEG, or TMS-EEG, either alone or in combination. In addition to changes in regional brain activity, functional brain imaging allows studying connectivity, i.e., communication between brain regions. Connectivity can be functional (FC), corresponding to an undirected statistical dependency between neurophysiological events within different neural populations, or synchrony in activity. Connectivity can also be effective (EC), when there exists a causal influence of the activity of one neural population over the activity of another. Connected brain regions organize into networks, where nodes and edges represent collections of brain tissue and their connectivity, respectively. Each of these network holds specific high-order brain functions. Some, like resting-state networks (RSNs), are active in awake, resting individuals who have their eyes closed and their mind is wandering. According to the graph theory, networks display several topological properties. The spatio-temporal dynamics of these networks continue to evolve over time and space [28]. Newly-appearing brain states, such as sleep or medication-associated sedation, are therefore associated with specific network property changes compared to the awake state. Many changes during sleep and sedation have yet to be characterized [5].

During sleep, the RSN architecture has been found to be the same as that during wakefulness, with no additional sleep-specific RSNs [29]. During NREM sleep, whole-brain metabolism and regional brain metabolism in the frontal and parietal

Table 3 Comparison of functional domains between sedation and sleep stages

Domain	Sedation	Sleep
Regional brain activity	GABA/DEX: decreased whole-brain activity, decreased frontal, parietal, thalamic and brain stem regional activity KET: Increased global brain activity, increased anterior cingulate, frontal, precuneus, parietal, and insula regional activity, decreased subgenual/subcallosal (anterior cingulate cortex), orbitofrontal and gyrus rectus regional activity	NREM: decreased whole-brain activity, decreased frontal, parietal, thalamic, and brain stem regional activity REM: higher brainstem, thalamus, extra-striate occipital cortex, hippocampus and amygdala activity as compared to NREM
Functional connectivity	Disruption of fronto-parietal connectivity and posterior 'hot zone' GABA: within- and between-network disruption in large-scale RSNs, thalamo-cortical FC disruption in higher-order networks, preserved in lower-order sensory networks DEX: similar to GABA and NREM, except for preserved FC between thalamus, anterior cingulate and meso-pontine area KET: global increase, disruptions in all higher-order RSNs except the ECN, fronto-parietal disruption, preserved in lower-order sensory networks	NREM: decreased global FC as NREM sleep deepens, higher-order connectivity patterns fade out but residual FC in RSNs, loss of widespread thalamo-cortical and hypothalamo-cortical FC during N1, high thalamo-cortical synchrony, hence strong thalamo-cortical FC during N2 and N3, attenuation of the anti-correlation between DMN and DAN, and between DMN and ECN REM: increased activity in the parietal posterior 'hot zone' during dreaming
Effective connectivity	GABA: impaired in large-scale networks and in lower-order sensory networks, reduced amplitude and complexity of long-distance cortical communication, directionality alteration, inhibition of long-latency evoked potentials DEX: inhibition of long-latency evoked potentials, increased cortical excitability KET: disturbed fronto-parietal anterior to posterior EC	NREM: progressive breakdown of trans-callosal long-range EC, increased cortical excitability, absent long-range temporal correlation in DMN and DAN during N3

(continued)

Table 3 (continued)

Domain	Sedation	Sleep
Network topology	GABA and DEX: connectivity strength reduction in large-scale networks, reduced global efficiency, increased clustering and modularity, reconfiguration of global brain network structure, disruption of the spatial balance between segregation and integration DEX: reduction in local and global large-scale network efficiency KET: network reorganization	RSN architecture identical to wakefulness N2 and N3: increased network modularity, increased network segregation NREM: reappearance of DMN nodes
Spatio-temporal dynamics	GABA and DEX: reduced complexity and repertoire of possible configurations, deviation from the critical point, disruption of metastability, disruption of the temporal balance between segregation and integration	Reduced and more stable repertoire of brain states N2 and N3: less frequent transitions between different FC topologies

REM = rapid-eye movement; NREM = non rapid-eye movement; N1, N2 and N3 = NREM sleep stages; GABA = mainly acting through a potentiation of γ-amino-butyric acid neurotransmission (propofol, benzodiazepines, barbiturates, and halogenated anesthetics); FC = functional connectivity; DMN = default-mode network; DAN = default attention network; ECN = executive control network; EC = effective connectivity; RSN = resting-state network; dex = dexmedetomidine; ket = ketamine

areas is reduced. Global FC decreases as NREM sleep deepens, with a loss of the widespread thalamo-cortical and hypothalamo-cortical FC during N1. Due to high thalamo-cortical synchrony during deeper NREM stages, this loss of widespread thalamo-cortical FC no longer exists at those stages [30, 31]. A growing body of evidence suggests residual FC during NREM sleep, even if higher-order connectivity patterns fade out [31, 32]. Indeed, the majority of RSN FC does not merely decrease in magnitude, but either reverses and increases in the opposite direction, or increases in amplitude. This is consistent with an altered rather than reduced FC during NREM sleep [33]. Long-range temporal correlations that are present in some RSNs during the waking state, and notably in the default mode network (DMN, thought to be responsible for self-awareness and internal thoughts) and the default attention network (DAN, responsible for switching attention from one element to the other), are diminished or even absent during N3 [34]. During wakefulness, DMN anti-correlates with DAN and the executive control network (ECN, responsible for attention to external environment), meaning that when one is active, the other is silent. This anti-correlation is attenuated during NREM sleep [30]. A breakdown of trans-callosal and long-range EC is also observed [35]. Another form of EC is cortical neurons' reactivity and response specificity to a stimulation, named cortical excitability, which corresponds to the strength of the response of cortical neurons to the stimulation. An endogenous-like response can be mimicked using TMS [36]. Cortical excitability varies across circadian rhythms, and increases during

NREM sleep [35], attentional lapses [37], and after sleep deprivation [38]. It reflects adequacy of local processing and reactivity of the cortex in time and space.

Compared to wakefulness, the transitions between different FC topologies are less frequent during N2 sleep [39]. NREM sleep has therefore a reduced and more stable repertoire of brain states [40]. Modularity, a spatial measure of functional segregation into networks, increases across the brain with the deepening of NREM sleep (stages N2 and N3). FC networks become more segregated during the deepest sleep phases [31, 41]. When dreaming during deep NREM sleep, the posterior "hot zone", a parietal hub within the DMN that has an extremely important role in information handling and dispatching, increases its activity [42]. During REM sleep, regional cerebral blood flow, a surrogate for regional activity, increases in the brainstem, the thalamus and the extra-striate occipital cortex that is consistent with PGO wave generation. It also increases in the hippocampus and amygdala, probably in relation with memory and emotion processes [30]. During REM sleep, the nodes of the DMN also reestablish their FC [31].

The effects of sedatives on brain function are predominantly agent-specific and dose-dependent. Overall, sedation seems to induce a reduced and more stable repertoire of brain states [40]. Propofol, the most studied GABAergic sedative in this area, produces a dose-dependent decrease in regional brain activity within the frontal cortex, cuneus/precuneus, thalamus, and brain stem [43]. It induces a disruption in within- and between-network FC in large-scale RSNs, particularly regarding the fronto-parietal connectivity and in the parietal "hot zone" [44–46]. Moreover, it disrupts the thalamo-cortical connectivity within higher order networks, while preserving FC within lower-order sensory networks [44]. Impairment in EC is present during propofol sedation, not only in large-scale networks, but also in lower-order sensory networks [28, 47–52]. Likewise, a reduction in the amplitude and complexity of long-distance cortical communication is observed [26, 52]. An alteration of the dynamics and directionality of EC, and a limitation of the connectivity configuration repertoire is also observed [47, 49, 51, 53, 54].

In contrast ketamine increases global and regional brain activity in a dose-dependent fashion in the anterior cingulate cortex, frontal lobe, precuneus, parietal lobe and insula [55]; activity is reduced in other regions (i.e., subgenual/subcallosal part of the anterior cingulate cortex, orbitofrontal cortex and gyrus rectus) [19]. Ketamine globally increases FC across the brain [56] leading to network reorganization and a preserved FC in lower-order sensory networks. However, FC disruptions are observed in all higher-order consciousness networks, except the ECN [2]. In addition, the fronto-parietal anterior to posterior EC fields are disturbed [46, 57].

Dexmedetomidine also provokes several FC alterations including within-network reductions in thalamic connectivity with higher-order RSNs but with preservation of lower-order sensory networks [58]. These observed FC changes resemble deep NREM sleep except the FC between the thalamus, the medial anterior cingulate cortex and meso-pontine area is better preserved than during sleep or propofol sedation. These regions pertain to the salience network (a collection of regions of the brain that select which stimuli require attention and then recruit relevant functional networks), and the observed FC preservation may be associated with the ability to awaken dexmedetomidine sedated patients upon stimulation more easily than during deep sleep or propofol sedation. Dexmedetomidine also induces a reduction in local and global large-scale network efficiency, and a reduction in large-scale network connectivity strength [59]. This agent produces an increase in cortical excitability as compared to the wake state, similar to what is observed during sleep (see https://www.biorxiv.org, under revision for the British Journal of Anaesthesia).

Finally, a set of functional changes common to all sedatives has been identified. Regarding FC and EC, these include reduced complexity and repertoire of possible configurations, disruption of fronto-parietal connectivity, and inhibition of long-latency evoked potentials. Regarding network structure, there is reduced global efficiency, increased clustering and modularity, disruption of the posterior "hot zone", reconfiguration of global brain network structure, and disruption of the spatial balance between segregation and integration. Regarding spatio-temporal dynamics, a deviation from the critical point (a state characterized by the largest ability to transfer information from one point of the network to the other), a disruption of metastability (apparently stable state within a dynamical system, where a perturbation can lead to an even more stable state), a constrained repertoire of temporal network configurations, and a disruption of the temporal balance between segregation and integration are observed [28]. These described changes may not apply to ketamine.

These purported comparisons between sleep and sedation in terms of brain functional changes remain preliminary because many connectivity and brain network properties have yet to be exhaustively studied, and studies directly comparing sleep and sedation remain scarce [5]. It is safe to summarize that during wakefulness the brain exhibits rapid, brilliant, and constantly changing configurations. These dynamic changes reflect the richness of mental activity. Conversely, the brain tends to exhibit more reduced, slower and more organized activity during NREM sleep and sedation. However, a lot of research work is still needed to further characterize the functional differences between REM, NREM sleep, and sedation, and to better define the brain states associated with dreaming, disconnectedness from the environment, responsiveness to external stimulation, episodes of conscious awareness during sedation, and the capacity of forming memories. The changes in specific aspects of brain function are probably more linked to the presence or absence of specific phenomenological elements (mental content, memory, perception of the environment, etc.) than to sedation or sleep themselves.

6 Sleep Outcomes

There are numerous core physiologic systems that are dependent on sleep for optimal function. It is not well understood whether some of these benefits are also gained under sedation (Table 4). For example, the ill-defined, subjective sense of restfulness associated with deep natural sleep has not been consistently reported after sedation. Studies of the critically ill have yielded poor patient-reported sleep with infusions of both propofol and dexmedetomidine. This may be the result of

Table 4 Comparison of outcomes between sleep and sedation

Domain	Sedation	Sleep
Restfulness, recovery sleep, and circadian rhythm	Not consistently reported after sedation Propofol and DEX decrease REM and N3 sleep Non-REM sleep debt can be repaid, but not REM sleep debt Alteration of the circadian system under sedation	Necessitates deep natural sleep
Learning (remembering and forgetting)	No sedation is known to improve memory GABA cause anterograde amnesia	Processing of input with previous knowledge and experience
Glymphatic system	May be enabled during infusion of sedatives that promote slow-wave oscillations (GABA and DEX, but not halogenated vapors)	NREM: astrocytes shrink to enhance lymphatic flow for the removal of waste products
Immune modulation, protein synthesis, emotional regulation, endocrine regulation	Not well studied Confounding effect of critical illness Effect of length and dose of sedation not known	Positive effect

NREM = non rapid-eye movement; GABA = mainly acting through a potentiation of γ-amino-butyric acid neurotransmission (propofol, benzodiazepines, barbiturates, and halogenated anesthetics); dex = dexmedetomidine

dexmedetomidine potentially still decreasing REM and N3 sleep despite its proven effect on improved N2 sleep (see chapter "Effects of Common ICU Medications on Sleep") [60, 61].

Recovery sleep refers to sleep that occurs after a period of sleep loss. Typically, over the course of several nights after a period of sleep loss, both REM and N3 NREM sleep will occur in higher-than-normal percent, suggesting what was lost with sleep must be regained. Under the influence of some sedative medications, NREM sleep debt can be repaid; however, this does not seem to be the case with REM sleep debt [62, 63]. Although the recovery of sleep under homeostatic control may occur in part, sedatives also influence the circadian system. (see chapter "Effects of Common ICU Medications on Sleep"). A late-afternoon 1-h infusion of propofol to simulate outpatient procedural sedation was found to result in delayed sleep latency [64].

While learning (both remembering and forgetting) is an essential function of sleep, sedatives, as a whole do not improve memory; the anterograde amnesia associated with GABAergic agonists like midazolam are well established. Under the influence of these sedatives, while information input may occur, the necessary brain processing of this input will not occur. Even under light, conscious sedation, memory may not be formed. This is in contradistinction to sleep where knowledge and experience assimilation will occur. The recall of survivors of a critical illness, however, is undoubtedly influenced by more than just the medications they received [65].

One interesting new area of research is of the dependence of the glymphatic system on sleep. During deep non-REM sleep, astrocytes shrink to enhance lymphatic flow for the removal of waste products such as amyloid protein [66]. This system is thought to be important to CNS nutrient delivery, long term cognitive function, and CNS drug delivery; dysfunction of this system has been proposed to be important to the development of neurodegenerative diseases including dementia [67]. In animal models, this function may be enabled during infusion of some sedatives, those that promote slow-wave oscillations, including the GABAergic agonists and α_2-agonists (but not inhalational anesthetics) [68, 69]. While this relationship is likely to be dose-dependent, the degree to which this occurs in humans is unknown and its mechanism is currently unknown.

The effects of extended infusions of sedating medications in critically ill patients on other sleep-dependent functions such as immune modulation, protein synthesis, emotional regulation, and endocrine regulation are not well studied for their clinical significance. It may be difficult to determine the effects under short-term infusions as with procedural sedation, or to separate the effects from those of critical illness for those on longer continuous infusions.

7 Conclusions

Despite multiple similarities between sleep and sedation, the altered state of consciousness produced by sedatives is clearly not the same as sleep. The most robust argument to assert that sedation is not the same as sleep is that sedatives are associated with specific EEG patterns that are different from those observed during sleep. Among different sedative pharmacologic classes, dexmedetomidine sedation most closely resembles sleep although important differences still exist. The use of sedation to treat some critically ill patients may be necessary in the ICU but the physiologic benefits of sleep may not be achieved during sedative infusions; therefore, the effects of sedatives on sleep have implications for recovery from critical illness.

References

1. Marechal H, Defresne A, Montupil J, Bonhomme V. Chapter 24 - Choice of sedation in neurointensive care. In: Prabhakar H, editor. Essentials of evidence-based practice of neuroanesthesia and neurocritical care [Internet]. Academic Press; 2022. p. 321–58. Available from: https://www.sciencedirect.com/science/article/pii/B978012821776400024X
2. Bonhomme V, Vanhaudenhuyse A, Demertzi A, Bruno MA, Jaquet O, Bahri MA, et al. Resting-state network-specific breakdown of functional connectivity during ketamine alteration of consciousness in volunteers. Anesthesiology. 2016;125(5):873–88.
3. Weerink MAS, Struys MMRF, Hannivoort LN, Barends CRM, Absalom AR, Colin P. Clinical pharmacokinetics and pharmacodynamics of dexmedetomidine. Clin Pharmacokinet [Internet]. 2017;56(8):893–913. https://doi.org/10.1007/s40262-017-0507-7.

4. Sanders RD, Tononi G, Laureys S, Sleigh JW. Unresponsiveness ≠ unconsciousness. Anesthesiology. 2012;116(4):946–59.

5. Bonhomme V, Staquet C, Montupil J, Defresne A, Kirsch M, Martial C, et al. General anesthesia: a probe to explore consciousness. Front Syst Neurosci. 2019;13:36.

6. Baird B, Mota-Rolim SA, Dresler M. The cognitive neuroscience of lucid dreaming. Neurosci Biobehav Rev. 2019;100:305–23.

7. Baird B, LaBerge S, Tononi G. Two-way communication in lucid REM sleep dreaming. Trends Cogn Sci. 2021;25(5):427–8.

8. Wamsley EJ, Stickgold R. Memory, sleep and dreaming: experiencing consolidation. Sleep Med Clin. 2011;6:97–108.

9. Zanos P, Moaddel R, Morris PJ, Riggs LM, Highland JN, Georgiou P, et al. Ketamine and ketamine metabolite pharmacology: insights into therapeutic mechanisms. Pharmacol Rev. 2018;70(3):621–60.

10. Brown EN, Purdon PL, Van Dort CJ. General anesthesia and altered states of arousal: a systems neuroscience analysis. Annu Rev Neurosci. 2011;34:601–28.

11. Moody OA, Zhang ER, Vincent KF, Kato R, Melonakos ED, Nehs CJ, et al. The neural circuits underlying general anesthesia and sleep. Anesthesia and Analgesia Lippincott Williams and Wilkins. 2021;132:1254–64.

12. Prerau MJ, Brown RE, Bianchi MT, Ellenbogen JM, Purdon PL. Sleep neurophysiological dynamics through the lens of multitaper spectral analysis. Physiology. 2017;32(1):60–92.

13. Adamantidis AR, Gutierrez Herrera C, Gent TC. Oscillating circuitries in the sleeping brain. Nat Rev Neurosci. 2019;20(12):746–62.

14. Nelson LE, Lu J, Guo T, Saper CB, Franks NP, Maze M. The alpha2-adrenoceptor agonist dexmedetomidine converges on an endogenous sleep-promoting pathway to exert its sedative effects. Anesthesiology. 2003;98(2):428–36.

15. Purdon PL, Sampson A, Pavone KJ, Brown EN. Clinical electroencephalography for anesthesiologists: part I: background and basic signatures. Anesthesiology. 2015;123(4):937–60.

16. Sleigh J, Harvey M, Voss L, Denny B. Ketamine - more mechanisms of action than just NMDA blockade. Trends Anaesth Crit Care [Internet]. 2014;4(2–3):76–81. https://doi.org/10.1016/j.tacc.2014.03.002.

17. Kokkinou M, Ashok AH, Howes OD. The effects of ketamine on dopaminergic function: meta-analysis and review of the implications for neuropsychiatric disorders. Mol Psychiatry. 2018;23(1):59–69.

18. Kraguljac NV, Frölich MA, Tran S, White DM, Nichols N, Barton-McArdle A, et al. Ketamine modulates hippocampal neurochemistry and functional connectivity: a combined magnetic resonance spectroscopy and resting-state fMRI study in healthy volunteers. Mol Psychiatry. 2017;22(4):562–9.

19. Höflich A, Hahn A, Küblböck M, Kranz GS, Vanicek T, Ganger S, et al. Ketamine-dependent neuronal activation in healthy volunteers. Brain Struct Funct. 2017;222(3):1533–42.

20. Franks NP, Zecharia AY. Sleep and general anesthesia. Can J Anesth. 2011;58(2):139–48.

21. Meuret P, Backman SBSB, Bonhomme V, Plourde G, Fiset P. Physostigmine reverses propofol-induced unconsciousness and attenuation of the auditory steady state response and bispectral index in human volunteers. Anesthesiology [Internet]. 2000;93(3):708–17. Available from: http://content.wkhealth.com/linkback/openurl?sid=WKPTLP:landingpage&an=00000542-200009000-00020.

22. Akeju O, Brown EN. Neural oscillations demonstrate that general anesthesia and sedative states are neurophysiologically distinct from sleep. Curr Opin Neurobiol. 2017;44:178–85.

23. Sarasso S, Rosanova M, Casali AG, Casarotto S, Fecchio M, Boly M, et al. Quantifying cortical EEG responses to TMS in (Un)consciousness. Clin EEG Neurosci. 2014;45(1):40–9.

24. Gaskell ALL, Hight DFF, Winders J, Tran G, Defresne A, Bonhomme V, et al. Frontal alpha-delta EEG does not preclude volitional response during anaesthesia: prospective cohort study of the isolated forearm technique. Br J Anaesth. 2017;119(4):664–73.

25. Purdon PL, Pierce ET, Mukamel EA, Prerau MJ, Walsh JL, Wong KFK, et al. Electroencephalogram signatures of loss and recovery of consciousness from propofol. Proc Natl Acad Sci [Internet]. 2013;110(12):E1142–51. https://doi.org/10.1073/pnas.1221180110.

26. Sarasso S, Boly M, Napolitani M, Gosseries O, Charland-Verville V, Casarotto S, et al. Consciousness and complexity during unresponsiveness induced by propofol, xenon, and ketamine. Curr Biol [Internet]. 2015;25(23):3099–105. https://doi.org/10.1016/j.cub.2015.10.014.

27. Purdon PL, Sampson A, Pavone KJ, Brown EN. Clinical electroencephalography for anesthesiologists- Part I- background and basic Signatures_Anesthesiology_2015.pdf - Google drive. Anesthesiology [Internet] 2015;123(4):937–60. Available from: https://drive.google.com/file/d/14_bPZ-wIZJ3-JrVsUN-2a5-b3_rDOw6u/view?ts=5aa038f3

28. Lee U, Mashour GA. Role of network science in the study of anesthetic state transitions. Anesthesiology [Internet]. 2018;129(5):1029–44. Available from: http://insights.ovid.com/crossref?an=00000542-900000000-96883.

29. Houldin E, Fang Z, Ray LB, Owen AM, Fogel SM. Toward a complete taxonomy of resting state networks across wakefulness and sleep: an assessment of spatially distinct resting state networks using independent component analysis. Sleep. 2019;42(3):1–9.

30. Picchioni D, Duyn JH, Horovitz SG. Sleep and the functional connectome. NeuroImage. 2013;80:387–96.

31. Tagliazucchi E, van Someren EJW. The large-scale functional connectivity correlates of consciousness and arousal during the healthy and pathological human sleep cycle. NeuroImage. 2017;160(June):55–72.

32. Sanz Perl Y, Pallavicini C, Pérez Ipiña I, Demertzi A, Bonhomme V, Martial C, et al. Perturbations in dynamical models of whole-brain activity dissociate between the level and stability of consciousness. PLoS Comput Biol. 2021;17(7):e1009139.

33. Houldin E, Fang Z, Ray LB, Stojanoski B, Owen AM, Fogel SM. Reversed and increased functional connectivity in non-REM sleep suggests an altered rather than reduced state of consciousness relative to wake. Sci Rep. 2021;11(1):1–15.

34. Tagliazucchi E, Von Wegner F, Morzelewski A, Brodbeck V, Jahnke K, Laufs H. Breakdown of long-range temporal dependence in default mode and attention networks during deep sleep. Proc Natl Acad Sci U S A. 2013;110(38):15419–24.

35. Massimini M, Ferrarelli F, Huber R, Esser SK. Breakdown of cortical effective connectivity during sleep. Science (80-). 2005;309(5744):2228–33.

36. Ly JQM, Gaggioni G, Chellappa SL, Papachilleos S, Brzozowski A, Borsu C, et al. Circadian regulation of human cortical excitability. Nat Commun. 2016;7(May):11828.

37. Cardone P, Egroo M, Van Chylinski D, Narbutas J, Gaggioni G, Vandewalle G. Increased cortical excitability and reduced brain response propagation during attentional lapses. medRxiv. 2020;2020.04.01.20049650.

38. Huber R, Mäki H, Rosanova M, Casarotto S, Canali P, Casali AG, et al. Human cortical excitability increases with time awake. Cereb Cortex. 2013;23(2):332–8.

39. Zhou S, Zou G, Xu J, Su Z, Zhu H, Zou Q, et al. Dynamic functional connectivity states characterize NREM sleep and wakefulness. Hum Brain Mapp. 2019;40(18):5256–68.

40. Del Pozo SM, Laufs H, Bonhomme V, Laureys S, Balenzuela P, Tagliazucchi E. Unconsciousness reconfigures modular brain network dynamics. Chaos. 2021 Sep;31(9):93117.

41. Tagliazucchi E, Laufs H. Decoding wakefulness levels from typical fMRI resting-state data reveals reliable drifts between wakefulness and sleep. Neuron. 2014;82(3):695–708.

42. Siclari F, Baird B, Perogamvros L, Bernardi G, LaRocque JJ, Riedner B, et al. The neural correlates of dreaming. Nat Neurosci. 2017;20(6):872–8.

43. Fiset P, Paus T, Daloze T, Plourde G, Meuret P, Bonhomme V, et al. Brain mechanisms of propofol-induced loss of consciousness in humans: a positron emission tomographic study. J Neurosci [Internet]. 1999;19(13):5506–13. Available from: http://eutils.ncbi.nlm.nih.gov/entrez/eutils/elink.fcgi?dbfrom=pubmed&id=10377359&retmode=ref&cmd=prlinks%5Cnpapers3://publication/uuid/18403EA6-98F9-4B0F-B8D3-538FDF747B51.

44. Boveroux P, Vanhaudenhuyse A, Bruno M-AA, Noirhomme Q, Lauwick S, Luxen A, et al. Breakdown of within- and between-network resting state functional magnetic resonance imaging connectivity during propofol-induced loss of consciousness. Anesthesiology [Internet]. 2010;113(5):1038–53. https://doi.org/10.1097/ALN.0b013e3181f697f5.

45. Ihalainen R, Gosseries O, de Steen F, Van Raimondo F, Panda R, Bonhomme V, et al. How hot is the hot zone? Computational modelling clarifies the role of parietal and frontoparietal connectivity during anaesthetic-induced loss of consciousness. NeuroImage. 2021;231:117841.

46. Lee U, Ku S, Noh G, Baek S, Choi B, Mashour G, a. Disruption of frontal – parietal communication. Anesthesiology. 2013;118(6):1264–75.

47. Lee U, Kim S, Noh GJ, Choi BM, Hwang E, Mashour GA. The directionality and functional organization of frontoparietal connectivity during consciousness and anesthesia in humans. Conscious Cogn [Internet]. 2009;18(4):1069–78. https://doi.org/10.1016/j.concog.2009.04.004.

48. Boly M, Moran R, Murphy M, Boveroux P, Bruno M-AM-A, Noirhomme Q, et al. Connectivity changes underlying spectral EEG changes during propofol-induced loss of consciousness. J Neurosci [Internet]. 2012;32(20):7082–90. https://doi.org/10.1523/JNEUROSCI.3769-11.2012.

49. Untergehrer G, Jordan D, Kochs EF, Ilg R, Schneider G. Fronto-parietal connectivity is a non-static phenomenon with characteristic changes during unconsciousness. PLoS One. 2014;9(1):e87498.

50. Guldenmund P, Gantner ISIS, Baquero K, Das T, Demertzi A, Boveroux P, et al. Propofol-induced frontal cortex disconnection: a study of resting-state networks, Total brain connectivity, and mean BOLD signal oscillation frequencies. Brain Connect [Internet]. 2016;6(3):225–37. https://doi.org/10.1089/brain.2015.0369.

51. Sanders RD, Banks MI, Darracq M, Moran R, Sleigh J, Gosseries O, et al. Propofol-induced unresponsiveness is associated with impaired feedforward connectivity in cortical hierarchy. Br J Anaesth [Internet]. 2018;121(5):1084–96. https://doi.org/10.1016/j.bja.2018.07.006.

52. Gómez F, Phillips C, Soddu A, Boly M, Boveroux P, Vanhaudenhuyse A, et al. Changes in effective connectivity by propofol sedation. PLoS One. 2013;8(8):e71370.

53. Barttfeld P, Uhrig L, Sitt JD, Sigman M, Jarraya B. Erratum: signature of consciousness in the dynamics of resting-state brain activity (Proceedings of the National Academy of Sciences of the United States of America (2015) 112 (887-892)). Proc Natl Acad Sci U S A. 2015;112(37):E5219–20.

54. Cavanna F, Vilas MG, Palmucci M, Tagliazucchi E. Dynamic functional connectivity and brain metastability during altered states of consciousness. Neuroimage [Internet]. 2018;180:383–95. Available from: https://doi.org/10.1016/j.neuroimage.2017.09.065.

55. Långsjö JW, Kaisti KK, Aalto S, Hinkka S, Aantaa R, Oikonen V, et al. Effects of subanesthetic doses of ketamine on regional cerebral blood flow, oxygen consumption, and blood volume in humans. Anesthesiology [Internet]. 2003;99(3):614–23. Available from: http://www.ncbi.nlm.nih.gov/pubmed/12960545.

56. Driesen NR, McCarthy G, Bhagwagar Z, Bloch M, Calhoun V, D'Souza DC, et al. Relationship of resting brain hyperconnectivity and schizophrenia-like symptoms produced by the NMDA receptor antagonist ketamine in humans. Mol Psychiatry [Internet]. 2013;18(11):1199–204. Available from: http://www.pubmedcentral.nih.gov/articlerender.fcgi?artid=3646075&tool=pmcentrez&rendertype=abstract.

57. Vlisides PE, Bel-Bahar T, Lee U, Li D, Kim H, Janke E, et al. Neurophysiologic correlates of ketamine sedation and anesthesia. Anesthesiology. 2017;127(1):58–69.

58. Guldenmund P, Vanhaudenhuyse A, Sanders RD, Sleigh J, Bruno MA, Demertzi A, et al. Brain functional connectivity differentiates dexmedetomidine from propofol and natural sleep. Br J Anaesth. 2017 Oct;119(4):674–84.

59. Hashmi JA, Loggia ML, Khan S, Gao L, Kim J, Napadow V, et al. Dexmedetomidine disrupts the local and global efficiencies of large-scale brain networks. Anesthesiology. 2017;126(3):419–30.

60. Treggiari-Venzi M, Borgeat A, Fuchs-Buder T, et al. Overnight sedation with midazolam or propofol in the ICU: effects on sleep quality, anxiety and depression. Intensive Care Med. 1996;22:1186–90.
61. Corbett SM, Rebuck JA, Greene CM, et al. Dexmedetomidine does not improve patient satisfaction when compared with propofol during mechanical ventilation. Crit Care Med. 2005;33:940–5.
62. Pal D, Lipinski WJ, Walker AJ, et al. State-specific effects of sevoflurane anesthesia on sleep homeostasis: selective recovery of slow wave but not rapid eye movement sleep. Anesthesiology. 2011;114:302–10.
63. Tung A, Bergmann BM, Herrara S, et al. Recovery from sleep deprivation occurs during propofol anesthesia. Anesthesiology. 2004;100:1419–26.
64. Ozone M, Itoh H, Wataru Y, et al. Changes in subjective sleepiness, subjective fatigue and nocturnal sleep after anaesthesia with propofol. Psychiatry Clin Neurosci. 2000;54:317–8.
65. Burry L, Cook D, Herridge M, et al. Recall of ICU stay in patients managed with a sedation protocol or a sedation protocol with daily interruption. Crit Care Med. 2015;43:210–90.
66. Xie L, Kang H, Xu Q, et al. Sleep drives metabolite clearance from the adult brain. Science. 2013;342:373–7.
67. Nedergaard M, Goldman SA. Glymphatic failure as a final common pathway to dementia. Science. 2020;370:50–6.
68. Lilius TO, Blomqvist K, Hauglund NL, et al. Dexmedetomidine enhances glymphatic brain delivery of intrathecally administered drugs. J Control Release. 2019;304:29–38.
69. Benveniste H, Heerdt P, Fontes M, et al. Glymphatic system function in relation to anesthesia and sleep states. Anesth Analg. 2019;128:747–58.

Biologic Effects of Disrupted Sleep

Makayla Cordoza, Christopher W. Jones, and David F. Dinges

1 Introduction

Sleep is a fundamental evolutionary activity that is observed across many animal species, especially mammals. A wealth of epidemiological, clinical, and laboratory-based evidence supports the importance of sleep as a regulator of homeostatic and neurobehavioral functions [1]. For adults, habitual high-quality sleep of 7–9 h per 24-h day is necessary to maintain health over the lifespan [1]. High quality sleep is best characterized as sleep that is continuous, efficient, appropriately timed, and adequate in physiologic stages and duration.

Disruption of sleep can negatively affect health and wellbeing. Sleep disruption, defined as sleep that is abnormal in duration (i.e., shorter or longer than recommended), timing, continuity, or quality, can occur from a variety of factors (see chapter "Risk Factors for Disrupted Sleep in the ICU") and may be acute or chronic. The effects of sleep disruption are extensive, and can adversely impact numerous biologic and behavioral systems both acutely (i.e., in the short-term) and chronically over time. The chronicity and severity of sleep disruption likely contributes to increased risk for numerous conditions, such as cardiometabolic disease and incident dementia [2, 3].

Critically ill adults in the intensive care unit (ICU) are at high risk for sleep disruption from the ICU environment, medications, and pathophysiologic conditions [4]. Extended hospital admissions and long recovery trajectories also increase the

M. Cordoza (✉)
School of Nursing, University of Pennsylvania, Philadelphia, PA, USA
e-mail: mcordoza@nursing.upenn.edu

C. W. Jones · D. F. Dinges
Division of Sleep and Chronobiology, Department of Psychiatry, University of Pennsylvania, Philadelphia, PA, USA
e-mail: Christopher.Jones@pennmedicine.upenn.edu; dinges@pennmedicine.upenn.edu

© The Author(s), under exclusive license to Springer Nature Switzerland AG 2022
G. L. Weinhouse, J. W. Devlin (eds.), *Sleep in Critical Illness*,
https://doi.org/10.1007/978-3-031-06447-0_5

risk for prolonged sleep disruption. Given the complex nature of critical illness, few studies have examined biologic changes in response to sleep disruption while in the ICU. As such, this chapter focuses primarily on established biologic effects of sleep disruption in healthy adults, with context for relevance in critically ill populations.

Describing all known biologic consequences of sleep disruption would require covering decades of research in a vast scientific field. The interplay between sleep and health is complex, and is influenced by a multitude of exogenous and endogenous factors. To frame this substantial field in the context of critical illness, this chapter will focus on the short-term, relevant biologic effects of sleep disruption for each major body system. It is important to recognize that the sleep-biology relationship is often bidirectional, meaning biologic responses also affect sleep quality. Furthermore, the biologic effects of sleep disruption can occur simultaneously, often interacting with multiple body systems to produce an overall response. Finally, differential vulnerability to the effects of sleep disruption may reflect the extent to which underlying biologic effects manifest between individuals [5].

2 Sleep Disruption and Neurobehavioral Functions

Sleep disruption, particularly the loss of sleep, has pronounced impacts on neurobehavioral functions, including mood and neurocognition (Table 1) [6–8]. During critical illness, the majority of evidence evaluating sleep loss and neurocognitive function has been in the context of ICU delirium. Chapters "Sleep Disruption and Its Relationship with Delirium: Electroencephalographic Perspectives" and "Sleep Disruption and Its Relationship with Delirium: Clinical Perspectives" discuss physiologic and clinical relationships, respectively, between sleep and ICU delirium, and thus will not be reviewed in this chapter. Instead, this section focuses on neurobehavioral responses to sleep disruption in healthy adults, which likely have relevance for patients in the ICU.

2.1 Mood

The relationship between sleep loss and mood is established [9, 10]. However, the specific components of mood adversely impacted by sleep loss appear to be a function of both the nature of the sleep lost (e.g. fragmented vs. restricted) and whether sleep is lost acutely (over one or a few days) or chronically (across multiple days or longer). For example, several days of restricted sleep largely effects the somatic components of mood (i.e., increased fatigue, reduced vigor) [7, 11], rather than the affective components of mood (e.g. anxiety, depressive symptoms). In comparison, acute sleep loss degrades both somatic and affective mood. Even one night without sleep is associated with greater symptoms of anxiety and depression [12, 13]. Further, acute sleep loss lowers the threshold of sensitivity to stressful situations,

Table 1 General effects of sleep disruption by major body system

Measured outcome	Change in response to sleep disruption
Neurobehavioral function	
Sleepiness	Higher
Fatigue	Worse
Vigor	Lower
Anxiety	Higher
Depression	Higher
Emotional regulation	Worse
Vigilant attention	Worse
Working/declarative memory	Worse
Immune function	
TNF-α	Higher[a]
IL-6	Higher[a]
CRP	Higher[a]
Endocrine function	
Cortisol	Higher[a]
Catecholamines	Higher[a]
Glucose	Higher
Insulin sensitivity	Lower
Cardiovascular function	
Heart rate variability	Lower
Left atrial function	Worse
QT interval	Longer
Propensity for arrhythmias	Higher
Reactive oxygen species	Higher
Endothelial function	Worse
Blood pressure	Higher
Pulmonary function	
Pulmonary functional capacity	Worse
Inspiratory endurance	Worse
Gastrointestinal function	
Ghrelin	Higher
Leptin	Lower
Caloric intake	Higher
Hunger	Higher
Musculoskeletal function	
Testosterone	Lower
Insulin-like growth factor-1	Lower
Growth hormone	Lower
Muscle protein synthesis	Lower
Bone mineral density	Lower[a]

[a]General response, although some studies show inconsistent findings related to changes in response to sleep loss

heightening reactivity to negative stimuli (i.e. when sleep deprived, it takes a smaller stress stimulus to produce elevated subjective stress, anxiety, and anger responses) [14, 15]. Patients in the ICU may therefore experience negative mood states resulting from one or more nights of disrupted sleep. This may be especially evident for ICU survivors who exhibit both prolonged sleep disruption and psychological conditions, such as anxiety and depression [16, 17]. Sleep recovery, an extended duration of sleep following partial or total sleep loss, has been shown to alleviate negative mood states, restoring mood to basal levels [7, 12]. Thus recovery sleep may be an important target in critical illness recovery.

2.2 *Vigilant Attention*

The most pronounced effect of sleep loss on neurobehavioral alertness is vigilant attention [18]. Vigilant attention, a fundamental component of attentional function, represents an individual's ability to respond quickly and accurately to a stimulus, such as reacting to a road hazard when driving [19, 20]. Sleep loss, whether through acute total deprivation or sustained chronic restriction, produces deficits in vigilant attention, including lapses of attention and slower response speeds, that are a function of the severity and timing of sleep loss (Fig. 1) [8, 18, 21].

The ability of individuals to subjectively self-evaluate neurobehavioral alertness is less clear. Subjective assessment of sleepiness and fatigue increase initially when sleep is restricted, and then level off across consecutive days of sleep loss; suggesting that subjective sleepiness and vigilant attention are distinct constructs, and/or that humans cannot accurately assess their deficits in vigilant attention [8, 22]. In the ICU, reduced vigilant attention from sleep loss may manifest as an inability to follow directions and keep eyes opened, or as delayed verbal or motor responses. These effects may be independent, or concomitant with impairments in attention from medications or pathology. When sleep is recovered, deficits in vigilant attention are usually resolved or attenuated [11, 22].

2.3 *Learning and Memory*

Sleep also plays an essential role in learning and memory [23], where the loss of sleep impairs both working memory, as well as declarative memory through disrupting memory encoding and consolidation [24, 25]. Critically ill patients experiencing acute sleep loss may therefore have difficulty retaining information and effectively participating in patient teaching activities. As with vigilant attention, deficits in memory performance (e.g. declarative memory) may not be fully restored following recovery sleep, at least in the short term [26, 27]. The restorative benefit of high-quality sleep on long-term memory and performance is less understood.

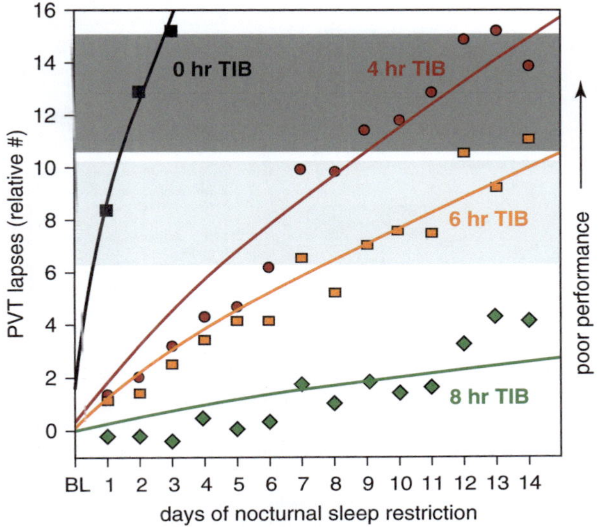

Fig. 1 Responses in vigilant attention to varying doses of daily sleep. PVT = psychomotor vigilance task; TIB = time in bed. Group averages are shown for subjects in the 8 h, 6 h, and 4 h chronic sleep period conditions across 14 days, and in the 0 h sleep condition across 3 days. Subjects were tested every 2 h each day; data points represent the daily average (07:30–23:30) expressed relative to baseline (BL). The y-axis shows PVT performance lapses. Upward corresponds to worse performance on the PVT. The curves through the data points represent statistical non-linear model-based best-fitting profiles of the response to sleep deprivation for subjects in each of the four experimental conditions. The mean = s.e. ranges of neurobehavioral functions for 1 and 2 days of 0 h sleep (total sleep deprivation) are shown as light and dark gray bands, respectively, allowing comparison of the 3-day total sleep deprivation condition and the 14-day chronic sleep restriction conditions. Adapted from: Van Dongen HPA et al. The Cumulative Cost of Additional Wakefulness: Dose-Response Effects on Neurobehavioral Functions and Sleep Physiology From Chronic Sleep Restriction and Total Sleep Deprivation. Sleep. 2003;26:117–126

3 Sleep Disruption and Immune Function

Sleep and the immune system are intimately intertwined through a bidirectional cross-talk between the brain and the immune system (Fig. 2) [28–30]. Mediators of the immune system (e.g., inflammatory cytokines) are involved in sleep regulation and exert influences at sleep onset and throughout the sleep period. Immunologic profiles are distinct during each sleep stage (i.e., non-rapid eye movement [REM] vs. REM sleep periods) [28, 31, 32]. Among the many inflammatory cytokines implicated in sleep regulation, interleukin-1β (IL-1β) and tumor necrosis factor-α (TNF-α) are primary contributors to non-REM sleep. Similar to endogenous sleep-wake cycles, the immune system exhibits a circadian dynamic where peripheral levels of inflammatory cytokines and immune markers display diurnal rhythms [30, 33].

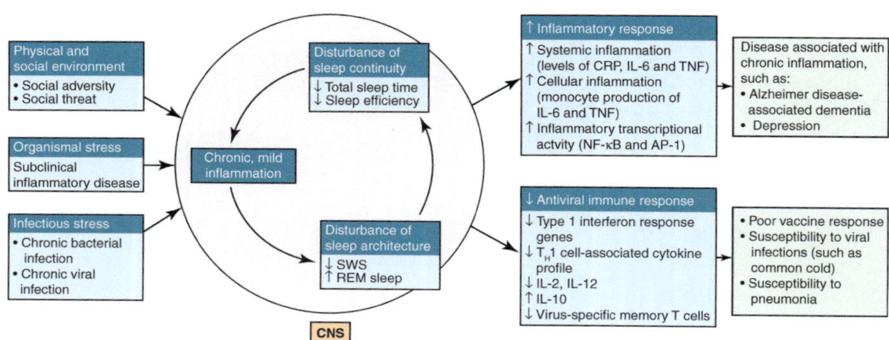

Fig. 2 Putative pathways linking chronic stress or inflammatory exposure to sleep disturbance and adverse outcomes. Social–environmental experiences that indicate potential social threat or adversity activate inflammatory activity at low levels, similar to that which occurs in the presence of subclinical inflammatory disease or chronic infection. However, when there is sustained engagement of these systems, owing to prolonged experiences of social threat or adversity, or from subclinical inflammatory states, levels of inflammation can further increase in the periphery and in areas of the brain that process social experiences. This model proposes that such chronic perceived stress, coupled with central inflammation, induces a biphasic shift in the regulation of sleep: initially, sleep continuity and slow wave sleep (SWS) are increased; later, total sleep time, sleep efficiency and SWS are decreased, with increases in rapid eye movement (REM) sleep, which together characterize sleep disturbance. This sleep disturbance shifts the transcriptional profile towards increased inflammatory activity and decreased antiviral responses. It is hypothesized that such an inflammatory transcriptional state might lead to clinical manifestations of inflammatory disorders and may also result in poor vaccine responses and increased susceptibility to infectious disease. AP-1, activator protein 1; CNS, central nervous system; CRP, C-reactive protein; NF-κB, nuclear factor-κB; T_H1 cell, T helper 1 cell; TNF, tumor necrosis factor. Reprinted with permission from: Irwin, M.R. Sleep and inflammation: partners in sickness and in health. Nat Rev Immunol 19, 702–715 (2019). https://doi.org/10.1038/s41577-019-0190-z

3.1 Cytokine Function

As with other neurobehavioral and biological systems, the impact of sleep loss on the immune system is dependent on whether sleep is lost acutely or chronically [34, 35]. In general, sleep loss is associated with a pro-inflammatory state [29, 36], although studies are mixed. For instance, acute total sleep deprivation across multiple days (i.e., 88 h without sleep) has been shown to elevate plasma levels of soluble TNF-α receptor I and interleukin-6 (IL-6) relative to partial sleep deprivation over the same time period [35].

A meta-analysis of sleep disruption and peripheral levels of systemic inflammation found that sleep disturbance was associated with elevated C-reactive protein (CRP) and IL-6, but not TNF-α [34]. Conversely, neither acute sleep deprivation nor sleep restriction, produced reliable changes in IL-6, or TNF-α levels, with only a small effect for CRP levels. Reasons for this contrast are unclear, but may represent underlying comorbidities in studies of sleep disturbance which usually include a wide range of community-based participants, whereas experimental sleep studies often only include healthy volunteers. Additionally, inconsistencies in experimental findings are also likely due to differences in study design, the tissue type studied, time of day effects (i.e., circadian influences), and immune targets. Although data relating to specific inflammatory cytokine activity and sleep loss are varied, epidemiological studies have robustly associated sleep loss with inflammatory-based diseases, such as cardiometabolic disease [2, 37].

3.2   Immunity and Illness Recovery

Sleep in response to acute illness, such as is common in the ICU, is poorly understood. In the few studies of sleep following an infectious challenge (e.g. exposure to rhinovirus), self-reported sleep duration increased in the immediate days after exposure [38]. However, one study assessing physiologic sleep demonstrated mild sleep disruption (shorter total sleep time and lower sleep efficiency) during the symptomatic phase of rhinovirus [39]. Further, experimental endotoxin exposure has shown a dose-response relationship, where mild host defense activation from a low exotoxin dose was associated with more non-REM sleep, and the highest endotoxin dose associated with sleep disruption [40]. Given that critically ill patients often present with a profound acute illness, it is likely that their pathophysiology contributes to sleep disruption, and the resulting sleep disruption further contributes to existing inflammation associated with their illness.

In relation to the role of sleep in host defense, several studies have shown that insufficient sleep is associated with an impaired host response, such as vaccine uptake for pathogens like influenza and hepatitis B [29]. For example, in a study of healthy subjects, individuals who slept less than 6 h per night on average had a lower secondary antibody response to hepatitis B antigen, and were significantly less likely to be protected from the virus compared to individuals who slept more than 7 h per night [41]. In addition, short sleep duration has been associated with increased risk for susceptibility to infectious pathogens such as the common cold [42]. The relationship between sleep and the immune system is also influenced by the potent anti-inflammatory effects of glucocorticoids. Cortisol (see Sect. 6.4) is tightly related to sleep-wake patterns [30], and organismal stress from acute illness can induce glucocorticoid resistance resulting in inhibition of the anti-inflammatory effects of cortisol [36, 43]. Overall, patients in the ICU exhibit complex immune profiles resulting from their critical illness, and the interaction with sleep is bi-directional. It is evident however that sleep plays an important role in immune response in health, and sleep disruption likely impairs the ability to respond to acute illness.

4 Sleep Disruption and Endocrine Function

The endocrine system is comprised of organs and glands that secrete hormones regulating metabolism, growth and repair, and maintenance of homeostasis [44]. Sleep and circadian rhythms play key roles in numerous signaling pathways controlling hormonal regulation. Indeed, endocrine dysfunction resulting from chronic sleep disruption is thought to be a contributing mechanism to the rising prevalence of metabolic disorders, such as obesity and diabetes [45, 46]. The endocrine system also largely regulates sleep and wake itself (see chapter "Atypical Sleep and Pathologic Wakefulness").

4.1 *Hypothalamic-Pituitary-Adrenal Axis*

The hypothalamic-pituitary-adrenal axis (HPA) is a primary stress response system that both modulates, and is affected by, sleep/wake and circadian rhythmicity [47]. Partial and total sleep loss have mixed effects on cortisol (primary end product of the HPA axis) patterns that depend on the timing of cortisol measurement and experimental model of sleep deprivation. Most studies of partial and total sleep loss show higher peripheral levels of cortisol in the afternoon/evening, and lower than expected cortisol levels in the morning [48–51]. This pattern reflects a dampening of circadian-regulated cortisol decline across the day, resulting in higher overall peripheral cortisol levels [52–55].

However, other cortisol patterns have been reported, with some studies showing no change, or even a slight decrease in peripheral cortisol levels [56–58]. These divergent findings are likely due to differences in study methodology such as length of sleep deprivation, the biofluid from which cortisol was measured (e.g. blood, urine, or saliva), timing of cortisol measurements, and other study variables (e.g. sleep opportunity periods, amount of physical activity, etc.). Importantly though, population-based studies have consistently shown that chronic insufficient sleep is associated with elevated cortisol levels [59, 60].

Timing, duration, and architectural composition of the sleep period also affects HPA axis activity. Inhibition of cortisol release is partially modulated by slow wave sleep (SWS) [61]. Frequent arousals from sleep that reduce the amount of SWS have been associated with elevated peripheral cortisol levels [62]. Further, a circadian misalignment of the sleep period (e.g. sleeping during the day) has also been associated with elevated peripheral cortisol levels [63, 64]. Patients in the ICU are known to experience fragmented sleep throughout the 24 h day with little to no SWS [65]. Thus, the specific sleep lost during critical illness (i.e. loss of deep [SWS] sleep) may contribute to the overall stress response and elevated cortisol secretion.

4.2 Catecholamines

Reports on the effect of sleep loss on catecholamine activity are also mixed. Several studies report elevated norepinephrine both during and after sleep loss [66–68]. Individuals with chronic sleep disturbance, such as insomnia, have also shown elevated nocturnal catecholamine levels [69]. However, some studies have not found changes in catecholamine activity with sleep loss [70, 71]. Similar to the inconsistencies seen with cortisol, this likely reflects differences in study methodologies. Patterns of elevated catecholamine and cortisol levels, similar to that of sleep loss, are also observed during critical illness for conditions such as sepsis [72]. Thus, sleep loss may exacerbate the already activated stress response during acute illness.

4.3 Metabolism and Thermoregulation

Sleep disruption affects metabolism (further described in Sect. 6.7) and thermoregulation. Acute sleep loss inhibits the normal nocturnal reduction in body temperature [73], which concomitantly is associated with increased thyroid stimulating hormone levels, and in some cases also increased free T3 and T4 [71, 74]. Similarly, sleep loss inhibits the normal release of growth hormone and testosterone for anabolic activities (see also Sect. 6.8), which are usually secreted most prominently during sleep [71, 75–77].

Both laboratory and epidemiologic studies have linked sleep loss and reduced insulin sensitivity [43, 51, 71, 78], which is thought to be an important risk factor for diabetes and obesity. Numerous studies demonstrate that sleep loss yields a lower rate of glucose clearance and an impaired insulin response, resulting in overall higher glucose levels and insulin resistance [56, 78, 79]. Similar to cortisol, glucose homeostasis is thought to be partly regulated by SWS [79, 80]. Thus, the amount of SWS achieved may be an important modulator of glucose activity. Sleep disruption, especially fragmented sleep, experienced in the ICU may therefore contribute to existing insulin and glucose dysregulation commonly observed during critical illness [81].

Importantly, sleep loss and endocrine function are intertwined in complex, bidirectional pathways. For example, cortisol and catecholamine activity affect glucose regulation and metabolism independent of sleep, and cortisol itself is an important sleep regulator. The duration and timing of the sleep period also influences endocrine regulation, with SWS being an important endocrine modulator. As critically ill patients in the ICU often have sleep periods throughout the 24 h day and are known to exhibit sleep fragmentation with a lack of adequate SWS [4, 65], it is possible that this sleep disruption may contribute to further endocrine dysregulation. However, direct effects of sleep disruption on endocrine activity in the ICU have not been rigorously evaluated.

5 Sleep Disruption and Cardiovascular Function

Insufficient and poor quality sleep have been identified as important risk factors for cardiovascular disease (Fig. 3) [79, 82]. In fact, a meta-analysis of 5,172,710 subjects across 153 studies showed that short sleep was associated with a 16% higher risk for cardiovascular disease compared to normal sleepers [83]. Sleep loss is associated with activation of the sympathetic nervous system [79], a key modulator of cardiac function. Most studies of sleep loss (either acute, chronic, or fragmented sleep) have demonstrated a reduction in overall heart rate variability, indicating a sympathovagal shift towards sympathetic predominance (or parasympathetic withdrawal) with a reduced capacity of the cardiovascular system to respond to stressors [79, 84, 85]. A concomitant blunting of baroreflex sensitivity in response to orthostatic position changes has also been reported [86].

Sleep loss has also been shown to affect cardiac function. Studies of healthy volunteers have demonstrated left atrial dysfunction (i.e. a reduction in early diastolic strain rate and reduction in passive emptying) following one night of sleep deprivation [87, 88]. Further, acute sleep loss has been associated with lengthening of the QT interval [89, 90], and other electrical changes, such as increased p-wave dispersion [91] and atrial electromechanical delay [92]. Among hospitalized patients, sleep disruption (measured by the frequency of nocturnal overhead emergency announcements causing awakenings from sleep) has been associated with increased frequency of ventricular ectopy and occurrence of cardiac arrest [93]. Thus, it is plausible that the electromechanical changes resulting from sleep disruption may promote cardiac dysfunction and development of cardiac arrhythmias, which may have serious implications for critically ill patients.

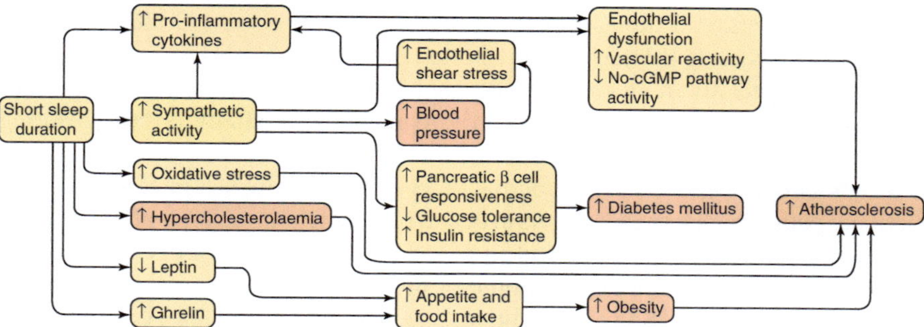

Fig. 3 Pathophysiological pathways linking short sleep duration and risk of cardiovascular disease. Short sleep duration induces alterations in several biological processes, such as the autonomic nervous system, inflammation, oxidative stress, and dyslipidaemia. These alterations lead to an increase in arterial blood pressure, endothelial dysfunction, diabetes mellitus, and accelerated atherosclerosis. NO, nitric oxide. Reprinted with permission from: Tobaldini, E., Fiorelli, E.M., Solbiati, M. et al. Short sleep duration and cardiometabolic risk: from pathophysiology to clinical evidence. Nat Rev Cardiol 16, 213–224 (2019). https://doi.org/10.1038/s41569-018-0109-6

One potential pathway through which sleep loss adversely impacts cardiac and vascular function is through oxidative stress. High levels of reactive oxygen species, indicative of oxidative stress, are known to impair cardiac and vascular function [94]. Sleep loss in animal models has been associated with increased oxidative stress [95]. Similarly, in humans, myeloperoxidase-modified low-density lipoprotein, an enzyme involved in the formation of oxidizing agents, has been shown to be elevated following sleep loss [96, 97].

Oxidative stress is postulated to promote endothelial dysfunction through a reduction in endothelial-dependent vasodilatation [98–102], and reductions in endothelial-dependent microvascular perfusion [85, 103]. Increased endothelin-1-mediated vascular tone following sleep loss has also been reported [104]. These alterations in vascular function, in addition to increased catecholamine activity, may, at least in part, account for higher blood pressure that is observed following sleep loss [105]. Normally during circadian-aligned sleep, blood pressure decreases in response to decreased sympathetic and increased parasympathetic activity [106]. However, sleep loss is associated with a blunting of this effect [107]. Although sleep loss profoundly affects cardiovascular stability, the extent to which these effects manifest and contribute to adverse outcomes in the ICU are unknown.

6 Sleep Disruption and Pulmonary Function

There are well established associations between pulmonary function and sleep disorders, such as sleep-related breathing disorders [108, 109]. The singular effects of sleep loss on the respiratory system however, are difficult to disentangle. For instance, the reductions in alertness and muscle function associated with sleep loss subsequently affects respiratory drive and pulmonary capacity. Nevertheless, acute sleep loss in healthy adults has been shown to impair pulmonary functional capacity, increase upper airway collapsibility, and reduce inspiratory endurance [110–115]. Self-reports of dyspnea, specifically air hunger, have also been reported following sleep deprivation [110]. For critically ill patients, respiratory complications resulting from sleep loss may have detrimental consequences for recovery, particularly as it relates to weaning from mechanical ventilation and for patients with underlying pulmonary comorbidities. In the ICU, several studies have investigated sleep disruption and breathing as it relates to mechanical ventilation, which are discussed in detail in chapter "Mechanical Ventilation and Sleep".

7 Sleep Disruption and Gastrointestinal Function

The gastrointestinal (GI) system is largely hormone and circadian regulated, and responsive to external cues such as food intake. Sleep disruption not only disturbs GI function through hormonal dysregulation, but also though alterations in meal timing and composition. Sleep disruption can also trigger the release of pro-inflammatory cytokines (as discussed in Sect. 6.2), an important mechanism in a number of GI disorders such as reflux, inflammatory bowel disease, and liver dysfunction [116–119]. Further, emerging evidence suggests a role for sleep in promoting diversity of the gut microbiome [120].

Appetite and caloric intake are affected by sleep disruption through a number of complex pathways. Sleep loss has been associated with increased levels of the appetite-stimulating hormone, ghrelin, and decreased levels of the appetite-suppressing hormone, leptin [121–123]. Not only do shorter sleep periods provide more opportunity for food intake, but individuals often report greater hunger following sleep loss [123]. Further, sleep loss is robustly associated with increased caloric intake, in particular from calorie-dense foods containing higher amounts of fat and sugar [124, 125]. This increased caloric intake tends to exceed the modest increased energy expenditure needed to maintain extended wakefulness [126, 127]. Similar patterns of food choices have also been observed from changes in sleep timing, such as when following a night shift work schedule, although not always associated with excessive caloric intake [128–130]. Notably, simulated night shift schedules with a daytime sleep opportunity have actually been associated with a lower 24 h energy expenditure [131].

The choice of food composition and calories consumed is also driven by neurobehavioral influences, gut-brain regulation, age, sex, and the environment. The profound effects sleep loss has on neurobehavioral functions (see Sect. 6.1) including mood, impulse control, and self-regulation, subsequently affect food choice. For example, sleep deprivation decreases frontal and insular cortical function that regulate appetitive behaviors and increases amygdalar activity, potentially resulting in an increased desire for calorie-dense foods [132, 133].

Overall, excessive caloric intake relative to 24 h energy expenditure can lead to a gain of free fat mass and contribute to obesity. Epidemiological and laboratory-based studies have consistently demonstrated relationships between sleep disruption and obesity or obesity-promoting behaviors [46, 134, 135]. In fact, a meta-analysis by Cappuccio et al. [136] found that for every 1 h reduction of daily sleep, body mass index increased by 0.35 kg/m^2. In the ICU, patient's dietary intake and food choices are often controlled, and changes in body weight are not always a result of caloric intake. However, it is possible that sleep disruption may further contribute to alterations in caloric demand and GI dysfunction commonly seen during critical illness.

8 Sleep Disruption and Musculoskeletal Function

Sleep loss may increase muscle atrophy and bone loss by disrupting normal patterns of hormone secretion. Following sleep loss, serum concentrations of anabolic hormones (e.g. testosterone), insulin, insulin-like growth factor-1, and growth hormone decrease, and catabolic hormones (e.g. cortisol) increase [49, 51, 54, 76, 137]. This hormonal profile represents dysregulation of the HPA and hypothalamic–pituitary–gonadal axes, and is consistent with a catabolic state where protein synthesis is reduced and protein degradation is increased. During critical illness, sleep disruption may therefore contribute to loss of muscle mass and impaired muscle recovery [138]. Even short periods of acute sleep loss (e.g. 1 night) are sufficient to induce anabolic resistance and promote a pro-catabolic state [139].

An association between sleep disruption and decreased bone mineral density (BMD) has been established in both animal and human studies [140–144]. Epidemiologic studies have shown both chronic short and long sleep duration, abnormal sleep timing (e.g. from nightshift work), and poor sleep quality to be associated with decreased BMD, abnormal bone turnover, and osteopenia and osteoporosis [142, 143, 145–147]. However, results have been inconsistent, with some studies finding no association between various aspects of sleep and bone health [142, 143, 148, 149]. These mixed results are likely, in part, due to differences in the population studied, method of BMD assessment, and inconsistent definitions of the type of sleep disruption. Regardless, this is an emerging field where further investigation is needed.

It is plausible that sleep disruption in the ICU, especially for prolonged critical illness, contributes to musculoskeletal impairment. Sleep-related musculoskeletal impairment may also play a role in long-term recovery from critical illness, and for conditions such post-intensive care syndrome [150]. Survivors of critical illness are at risk for developing ICU-acquired weakness [151] and may have decreased BMD [152], with evidence of ongoing sleep disruption up to 1 year post-hospitalization [16, 153, 154]. However, the extent and duration to which these relationships exist across the critical illness trajectory are less clear.

9 Inter-Individual Vulnerability to Sleep Loss

This chapter has described biologic consequences of sleep loss. However, significant variations in individual responses to sleep loss exist [155]. For example, some individuals display resilience to sleep loss, maintaining neurobehavioral and cognitive function, while others may be especially vulnerable to the effects of sleep loss. Further, genetic variation may pre-dispose individuals to shorter sleep durations (e.g. less than 6 h per night) with no distinguishable impairments in neurobehavioral function [156]. Importantly, the optimal amount of sleep needed for recovery from acute illness has not been established. Therefore, although individuals may respond differently to sleep loss, promoting high quality sleep in the ICU remains an important component of health promotion and recovery.

10 Conclusion

The biologic consequences of sleep disruption are widespread. With sleep loss responses being both integrated and interdependent within individual body systems, the effects of sleep disruption on biologic systems must be considered from both a global and individual body systems approach (Fig. 4). The interdependence of these relationships makes establishing cause and effect associations challenging, and is further complicated by the often bi-directional interactions between sleep and physiologic systems. Nevertheless, it is clear that adequate sleep is fundamental to maintain health, and the lack of sufficient, high quality, sleep can lead to increased disease risk and poorer overall functioning. Although many of the consequences of sleep disruption have not been investigated in critically ill individuals, it is reasonable to consider that patients in the ICU who are at high risk for sleep disruption may experience similar effects which could negatively impact recovery.

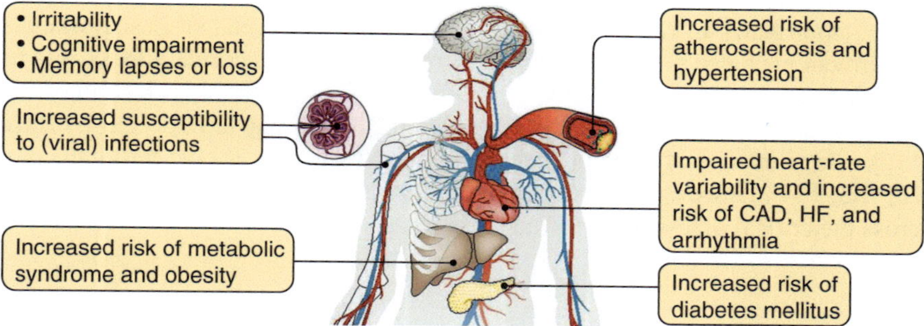

Fig. 4 General effects of short sleep duration on different organs and systems. Short sleep duration can affect cognitive function and immune responses, increase the risk of metabolic disorders (diabetes mellitus, obesity, and metabolic syndrome), and affect cardiovascular function, with accelerated atherosclerosis, increased blood pressure, and increased risk of cardiovascular events. CAD, coronary artery disease; HF, heart failure. Reprinted with permission from: Tobaldini, E., Fiorelli, E.M., Solbiati, M. et al. Short sleep duration and cardiometabolic risk: from pathophysiology to clinical evidence. Nat Rev Cardiol 16, 213–224 (2019). https://doi.org/10.1038/s41569-018-0109-6

References

1. Watson NF, Badr MS, Belenky G, Bliwise DL, Buxton OM, Buysse D, et al. Joint Consensus Statement of the American Academy of Sleep Medicine and Sleep Research Society on the recommended amount of sleep for a healthy adult: methodology and discussion. Sleep. 2015;38(8):1161–83.
2. Beccuti G, Pannain S. Sleep and obesity. Curr Opin Clin Nutr Metab Care. 2011;14(4):402–12.
3. Sabia S, Fayosse A, Dumurgier J, van Hees VT, Paquet C, Sommerlad A, et al. Association of sleep duration in middle and old age with incidence of dementia. Nat Commun. 2021;12(1):2289.
4. Pisani MA, Friese RS, Gehlbach BK, Schwab RJ, Weinhouse GL, Jones SF. Sleep in the intensive care unit. Am J Respir Crit Care Med. 2015;191(7):731–8.
5. Tkachenko O, Dinges DF. Interindividual variability in neurobehavioral response to sleep loss: a comprehensive review. Neurosci Biobehav Rev. 2018;89:29–48.
6. Banks S. Behavioral and physiological consequences of sleep restriction. J Clin Sleep Med. 2007;3(05):519–28.
7. Dinges DF, Pack F, Williams K, Gillen KA, Powell JW, Ott GE, et al. Cumulative sleepiness, mood disturbance, and psychomotor vigilance performance decrements during a week of sleep restricted to 4–5 hours per night. Sleep. 1997;20(4):267–77.
8. Van Dongen H, Maislin G, Mullington JM, Dinges DF. The cumulative cost of additional wakefulness: dose-response effects on neurobehavioral functions and sleep physiology from chronic sleep restriction and total sleep deprivation. Sleep. 2003;26(2):117–26.
9. Goldstein AN, Walker MP. The role of sleep in emotional brain function. Annu Rev Clin Psychol. 2014;10:679–708.
10. Pilcher JJ, Huffcutt AI. Effects of sleep deprivation on performance: a meta-analysis. Sleep. 1996;19(4):318–26.
11. Banks S, Van Dongen HPA, Maislin G, Dinges DF. Neurobehavioral dynamics following chronic sleep restriction: dose-response effects of one night for recovery. Sleep. 2010;33(8):1013–26.
12. Kahn-Greene ET, Killgore DB, Kamimori GH, Balkin TJ, Killgore WD. The effects of sleep deprivation on symptoms of psychopathology in healthy adults. Sleep Med. 2007;8(3):215–21.
13. Simon EB, Rossi A, Harvey AG, Walker MP. Overanxious and underslept. Nat Hum Behav. 2020;4(1):100–10.
14. Minkel JD, Banks S, Htaik O, Moreta MC, Jones CW, McGlinchey EL, et al. Sleep deprivation and stressors: evidence for elevated negative affect in response to mild stressors when sleep deprived. Emotion. 2012;12(5):1015.
15. Gruber R, Cassoff J. The interplay between sleep and emotion regulation: conceptual framework empirical evidence and future directions. Curr Psychiatry Rep. 2014;16(11):500.
16. Altman MT, Knauert MP, Pisani MA. Sleep disturbance after hospitalization and critical illness: a systematic review. Ann Am Thorac Soc. 2017;14(9):1457–68.
17. Hatch R, Young D, Barber V, Griffiths J, Harrison DA, Watkinson P. Anxiety, depression and post traumatic stress disorder after critical illness: a UK-wide prospective cohort study. Crit Care. 2018;22(1):310.
18. Lim JL, Dinges DF. Sleep deprivation and vigilant attention. In: Pfaff DW, Kieffer BL, editors. Molecular and biophysical mechanisms of arousal, alertness, and attention. Annals of the New York Academy of Sciences. 11292008. p. 305–22.
19. Dinges DF, Powell JW. Microcomputer analyses of performance on a portable, simple visual RT task during sustained operations. Behav Res Methods Instrum Comput. 1985;17(6):652–5.
20. Dinges DF. An overview of sleepiness and accidents. J Sleep Res. 1995;4:4–14.
21. McHill AW, Hull JT, Wang W, Czeisler CA, Klerman EB. Chronic sleep curtailment, even without extended (> 16-h) wakefulness, degrades human vigilance performance. Proc Natl Acad Sci. 2018;115(23):6070–5.

22. Franzen PL, Siegle GJ, Buysse DJ. Relationships between affect, vigilance, and sleepiness following sleep deprivation. J Sleep Res. 2008;17(1):34–41.
23. Stickgold R, Hobson JA, Fosse R, Fosse M. Sleep, learning, and dreams: off-line memory reprocessing. Science. 2001;294(5544):1052–7.
24. Stickgold R. Sleep-dependent memory consolidation. Nature. 2005;437(7063):1272–8.
25. Killgore WD. Effects of sleep deprivation on cognition. Prog Brain Res. 2010;185:105–29.
26. Chai Y, Fang Z, Yang FN, Xu S, Deng Y, Raine A, et al. Two nights of recovery sleep restores hippocampal connectivity but not episodic memory after total sleep deprivation. Sci Rep. 2020;10(1):1–11.
27. Zhao Z, Zhao X, Veasey SC. Neural consequences of chronic short sleep: reversible or lasting? Front Neurol. 2017;8:235.
28. Imeri L, Opp MR. How (and why) the immune system makes us sleep. Nat Rev Neurosci. 2009;10(3):199–210.
29. Besedovsky L, Lange T, Haack M. The sleep-immune crosstalk in health and disease. Physiol Rev. 2019;99(3):1325–80.
30. Lange T, Dimitrov S, Born J. Effects of sleep and circadian rhythm on the human immune system. Ann N Y Acad Sci. 2010;1193(1):48–59.
31. Krueger JM, Obál F Jr, Fang J, Kubota T, Taishi P. The role of cytokines in physiological sleep regulation. Ann N Y Acad Sci. 2001;933(1):211–21.
32. Irwin MR, Cole SW. Reciprocal regulation of the neural and innate immune systems. Nat Rev Immunol. 2011;11(9):625–32.
33. Irwin MR. Sleep and inflammation: partners in sickness and in health. Nat Rev Immunol. 2019;19(11):702–15.
34. Irwin MR, Olmstead R, Carroll JE. Sleep disturbance, sleep duration, and inflammation: a systematic review and meta-analysis of cohort studies and experimental sleep deprivation. Biol Psychiatry. 2016;80(1):40–52.
35. Shearer WT, Reuben JM, Mullington JM, Price NJ, Lee B-N, Smith EB, et al. Soluble TNF-α receptor 1 and IL-6 plasma levels in humans subjected to the sleep deprivation model of spaceflight. J Allergy Clin Immunol. 2001;107(1):165–70.
36. Irwin MR, Opp MR. Sleep health: reciprocal regulation of sleep and innate immunity. Neuropsychopharmacology. 2017;42(1):129–55.
37. Ruparelia N, Chai JT, Fisher EA, Choudhury RP. Inflammatory processes in cardiovascular disease: a route to targeted therapies. Nat Rev Cardiol. 2017;14(3):133–44.
38. Smith A. Sleep, arousal, and performance. Boston: Birkhäuser; 1992.
39. Drake CL, Roehrs TA, Royer H, Koshorek G, Turner RB, Roth T. Effects of an experimentally induced rhinovirus cold on sleep, performance, and daytime alertness. Physiol Behav. 2000;71(1–2):75–81.
40. Mullington J, Korth C, Hermann DM, Orth A, Galanos C, Holsboer F, et al. Dose-dependent effects of endotoxin on human sleep. Am J Physiol Regul Integr Comp Physiol. 2000;278(4):R947–55.
41. Prather AA, Hall M, Fury JM, Ross DC, Muldoon MF, Cohen S, et al. Sleep and antibody response to hepatitis B vaccination. Sleep. 2012;35(8):1063–9.
42. Prather AA, Janicki-Deverts D, Hall MH, Cohen S. Behaviorally assessed sleep and susceptibility to the common cold. Sleep. 2015;38(9):1353–9.
43. Hirotsu C, Tufik S, Andersen ML. Interactions between sleep, stress, and metabolism: from physiological to pathological conditions. Sleep Sci. 2015;8(3):143–52.
44. Silverthorn D. Human physiology: an integrated approach. 6th ed. San Francisco: Pearson/Benjamin Cummings; 2013.
45. Knutson KL, Spiegel K, Penev P, Van Cauter E. The metabolic consequences of sleep deprivation. Sleep Med Rev. 2007;11(3):163–78.
46. Ogilvie RP, Patel SR. The epidemiology of sleep and obesity. Sleep Health. 2017;3(5):383–8.

47. Buckley TM, Schatzberg AF. On the interactions of the hypothalamic-pituitary-adrenal (HPA) axis and sleep: normal HPA axis activity and circadian rhythm, exemplary sleep disorders. J Clin Endocrinol Metab. 2005;90(5):3106–14.
48. Omisade A, Buxton OM, Rusak B. Impact of acute sleep restriction on cortisol and leptin levels in young women. Physiol Behav. 2010;99(5):651–6.
49. Leproult R, Copinschi G, Buxton O, Van Cauter E. Sleep loss results in an elevation of cortisol levels the next evening. Sleep. 1997;20(10):865–70.
50. Guyon A, Balbo M, Morselli LL, Tasali E, Leproult R, L'Hermite-Balériaux M, et al. Adverse effects of two nights of sleep restriction on the hypothalamic-pituitary-adrenal axis in healthy men. J Clin Endocrinol Metab. 2014;99(8):2861–8.
51. Spiegel K, Leproult R, Van Cauter E. Impact of sleep debt on metabolic and endocrine function. Lancet (Lond, Engl). 1999;354(9188):1435–9.
52. Song HT, Sun XY, Yang TS, Zhang LY, Yang JL, Bai J. Effects of sleep deprivation on serum cortisol level and mental health in servicemen. Int J Psychophysiol. 2015;96(3):169–75.
53. Wright KP Jr, Drake AL, Frey DJ, Fleshner M, Desouza CA, Gronfier C, et al. Influence of sleep deprivation and circadian misalignment on cortisol, inflammatory markers, and cytokine balance. Brain Behav Immun. 2015;47:24–34.
54. Minkel J, Moreta M, Muto J, Htaik O, Jones C, Basner M, et al. Sleep deprivation potentiates HPA axis stress reactivity in healthy adults. Health Psychol. 2014;33(11):1430–4.
55. Joo EY, Yoon CW, Koo DL, Kim D, Hong SB. Adverse effects of 24 hours of sleep deprivation on cognition and stress hormones. J Clin Neurol (Seoul, Korea). 2012;8(2):146–50.
56. González-Ortiz M, Martínez-Abundis E, Balcázar-Muñoz BR, Pascoe-González S. Effect of sleep deprivation on insulin sensitivity and cortisol concentration in healthy subjects. Diabetes Nutr Metab. 2000;13(2):80–3.
57. Vgontzas AN, Zoumakis E, Bixler EO, Lin HM, Follett H, Kales A, et al. Adverse effects of modest sleep restriction on sleepiness, performance, and inflammatory cytokines. J Clin Endocrinol Metab. 2004;89(5):2119–26.
58. Klumpers UM, Veltman DJ, van Tol MJ, Kloet RW, Boellaard R, Lammertsma AA, et al. Neurophysiological effects of sleep deprivation in healthy adults, a pilot study. PLoS One. 2015;10(1):e0116906.
59. Kumari M, Badrick E, Ferrie J, Perski A, Marmot M, Chandola T. Self-reported sleep duration and sleep disturbance are independently associated with cortisol secretion in the Whitehall II study. J Clin Endocrinol Metab. 2009;94(12):4801–9.
60. Abell JG, Shipley MJ, Ferrie JE, Kivimäki M, Kumari M. Recurrent short sleep, chronic insomnia symptoms and salivary cortisol: a 10-year follow-up in the Whitehall II study. Psychoneuroendocrinology. 2016;68:91–9.
61. Follenius M, Brandenberger G, Bandesapt JJ, Libert JP, Ehrhart J. Nocturnal cortisol release in relation to sleep structure. Sleep. 1992;15(1):21–7.
62. Vgontzas AN, Bixler EO, Papanicolaou DA, Kales A, Stratakis CA, Vela-Bueno A, et al. Rapid eye movement sleep correlates with the overall activities of the hypothalamic-pituitary-adrenal axis and sympathetic system in healthy humans. J Clin Endocrinol Metab. 1997;82(10):3278–80.
63. Li J, Bidlingmaier M, Petru R, Pedrosa Gil F, Loerbroks A, Angerer P. Impact of shift work on the diurnal cortisol rhythm: a one-year longitudinal study in junior physicians. J Occup Med Toxicol (Lond, Engl). 2018;13:23.
64. Cannizzaro E, Cirrincione L, Mazzucco W, Scorciapino A, Catalano C, Ramaci T, et al. Night-time shift work and related stress responses: a study on security guards. Int J Environ Res Public Health. 2020;17(2).
65. Elliott R, McKinley S, Cistulli P, Fien M. Characterisation of sleep in intensive care using 24-hour polysomnography: an observational study. Crit Care. 2013;17(2):R46.
66. Irwin M, Thompson J, Miller C, Gillin JC, Ziegler M. Effects of sleep and sleep deprivation on catecholamine and interleukin-2 levels in humans: clinical implications. J Clin Endocrinol Metab. 1999;84(6):1979–85.

67. Tochikubo O, Ikeda A, Miyajima E, Ishii M. Effects of insufficient sleep on blood pressure monitored by a new multibiomedical recorder. Hypertension (Dallas, Tex: 1979). 1996;27(6):1318–24.
68. Lusardi P, Zoppi A, Preti P, Pesce RM, Piazza E, Fogari R. Effects of insufficient sleep on blood pressure in hypertensive patients: a 24-h study. Am J Hypertens. 1999;12(1 Pt 1):63–8.
69. Irwin M, Clark C, Kennedy B, Christian Gillin J, Ziegler M. Nocturnal catecholamines and immune function in insomniacs, depressed patients, and control subjects. Brain Behav Immun. 2003;17(5):365–72.
70. Schmid SM, Hallschmid M, Jauch-Chara K, Bandorf N, Born J, Schultes B. Sleep loss alters basal metabolic hormone secretion and modulates the dynamic counterregulatory response to hypoglycemia. J Clin Endocrinol Metab. 2007;92(8):3044–51.
71. Mullington JM, Haack M, Toth M, Serrador JM, Meier-Ewert HK. Cardiovascular, inflammatory, and metabolic consequences of sleep deprivation. Prog Cardiovasc Dis. 2009;51(4):294–302.
72. Annane D. The role of ACTH and corticosteroids for sepsis and septic shock: an update. Front Endocrinol. 2016;7:70.
73. Harding EC, Franks NP, Wisden W. The temperature dependence of sleep. Front Neurosci. 2019;13:336.
74. Gary KA, Winokur A, Douglas SD, Kapoor S, Zaugg L, Dinges DF. Total sleep deprivation and the thyroid axis: effects of sleep and waking activity. Aviat Space Environ Med. 1996;67(6):513–9.
75. Redwine L, Hauger RL, Gillin JC, Irwin M. Effects of sleep and sleep deprivation on interleukin-6, growth hormone, cortisol, and melatonin levels in humans. J Clin Endocrinol Metab. 2000;85(10):3597–603.
76. Everson CA, Crowley WR. Reductions in circulating anabolic hormones induced by sustained sleep deprivation in rats. Am J Physiol Endocrinol Metab. 2004;286(6):E1060–70.
77. Leproult R, Van Cauter E. Effect of 1 week of sleep restriction on testosterone levels in young healthy men. JAMA. 2011;305(21):2173–4.
78. Donga E, van Dijk M, van Dijk JG, Biermasz NR, Lammers GJ, van Kralingen KW, et al. A single night of partial sleep deprivation induces insulin resistance in multiple metabolic pathways in healthy subjects. J Clin Endocrinol Metab. 2010;95(6):2963–8.
79. Tobaldini E, Fiorelli EM, Solbiati M, Costantino G, Nobili L, Montano N. Short sleep duration and cardiometabolic risk: from pathophysiology to clinical evidence. Nat Rev Cardiol. 2019;16(4):213–24.
80. Aldabal L, Bahammam AS. Metabolic, endocrine, and immune consequences of sleep deprivation. Open Respir Med J. 2011;5:31–43.
81. Robinson LE, van Soeren MH. Insulin resistance and hyperglycemia in critical illness: role of insulin in glycemic control. AACN Clin Issues. 2004;15(1):45–62.
82. Yin J, Jin X, Shan Z, Li S, Huang H, Li P, et al. Relationship of sleep duration with all-cause mortality and cardiovascular events: a systematic review and dose-response meta-analysis of prospective cohort studies. J Am Heart Assoc. 2017;6(9)
83. Itani O, Jike M, Watanabe N, Kaneita Y. Short sleep duration and health outcomes: a systematic review, meta-analysis, and meta-regression. Sleep Med. 2017;32:246–56.
84. Bourdillon N, Jeanneret F, Nilchian M, Albertoni P, Ha P, Millet GP. Sleep deprivation deteriorates heart rate variability and photoplethysmography. Front Neurosci. 2021;15:642548.
85. Sauvet F, Leftheriotis G, Gomez-Merino D, Langrume C, Drogou C, Van Beers P, et al. Effect of acute sleep deprivation on vascular function in healthy subjects. J Appl Physiol (Bethesda, Md: 1985). 2010;108(1):68–75.
86. Zhong X, Hilton HJ, Gates GJ, Jelic S, Stern Y, Bartels MN, et al. Increased sympathetic and decreased parasympathetic cardiovascular modulation in normal humans with acute sleep deprivation. J Appl Physiol (Bethesda, Md : 1985). 2005;98(6):2024–32.

87. Açar G, Akçakoyun M, Sari I, Bulut M, Alizade E, Özkan B, et al. Acute sleep deprivation in healthy adults is associated with a reduction in left atrial early diastolic strain rate. Sleep Breathing = Schlaf & Atmung. 2013;17(3):975–83.

88. Cincin A, Sari I, Sunbul M, Kepez A, Oguz M, Sert S, et al. Effect of acute sleep deprivation on left atrial mechanics assessed by three-dimensional echocardiography. Sleep Breathing = Schlaf & Atmung. 2016;20(1):227–35. discussion 35

89. Cakici M, Dogan A, Cetin M, Suner A, Caner A, Polat M, et al. Negative effects of acute sleep deprivation on left ventricular functions and cardiac repolarization in healthy young adults. Pacing Clin Electrophysiol. 2015;38(6):713–22.

90. Ozer O, Ozbala B, Sari I, Davutoglu V, Maden E, Baltaci Y, et al. Acute sleep deprivation is associated with increased QT dispersion in healthy young adults. Pacing Clin Electrophysiol. 2008;31(8):979–84.

91. Sari I, Davutoglu V, Ozbala B, Ozer O, Baltaci Y, Yavuz S, et al. Acute sleep deprivation is associated with increased electrocardiographic P-wave dispersion in healthy young men and women. Pacing Clin Electrophysiol. 2008;31(4):438–42.

92. Esen Ö, Akçakoyun M, Açar G, Bulut M, Alızade E, Kargin R, et al. Acute sleep deprivation is associated with increased atrial electromechanical delay in healthy young adults. Pacing Clin Electrophysiol. 2011;34(12):1645–51.

93. Miner SE, Pahal D, Nichols L, Darwood A, Nield LE, Wulffhart Z. Sleep disruption is associated with increased ventricular ectopy and cardiac arrest in hospitalized adults. Sleep. 2016;39(4):927–35.

94. Münzel T, Camici GG, Maack C, Bonetti NR, Fuster V, Kovacic JC. Impact of oxidative stress on the heart and vasculature: part 2 of a 3-part series. J Am Coll Cardiol. 2017;70(2):212–29.

95. Villafuerte G, Miguel-Puga A, Rodríguez EM, Machado S, Manjarrez E, Arias-Carrión O. Sleep deprivation and oxidative stress in animal models: a systematic review. Oxidative Med Cell Longev. 2015;2015:234952.

96. Boudjeltia KZ, Faraut B, Esposito MJ, Stenuit P, Dyzma M, Antwerpen PV, et al. Temporal dissociation between myeloperoxidase (MPO)-modified LDL and MPO elevations during chronic sleep restriction and recovery in healthy young men. PLoS One. 2011;6(11):e28230.

97. Faraut B, Boudjeltia KZ, Vanhamme L, Kerkhofs M. Immune, inflammatory and cardiovascular consequences of sleep restriction and recovery. Sleep Med Rev. 2012;16(2):137–49.

98. Sauvet F, Drogou C, Bougard C, Arnal PJ, Dispersyn G, Bourrilhon C, et al. Vascular response to 1 week of sleep restriction in healthy subjects. A metabolic response? Int J Cardiol. 2015;190:246–55.

99. Dettoni JL, Consolim-Colombo FM, Drager LF, Rubira MC, Souza SB, Irigoyen MC, et al. Cardiovascular effects of partial sleep deprivation in healthy volunteers. J Appl Physiol (Bethesda, Md: 1985). 2012;113(2):232–6.

100. Bain AR, Weil BR, Diehl KJ, Greiner JJ, Stauffer BL, DeSouza CA. Insufficient sleep is associated with impaired nitric oxide-mediated endothelium-dependent vasodilation. Atherosclerosis. 2017;265:41–6.

101. Calvin AD, Covassin N, Kremers WK, Adachi T, Macedo P, Albuquerque FN, et al. Experimental sleep restriction causes endothelial dysfunction in healthy humans. J Am Heart Assoc. 2014;3(6):e001143.

102. Higashi Y, Maruhashi T, Noma K, Kihara Y. Oxidative stress and endothelial dysfunction: clinical evidence and therapeutic implications. Trends Cardiovasc Med. 2014;24(4):165–9.

103. Cherubini JM, Cheng JL, Williams JS, MacDonald MJ. Sleep deprivation and endothelial function: reconciling seminal evidence with recent perspectives. Am J Physiol Heart Circ Physiol. 2021;320(1):H29–h35.

104. Weil BR, Mestek ML, Westby CM, Van Guilder GP, Greiner JJ, Stauffer BL, et al. Short sleep duration is associated with enhanced endothelin-1 vasoconstrictor tone. Can J Physiol Pharmacol. 2010;88(8):777–81.

105. Covassin N, Bukartyk J, Singh P, Calvin AD, St Louis EK, Somers VK. Effects of experimental sleep restriction on ambulatory and sleep blood pressure in healthy young adults: a randomized crossover study. Hypertension (Dallas, Tex : 1979). 2021;78(3):859–70.

106. Sherwood A, Steffen PR, Blumenthal JA, Kuhn C, Hinderliter AL. Nighttime blood pressure dipping: the role of the sympathetic nervous system. Am J Hypertens. 2002;15(2 Pt 1):111–8.

107. Yang H, Haack M, Gautam S, Meier-Ewert HK, Mullington JM. Repetitive exposure to shortened sleep leads to blunted sleep-associated blood pressure dipping. J Hypertens. 2017;35(6):1187–94.

108. Budhiraja R, Siddiqi TA, Quan SF. Sleep disorders in chronic obstructive pulmonary disease: etiology, impact, and management. J Clin Sleep Med. 2015;11(3):259–70.

109. Adir Y, Humbert M, Chaouat A. Sleep-related breathing disorders and pulmonary hypertension. Eur Respir J. 2021;57(1)

110. Rault C, Heraud Q, Ragot S, Robert R, Drouot X. Sleep deprivation increases air hunger rather than breathing effort. Am J Respir Crit Care Med. 2021;203(5):642–5.

111. Rault C, Sangaré A, Diaz V, Ragot S, Frat JP, Raux M, et al. Impact of sleep deprivation on respiratory motor output and endurance. A physiological study. Am J Respir Crit Care Med. 2020;201(8):976–83.

112. Cooper KR, Phillips BA. Effect of short-term sleep loss on breathing. J Appl Physiol Respir Environ Exerc Physiol. 1982;53(4):855–8.

113. Chen HI, Tang YR. Sleep loss impairs inspiratory muscle endurance. Am Rev Respir Dis. 1989;140(4):907–9.

114. Westphal WP, Rault C, Robert R, Ragot S, Neau JP, Fernagut PO, et al. Sleep deprivation reduces vagal tone during an inspiratory endurance task in humans. Sleep. 2021;44(10):zsab105.

115. Sériès F, Roy N, Marc I. Effects of sleep deprivation and sleep fragmentation on upper airway collapsibility in normal subjects. Am J Respir Crit Care Med. 1994;150(2):481–5.

116. Khanijow V, Prakash P, Emsellem HA, Borum ML, Doman DB. Sleep dysfunction and gastrointestinal diseases. Gastroenterol Hepatol. 2015;11(12):817–25.

117. Huang ZP, Li SM, Shen T, Zhang YY. Correlation between sleep impairment and functional dyspepsia. J Int Med Res. 2020;48(7):300060520937164.

118. Grover M, Kolla BP, Pamarthy R, Mansukhani MP, Breen-Lyles M, He JP, et al. Psychological, physical, and sleep comorbidities and functional impairment in irritable bowel syndrome: results from a national survey of U.S. adults. PLoS One. 2021;16(1):e0245323.

119. Bruyneel M, Sersté T. Sleep disturbances in patients with liver cirrhosis: prevalence, impact, and management challenges. Nat Sci Sleep. 2018;10:369–75.

120. Smith RP, Easson C, Lyle SM, Kapoor R, Donnelly CP, Davidson EJ, et al. Gut microbiome diversity is associated with sleep physiology in humans. PLoS One. 2019;14(10):e0222394.

121. Lin J, Jiang Y, Wang G, Meng M, Zhu Q, Mei H, et al. Associations of short sleep duration with appetite-regulating hormones and adipokines: a systematic review and meta-analysis. Obes Rev. 2020;21(11):e13051.

122. Taheri S, Lin L, Austin D, Young T, Mignot E. Short sleep duration is associated with reduced leptin, elevated ghrelin, and increased body mass index. PLoS Med. 2004;1(3):e62.

123. Spiegel K, Tasali E, Penev P, Van Cauter E. Brief communication: sleep curtailment in healthy young men is associated with decreased leptin levels, elevated ghrelin levels, and increased hunger and appetite. Ann Intern Med. 2004;141(11):846–50.

124. Spaeth AM, Goel N, Dinges DF. Caloric and macronutrient intake and meal timing responses to repeated sleep restriction exposures separated by varying intervening recovery nights in healthy adults. Nutrients. 2020;12(9)

125. Spaeth AM, Dinges DF, Goel N. Effects of experimental sleep restriction on weight gain, caloric intake, and meal timing in healthy adults. Sleep. 2013;36(7):981–90.

126. Shechter A, Rising R, Albu JB, St-Onge MP. Experimental sleep curtailment causes wake-dependent increases in 24-h energy expenditure as measured by whole-room indirect calorimetry. Am J Clin Nutr. 2013;98(6):1433–9.

127. Markwald RR, Melanson EL, Smith MR, Higgins J, Perreault L, Eckel RH, et al. Impact of insufficient sleep on total daily energy expenditure, food intake, and weight gain. Proc Natl Acad Sci U S A. 2013;110(14):5695–700.
128. Chen C, ValizadehAslani T, Rosen GL, Anderson LM, Jungquist CR. Healthcare shift workers' temporal habits for eating, sleeping, and light exposure: a multi-instrument pilot study. J Circadian Rhythms. 2020;18:6.
129. Chen Y, Lauren S, Chang BP, Shechter A. Objective food intake in night and day shift workers: a laboratory study. Clocks & Sleep. 2018;1(1):42–9.
130. Lauren S, Chen Y, Friel C, Chang BP, Shechter A. Free-living sleep, food intake, and physical activity in night and morning shift workers. J Am Coll Nutr. 2020;39(5):450–6.
131. McHill AW, Melanson EL, Higgins J, Connick E, Moehlman TM, Stothard ER, et al. Impact of circadian misalignment on energy metabolism during simulated nightshift work. Proc Natl Acad Sci U S A. 2014;111(48):17302–7.
132. Greer SM, Goldstein AN, Walker MP. The impact of sleep deprivation on food desire in the human brain. Nat Commun. 2013;4:2259.
133. Rihm JS, Menz MM, Schultz H, Bruder L, Schilbach L, Schmid SM, et al. Sleep deprivation selectively upregulates an amygdala-hypothalamic circuit involved in food reward. J Neurosci. 2019;39(5):888–99.
134. St-Onge MP. Sleep-obesity relation: underlying mechanisms and consequences for treatment. Obes Rev. 2017;18(Suppl 1):34–9.
135. Zhu B, Shi C, Park CG, Zhao X, Reutrakul S. Effects of sleep restriction on metabolism-related parameters in healthy adults: a comprehensive review and meta-analysis of randomized controlled trials. Sleep Med Rev. 2019;45:18–30.
136. Cappuccio FP, Taggart FM, Kandala NB, Currie A, Peile E, Stranges S, et al. Meta-analysis of short sleep duration and obesity in children and adults. Sleep. 2008;31(5):619–26.
137. Andersen ML, Martins PJ, D'Almeida V, Bignotto M, Tufik S. Endocrinological and catecholaminergic alterations during sleep deprivation and recovery in male rats. J Sleep Res. 2005;14(1):83–90.
138. Dattilo M, Antunes HK, Medeiros A, Mônico Neto M, Souza HS, Tufik S, et al. Sleep and muscle recovery: endocrinological and molecular basis for a new and promising hypothesis. Med Hypotheses 2011;77(2):220–2.
139. Lamon S, Morabito A, Arentson-Lantz E, Knowles O, Vincent GE, Condo D, et al. The effect of acute sleep deprivation on skeletal muscle protein synthesis and the hormonal environment. Physiol Rep. 2021;9(1):e14660.
140. Xu X, Wang L, Chen L, Su T, Zhang Y, Wang T, et al. Effects of chronic sleep deprivation on bone mass and bone metabolism in rats. J Orthop Surg Res. 2016;11(1):87.
141. Everson CA, Folley AE, Toth JM. Chronically inadequate sleep results in abnormal bone formation and abnormal bone marrow in rats. Exp Biol Med (Maywood). 2012;237(9):1101–9.
142. Lucassen EA, de Mutsert R, le Cessie S, Appelman-Dijkstra NM, Rosendaal FR, van Heemst D, et al. Poor sleep quality and later sleep timing are risk factors for osteopenia and sarcopenia in middle-aged men and women: the NEO study. PLoS One. 2017;12(5):e0176685.
143. Swanson CM. Sleep disruptions and bone health: what do we know so far? Curr Opin Endocrinol Diabetes Obes. 2021;28(4):348–53.
144. Wang D, Ruan W, Peng Y, Li W. Sleep duration and the risk of osteoporosis among middle-aged and elderly adults: a dose-response meta-analysis. Osteoporosis Int. 2018;29(8):1689–95.
145. Foley D, Ancoli-Israel S, Britz P, Walsh J. Sleep disturbances and chronic disease in older adults: results of the 2003 National Sleep Foundation Sleep in America Survey. J Psychosom Res. 2004;56(5):497–502.
146. Feskanich D, Hankinson SE, Schernhammer ES. Nightshift work and fracture risk: the Nurses' Health Study. Osteoporosis Int. 2009;20(4):537–42.
147. Moradi S, Shab-Bidar S, Alizadeh S, Djafarian K. Association between sleep duration and osteoporosis risk in middle-aged and elderly women: a systematic review and meta-analysis of observational studies. Metab Clin Exp. 2017;69:199–206.

148. Swanson CM, Blatchford PJ, Stone KL, Cauley JA, Lane NE, Rogers-Soeder TS, et al. Sleep duration and bone health measures in older men. Osteoporosis Int. 2021;32(3):515–27.
149. Santhanam P, Khthir R, Dial L, Driscoll HK, Gress TW. Femoral neck bone mineral density in persons over 50 years performing shiftwork: an epidemiological study. J Occup Environ Med. 2016;58(3):e63–5.
150. Rawal G, Yadav S, Kumar R. Post-intensive care syndrome: an overview. J Transl Int Med. 2017;5(2):90–2.
151. Jolley SE, Bunnell AE, Hough CL. ICU-acquired weakness. Chest. 2016;150(5):1129–40.
152. Orford NR, Lane SE, Bailey M, Pasco JA, Cattigan C, Elderkin T, et al. Changes in bone mineral density in the year after critical illness. Am J Respir Crit Care Med. 2016;193(7):736–44.
153. Alexopoulou C, Bolaki M, Akoumianaki E, Erimaki S, Kondili E, Mitsias P, et al. Sleep quality in survivors of critical illness. Sleep & breathing = Schlaf & Atmung. 2019;23(2):463–71.
154. Solverson KJ, Easton PA, Doig CJ. Assessment of sleep quality post-hospital discharge in survivors of critical illness. Respir Med. 2016;114:97–102.
155. Dennis LE, Wohl RJ, Selame LA, Goel N. Healthy adults display long-term trait-like neurobehavioral resilience and vulnerability to sleep loss. Sci Rep. 2017;7(1):14889.
156. He Y, Jones CR, Fujiki N, Xu Y, Guo B, Holder JL Jr, et al. The transcriptional repressor DEC2 regulates sleep length in mammals. Science (New York, NY). 2009;325(5942):866–70.

Risk Factors for Disrupted Sleep in the ICU

Kimia Honarmand and Karen J. Bosma

1   Introduction

Sleep disruption is a pervasive and distressing problem for critically ill patients [1–3]. Patients in the intensive care unit (ICU) often experience disrupted circadian rhythms, sleep fragmentation, decreased slow-wave sleep and almost absent rapid eye movement (REM) sleep [4, 5]. Despite the evaluation of multiple different interventions to improve ICU sleep, many strategies have met with limited success in improving patient-perceived sleep quality [6–8]. A failure to understand and recognize underlying factors that disrupt our patients' sleep is an important contributor to the failure of many sleep improvement initiatives. One large ICU cohort study [9] found that light, noise, and care activities explain only 30% of sleep fragmentation therefore leaving 70% of sleep arousals and awakenings unexplained. It may also be that the factors disrupting sleep are so numerous that a single intervention, even if multi-faceted, may not be able to reverse all underlying sleep disrupting factors. Risk factors for sleep disruption may also vary from night to night. Finally, sleep risk factors intrinsic to the patient may not be modifiable. For these reasons, to successfully improve sleep in the ICU, it is imperative that we understand as much as possible about the predisposing and precipitating factors that disrupt sleep and circadian rhythms in our critically ill patients.

This chapter will highlight those factors shown to disrupt sleep in the ICU, provide an overview of the methodological approaches used to identify and evaluate sleep risk factors, and examine the prevalence and impact of patient-reported factors

K. Honarmand · K. J. Bosma (✉)
Department of Medicine, Division of Critical Care Medicine, Schulich School of Medicine and Dentistry, University of Western Ontario, London, ON, Canada
e-mail: kimia.honarmand@medportal.ca; karenj.bosma@lhsc.on.ca

G. L. Weinhouse, J. W. Devlin (eds.), *Sleep in Critical Illness*,
https://doi.org/10.1007/978-3-031-06447-0_6

associated with poor sleep. We will also consider risk factors for disrupted sleep in special ICU populations, explore inter-patient risk factor variability, and lay foundations for both future research and clinical quality improvement interventions focused on improving not only sleep but also discomfort, agitation, and delirium.

2 Characterizing and Identifying Risk Factors for Disrupted Sleep

2.1 Risk Factor Characterization

A risk factor is defined as any attribute, characteristic, or exposure that precedes and is associated with an increased likelihood of an adverse outcome or event [10]. Risk factors may be classified as: (1) a fixed marker i.e., a non-modifiable attribute or characteristic (e.g., sex, age), (2) a variable marker i.e., a modifiable variable but its modification does not change the risk of the outcome of interest, or (3) a causal risk factor i.e., where modification of the variable changes the likelihood of the outcome. Predisposing factors are those patient-intrinsic factors that exist prior to ICU admission that place patients at risk of poor sleep. Precipitating factors are those risk factors that occur in the ICU, and may be related to the ICU environment, and/or the physiologic and/or psychologic impact of critical illness. As described in chapter "Biologic Effects of Disrupted Sleep", the complex biological mechanisms of disrupted sleep in the ICU suggests sleep disruption involves an interplay between intrinsic (patient-related) and extrinsic (external) factors and that various protective factors have an important mitigating effect. As such, identifying risk factors for sleep disruption in ICU patients is best achieved by reviewing studies having diverse designs.

2.2 Risk Factor Identification

2.2.1 Patient Perceived

Various approaches have been used to identify risk factors for disrupted sleep in critically ill patients. Some factors are best identified by the patient themselves. These descriptive ('self-report') studies typically rely on the administration of questionnaires to determine the proportion of patients who report whether a particular factor is perceived by the patient to be either detrimental or beneficial to sleep quality. Subjective methods that can be used to measure ICU sleep are reviewed in chapter "Methods for Routine Sleep Assessment and Monitoring". In some 'patient-reported' studies, patients are asked in an open-ended fashion to communicate those factors they believed adversely affected their sleep. In others, patients are asked to select risk factors from a pre-specified list of factors known to influence sleep; the proportion of patients endorsing each risk factor are subsequently reported. And still other studies use questionnaires where patients are asked to numerically rate the perceived impact of each factor (vs. simply providing a yes or no).

2.2.2 Objective

Other risk factors (e.g., patient characteristics and clinical history, ICU interventions) are best identified using analytical studies, which estimate the strength of association between each potential sleep risk factor and sleep quality, usually using multivariable methods. Both intrinsic (i.e., patient-related or illness-related) and extrinsic (i.e., ICU-acquired) factors for sleep disruption can be considered. Sleep quality outcomes can be assessed by either subjective (i.e., patient self-report instruments) or objective (e.g., polysomnography [PSG], actigraphy, or bispectral index [BIS]) measures. Please see "objective sleep assessment" in the chapter "Methods for Routine Sleep Assessment and Monitoring". Based on the resulting risk estimate (i.e., association) each potential sleep risk factor will then fall into one of three categories: (1) sleep-disruptive, (2) sleep-protective, or (3) not associated with a change in sleep. A subset of analytical studies that have utilized PSG have the advantage of providing data on the degree of temporal association between a risk factor and arousal or awakening from sleep, allowing for basic causal inferences to be made.

2.3 A Systematic Approach to Summarizing the Sleep Risk Factor Literature

In the next two sections, we summarize the results of multiple studies that have evaluated patient-related, illness-related, and ICU-acquired risk factors for disrupted sleep in ICU. Our approach is informed by a systematic review [11] we conducted of 63 original ICU studies evaluating potential risk factors for disrupted sleep. To synthesize this broad and heterogeneous body of literature, in the updated search we completed for this chapter, we categorize studies into: (1) *patient-reported studies* where risk factors identified or endorsed by patients as sleep-disruptive were reported; (2) *impact rating studies* where patients ranked various risk factors based on their impact on sleep; (3) *association studies* where the association between potential risk factors and measures of sleep was reported (and separated into premorbid, illness-related, and ICU-acquired factors). Of note, these categories were not treated as mutually exclusive, as some studies evaluated potential risk factors across more than one of these three categories.

3 Patient-Reported Risk Factors

3.1 *Illness-Associated*

Critical illness is often associated with debilitating physical and psychological sequelae that may adversely impact sleep in ICU. Figure 1 demonstrates the patient-reported physiologic (1a) and psychologic (1b) risk factors for sleep disruption in this setting. Among the physiologic sequelae of critical illness, patients most frequently endorsed pain [3, 12–16] and discomfort [12–17] as disruptive to their sleep among a general cohort of ICU survivors irrespective of their self-reported sleep quality. Among patients who reported poor sleep quality in ICU, pain remained the most frequently reported risk factor [3, 18, 19]. Among the psychological sequelae, anxiety, worry, or stress [3, 12, 13, 15, 16], being in an unfamiliar environment [3, 12, 20], and loneliness [3, 21] were frequently reported as contributing to poor sleep in ICU. Other patient-reported risk factors related to critical illness are shown in Fig. 1.

3.2 *ICU-Related*

Figure 1c shows the patient-reported risk factors related to the ICU environment and therapies. Among these, noise [3, 12–18, 20–24], care activities such as medication administration, tests, and procedures [3, 12, 15–17, 20–23, 25], and ambient light [12, 14–17, 20, 23] were the most frequently reported ICU-related risk factors for sleep disruption. Among patients who reported poor sleep quality in ICU, noise remained the most frequently reported risk factor [3, 18, 19, 26].

3.3 *Impact/Severity-Rated*

Among studies reporting patient ratings of the impact/severity of different factors on sleep (Fig. 2), patients rated noise, ambient light, and care activities as the highest (most impactful) sleep-disruptive factors. Of note, aggregate patient ratings across four studies were relatively low (4 to 4.5 on the 10-point scale questionnaire designed by Freedman et al. [27]), suggesting that although patients endorse these factors to be sleep-disruptive, patients tend to give only modest attribution to individual factors.

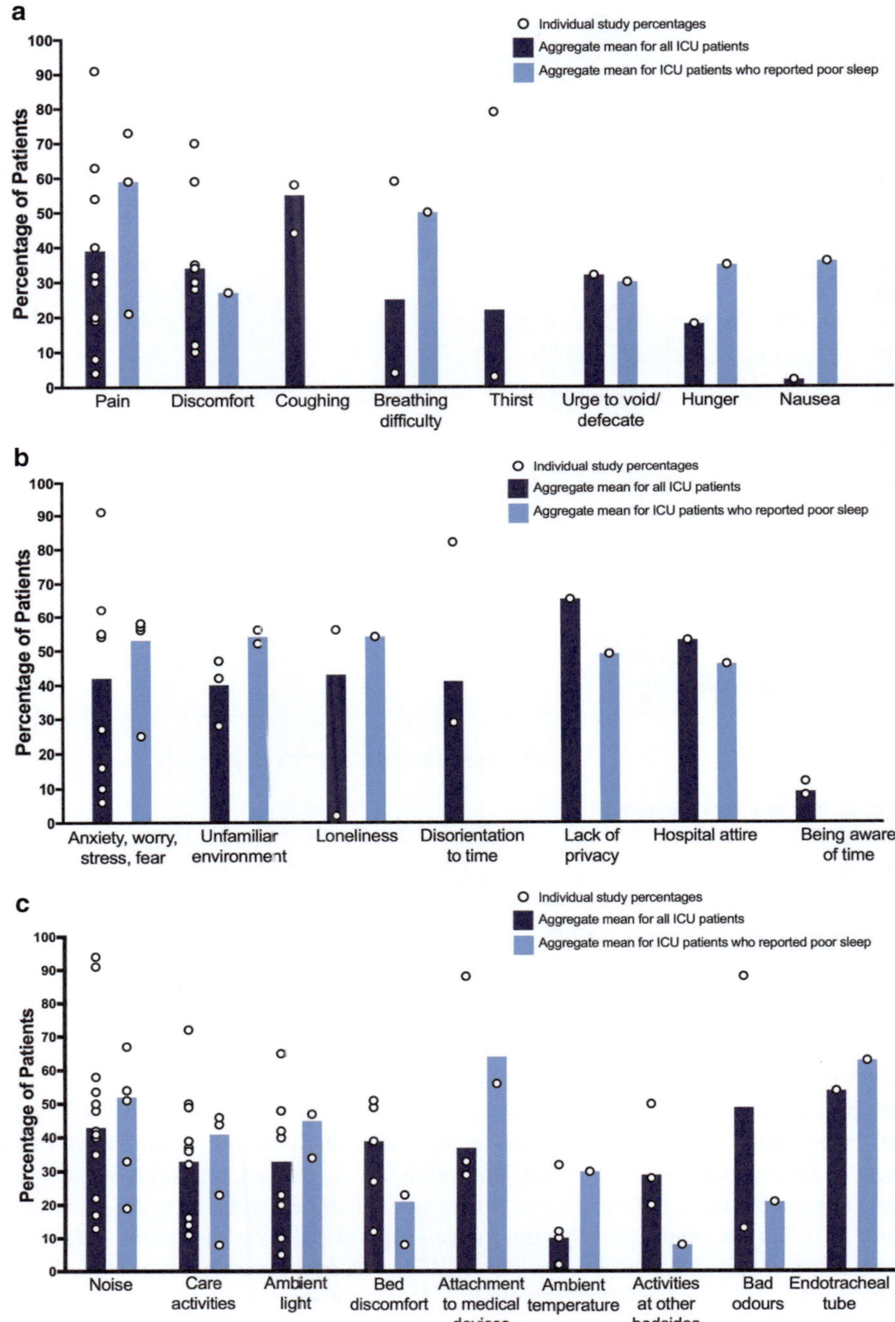

Fig. 1 (**a, b, c**) Patient-reported risk factors. (**a**) Frequency of patient-reported physiological risk factors. (**b**) Frequency of patient-reported psychological risk factors. (**c**) Frequency of patient-reported ICU-related risk factors

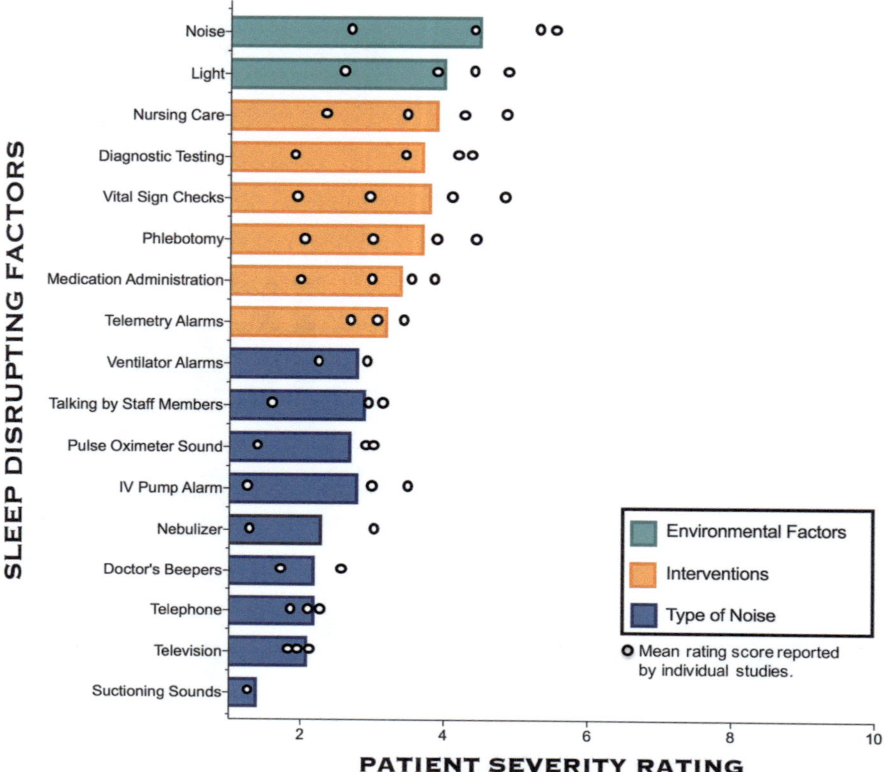

Fig. 2 Patient severity/impact rating

4 Patient-Related Risk Factors for Sleep Disruption

4.1 Baseline (Premorbid)

Although patient characteristics and health history factors are non-modifiable in the ICU setting, recognizing such risk factors is critical to identifying patients at high risk for sleep disruption. The prognostic value of patient-related (premorbid) factors are best identified using multivariate association studies (Fig. 3). Here, the balance of the evidence suggests that patient demographic characteristics such as age and gender are not associated with sleep disruption in ICU. In fact, one study identified an age-gender interaction, with older women *less* likely to experience sleep disruption [28]. On the other hand, having multiple pre-existing comorbidities [29, 30], poor sleep quality prior to hospitalization [28, 31], and possibly the use of sleep medications at home (shown in one study [31] but not shown in another study [28]) have been associated with sleep disruption and may represent potential prognostic indicators to identify patients at high-risk for sleep disruption in ICU.

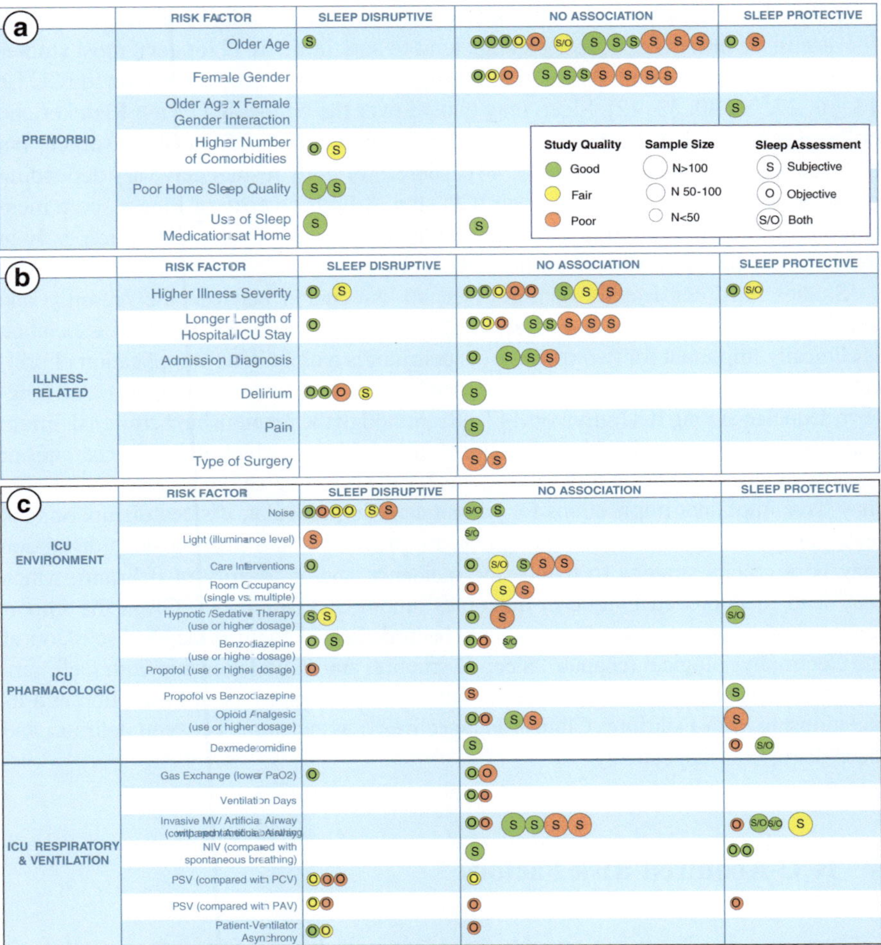

Fig. 3 (**a**, **b**, **c**) Statistical or temporal associations. (**a**) Premorbid risk factors. (**b**) Illness-related risk factors. (**c**) ICU-related risk factors

4.2 Illness-Associated

Similar to patient-related risk factors, illness-associated variables are generally non-modifiable but may help ICU clinicians identify those patients at high-risk for disrupted sleep (Fig. 3b). Neither ICU admission diagnosis [7, 32–34] nor type of surgery (for surgical patients) [15, 16] have been shown to be associated with sleep disruption. However, the relationship between severity of illness and sleep disruption is less clear. While many studies report no association between illness severity score and sleep quality [9, 14, 28, 35–39], two studies report that sleep disruption is worse in patients who are sicker [29, 34], while two others describe better sleep in patients with higher severity of illness [40, 41]. Length of ICU stay may be considered an indirect metric for disease severity (i.e., sicker patients tend to stay in the ICU longer); most studies have found no association between ICU length of stay and sleep disruption in ICU [9, 13, 16, 27, 28, 30, 33, 42]. Sleep may evolve over the course ICU stay: Redeker and colleagues found that sleep was highly fragmentated initially after cardiac surgery but decreased in the days following [43, 44]. Therefore, study results may vary depending on when sleep is assessed during the ICU stay. A high severity of illness score measured at ICU admission may correlate with a high degree of sleep disruption early in the ICU stay but good sleep later in the ICU stay.

Studies have consistently demonstrated an association between the presence and severity of delirium and disrupted sleep in ICU (Fig. 3b) [34, 35, 38, 45]. This association is clinically important for two reasons: (1) delirium is a ubiquitous complication of critical illness [46] and (2) delirium is an independent risk factor for adverse short- and long-term sequelae among ICU survivors [47, 48]. Although the relationship between delirium and sleep disruption is likely bi-directional, the degree to which the presence and/ or severity of sleep disruption in ICU accounts for the presence and/or severity of delirium may have important implications for patient care. In particular, if sleep disruption is at least partly causally associated with delirium, preventing and treating sleep disruption may be a crucial strategy to reduce the incidence and/or severity of delirium, which may lead to improved long-term outcomes among ICU survivors. Given the importance of this question, two chapters have been dedicated to an in-depth discussion of the electrophysiological (chapter "Sleep Disruption and Its Relationship with Delirium: Electroencephalographic Perspectives") and clinical (chapter "Sleep Disruption and Its Relationship with Delirium: Clinical Perspectives") associations between delirium and sleep disruption, respectively.

5 ICU-Acquired Risk Factors

ICU-acquired risk factors are arguably the most modifiable risk factors for poor sleep in the ICU and recognition and resolution of these factors serve as the foundation for sleep-improvement efforts in this setting (please see chapter "Best Practices for Improving Sleep in the ICU. Part I: Non-pharmacologic"). Figure 3 presents the ICU-acquired risk factors, stratified into three categories: (1) the ICU environment, (2) pharmacological agents used to treat critical illness and its sequelae, and (3) respiratory therapies.

5.1 *ICU Environment*

The typical ICU environment is not conducive to sleep promotion. The degree to which specific environmental risk factors affect sleep in the ICU is challenging to characterize given the potential inter-relationship of factors (e.g., light and noise), the multiple methods by which these factors can be evaluated and the degree by which they vary over the course of 24 h and between patients. Studies evaluating the potential effect of ambient noise and light in the ICU environment have been highly variable in methodological quality and conclusions, with some reporting more sleep disruption with higher levels of noise [9, 24, 31, 38, 41, 42, 45, 49, 50] and illuminance [24] and others reporting no association [noise: 13, 51; light: 52]. Although nursing care/number of care interventions are commonly believed to exacerbate disrupted sleep, the balance of the evidence does not support this assumption [15, 25, 36, 40, 53]; making it likely patient care activities account for only one of many factors that may disrupt sleep in the ICU. Some potential factors that may influence sleep are elusive to identify and/or challenging to measure (e.g., activities at other bedsides). Despite these inconsistent results and the methodo-logic challenges associated with research in this area, patients rate noise, ambient light, and care activities as the highest (most impactful) sleep-disruptive factors in their subjective experience and thus these factors should still be modified whenever possible.

5.2   *ICU Medications*

As outlined in chapter "Effects of Common ICU Medications on Sleep", many commonly used ICU medications have been shown to disrupt sleep, often in a dose-related fashion. When clinically possible, ICU clinicians should consider the effect of drugs on sleep when making prescribing decisions. Studies evaluat-ing the association between different pharmacological agents and sleep disrup-tion have yielded inconsistent results [Fig. 3c], possibly related to the varying measurement tools used to assess sleep quality. The most divergent finding is that opioid analgesics are not sleep disruptive [28, 34, 42, 54] and may in fact be sleep protective [18], although the effect of opiates on sleep quality likely depends on the extent to which pain is contributing to sleep disruption in a particular patient. When patients are asked to rate their sleep quality, they may note reduced insom-nia and sleep latency with opiates and hypnotics, and therefore rank their sleep quality higher than with placebo, whereas if sleep is assessed with polysomnogra-phy, suppression of REM sleep may result in overall worse sleep quality. Studies of fair and good methodological quality have shown that hypnotic and sedative agents [13, 29], particularly benzodiazepines [28, 34], tend to be sleep disrup-tive. Dexmedetomidine, known to increase stage N2 and N3 sleep, was not shown to influence patient-reported sleep quality in one study (even though it reduced incidence of delirium) [8] but was found to be sleep protective by subjective (patient-reported) measures in two studies [55, 56]. The chapter "Best Practices for Improving Sleep in the ICU. Part II: Pharmacologic" highlights medication-based strategies shown to improve sleep in the ICU.

5.3 Ventilatory Support Therapies

Acute respiratory illness is among the most common conditions in the ICU setting and management of critically ill patients often involves invasive and non-invasive ventilation. Figure 3c outlines the results of studies that have evaluated the association between respiratory therapies and sleep disruption in the ICU. Most studies have found no association between sleep disruption and invasive [7, 14, 27, 28, 41, 42] or non-invasive [38] mechanical ventilation. In fact, some studies have reported that ventilatory support may be sleep protective compared with spontaneous breathing [38, 51, 52, 57, 58].

Conversely, several studies have found that the mode of invasive ventilation may affect sleep disruption occurrence. Current evidence suggests pressure-support ventilation [PSV] may be more sleep disruptive than pressure control ventilation (PCV; [59–61]) or proportional assist ventilation (PAV; [62, 63]). In the small number of studies evaluating the effect of respiratory parameters on sleep, patient-ventilator dysynchrony was associated with sleep disruption by increasing fragmentation index [57, 63], with apnea-related arousals and ineffective efforts accounting for 7% and 8% of the total amount of arousals and awakenings (fragmentation index), respectively [49]. The literature evaluating these respiratory parameters remains limited: trials are small and generally have a moderate risk of bias, primarily due to issues related to allocation concealment and absence of blinding (generally unavoidable in studies comparing different modes of mechanical ventilation). Despite potential limitations, these studies often employ continuous measures of respiratory parameters and sleep quality (via PSG) and thereby, provide valuable data on potential temporal associations between patient-ventilatory dysynchrony and sleep quality. The chapter "Mechanical Ventilation and Sleep" provides a comprehensive overview of the impact of mechanical ventilation on sleep in ICU.

6 Special Populations

6.1 Neurological Injury

Special challenges exist when identifying risk factors for disrupted sleep in neurologically injured adults (e.g., head trauma, stroke, subarachnoid or intracranial hemorrhage). First, the need to frequently clinically assess neurological status, sometimes hourly, requires the patient to be woken up from sleep. Second, this population often does not have capacity to self-report on their sleep quality, comfort/pain, sleep habits, preferences, or those factors keeping them from sleep. Third, critically ill neurologic patients often receive short-acting sedatives like propofol, known to disrupt sleep. Fourth, the results of polysomnography and EEG-based sleep assessments are often uninterpretable based on American Academy of Sleep Medicine standard scoring criteria, thus making the objective determination of sleep disrupting risk factors challenging. Finally, the spontaneous or induced hyperventilation that occurs in this population may lead to periodic breathing which has been shown to induce sleep fragmentation in non-neurologic populations.

In the acute phase of neurologic injury, essential patient care activities, including frequent neurological assessments, must take precedence, even at the expense of sleep disruption. However, once the patient has been stabilized, optimizing the environment and consolidating patient care activities to promote undisturbed nocturnal sleep should be considered. Indeed, in a population of subacute post-traumatic coma patients the presence of organized sleep-wake patterns, based on polysomnography assessment, and after other variables affecting sleep were considered, was highly predictive of a good outcome as measured by the Glasgow Outcome Scale (i.e., complete recovery without disability or regaining autonomy despite minor neurological deficits) [64]. However, it remains unclear whether sleep promotion efforts in this population improves outcomes, given that use of sleep improvement bundles have not been well evaluated in neurologic ICUs. Nonetheless, since sleep promotion techniques have been shown to reduce days of delirium, and neurologically injured patients are at high risk of delirium, there is rationale for improving sleep when possible in this high-risk population. For a complete review of sleep promotion techniques, please see chapters "Best Practices for Improving Sleep in the ICU. Part I: Non-pharmacologic" and "Best Practices for Improving Sleep in the ICU. Part II: Pharmacologic".

6.2 Coronavirus Disease 2019

The global pandemic of coronavirus disease 2019 (COVID-19) has presented new challenges and risks for sleep disruption in critically ill patients. Compared to pre-COVID periods, the general population has been shown to have greater sleep disturbances (termed "COVID-somnia" by some sleep neurologists [65]), most commonly related to insomnia, night terrors/disturbing dreams, and the misuse of sleep medications. An online survey of 5641 adults living in China during the peak spread of the coronavirus in February, 2020, reported high rates of clinically significant insomnia (20%), stress (16%) and anxiety (18%); insomnia was found to increase by 25% from late 2019 [66]. This increased insomnia has been attributable to increased Covid-19 infection [67] and greater sleep disturbance during hospitalization, particularly if patients relied on hypnotic use to combat insomnia [68]. Across six observational studies, the incidence of sleep disturbance in hospitalized COVID-19 patients has ranged from 33 to 85%; one study reported 60% of hospitalized COVID-19 patients had been taking sleeping pills in the prior 12 months [68].

For patients admitted to the ICU with COVID-19, the fear, anxiety, foreign surroundings, and isolation experienced by most patients due to visitor restrictions and the mandatory use of personal protective equipment (PPE) by all clinicians may further exacerbate insomnia and loss of circadian rhythm. Although COVID-related reductions in room entry by ICU clinicians could theoretically promote sleep consolidation, many patients find comfort in knowing their nurse is nearby to respond to alarms and help them as needed. Invasively ventilated patients with COVID-19 pneumonia and/or ARDS often have a high respiratory drive, necessitating the administration of large amounts of sedatives to ensure lung protective ventilation. As highlighted in chapter "Effects of Common ICU Medications on Sleep", benzodiazepines and propofol suppress REM sleep and favor Stage 1 and 2 sleep over deep Stage 3 sleep. On the flip side, inadequate mechanical support for the COVID-19 patient having worsening respiratory failure and the high work of breathing that results is also an important risk factor for poor sleep quality. As outlined in chapter "Long-Term Outcomes: Sleep in Survivors of Critical Illness", sleep disturbances continue to plague COVID-19 survivors for weeks to months post hospital discharge, indicating factors other than just the ICU environment affect sleep in this population.

7   Inter-patient Sleep Risk Factor Variability

Tremendous variability exists between individual patients with respect to their risk factors for sleep and circadian rhythm disturbance. Patients with poor sleep at home [7, 28], using sleep medications to aid sleep at home prior to admission, and with higher number of comorbidities [29, 30] are more likely to rate their sleep poor relative to their peers in ICU [11]. Furthermore, there is variability in terms of what patients find comforting and sleep-inducing versus noxious and sleep-disrupting, depending on their sleep habits and personal preferences. For example, some patients are reassured by hearing nearby voices and footsteps, knowing their nurse was close by, while others report overhearing nurses' conversations as disruptive to their sleep [12]. White noise or music may be relaxing to some patients, while others prefer silence, or find some genres of music disruptive [69, 70]. Moreover, risk factors for sleep disruption may change over time in the ICU, as critical illness dissipates, sedatives are reduced, and patients become more aware and acclimatized to their surroundings. Factors they perceived to bother them (and interrupt their sleep) on the first day of ICU admission may be no longer relevant on fifth day of ICU admission. Finally, polysomnography studies may detect, or patients may recall, only the most noxious, proximal factor prompting awakenings from sleep. Removal of this factor (e.g., silencing of an alarm) may lead to the emergence of other factors that then take precedence as being more noticeably sleep disruptive by the patient (e.g., uncomfortable bed or room temperature). One ICU study found that patients ranked an average of 11 different factors (among a list of 33 possible factors) as being sleep-disruptive during their ICU stay [16]. This suggests that a multitude of risk factors disrupt sleep, and that individual patients are likely to differ in the factors they find most intrusive to sleep.

8 Risk Reduction and Sleep Improvement

With the large number of premorbid, ICU-acquired or illness-related factors known to interrupt sleep, and the inter-patient variability and temporal heterogeneity of these factors, it is no wonder that many sleep interventions have had limited impact on improving patient-perceived sleep quality. The myriad risk factors, which may evolve from night to night, and vary between patients, point to the need for sleep promotion interventions to be tailored to individual patient preference and holistic, multi-component bundles (i.e. it is insufficient to provide eye mask and ear plugs to patients but leave the room too hot or too cold, or neglect to address the patient's fears and questions before turning out the lights). Please see chapters "Best Practices for Improving Sleep in the ICU. Part I: Non-pharmacologic" and "Best Practices for Improving Sleep in the ICU. Part II: Pharmacologic" for a detailed review of these approaches. Additionally, there is significant overlap between risk factors for pain, agitation, delirium, and sleeplessness. When modifiable risk factors for sleep disturbance are identified, they should be considered not only for a sleep improvement plan but also as part of the patient's holistic plan to manage pain, agitation, delirium, immobility and sleep disruption (PADIS) according to recently published guidelines [6]. Indeed, despite not improving sleep quality as measured subjectively by validated patient-rated scales, some studies have demonstrated an improvement in delirium-free days by use of a sleep improvement bundle [7] or nocturnal dexmedetomidine [8]. This may reflect deficiencies and/or imprecision of subjective measurement tools more so than inability to improve sleep quality from a brain- and cognition-restorative perspective.

9 Research Opportunities and Future Directions

Research opportunities abound to identify and further understand risk factors for sleep disruption and the mechanisms by which certain factors impede restorative sleep. Table 1 presents several methodological issues pertaining to ICU sleep risk factor studies and offers potential solutions on how they can be addressed. Future research should seek to identify previously undescribed risk factors, establish causality and mechanism between potential risk factors and poor sleep, and evaluate the impact of risk mitigation techniques on improving not only sleep quality/quantity and circadian rhythm but also on potentially related outcomes such as delirium-, ventilator- and ICU-free days. Sleep is intricately complex and our tools to measure it in ICU are dull; thus, research efforts to evaluate risk of sleep disruption and risk reduction techniques will also need to encompass honing of measurement tools, or perhaps redefining "good sleep" and "poor sleep" according to its relevance to patient-important outcomes. Finally, evaluation of risk factors requires adequately

Table 1 Methodological considerations for the design and interpretation of research evaluating risk factors for sleep disruption

Potential source of bias in risk factor studies	Bias description	Potential mitigation strategies in study design
Risk of bias due to study design		
Selection bias	Systematic error due to non-random sampling. Although unavoidable in risk factor studies, this may result in a non-representative sample of patients, leading to a selection effect	Compare an exposed cohort (those with exposure to the potential risk factor) and unexposed individuals
Confounding bias	Unevaluated variables that influence both the potential risk factor and the outcome variable may lead to spurious associations between the risk factor and sleep outcomes	Stratification (reporting of findings stratified by patient subgroups) will reduce the impact of confounding by patient subtype (e.g., stratified reporting for medical versus surgical ICU patients, older vs. younger patients, etc.)
		Report multivariable analysis to control for potential confounders in larger datasets
Recall bias (for patient-reported studies)	A non-random misclassification bias that may arise in patient-reported studies	Attempt to evaluate risk factors using objective measures whenever possible (e.g., sound levels) If feasible, consider administering self-reported sleep assessments as close to ICU stay as possible
Risk of bias related to interpretation		
Incorrect causal inference	Inaccurate conclusions about a causal association between a risk factor and sleep outcomes based on the presence of a statistical association	Avoid drawing conclusions about efficacy of interventions from studies designed to identify potential risk factors Evaluate the efficacy of risk factor reduction/mitigation strategies in randomized trials; avoid use of observational data to draw conclusions about efficacy of interventions
Weak associations	A small or weak statistical association between a risk factor and sleep metric does not indicate lack of causality but is a consequence of the background rate of the outcome in the population	Evaluate risk factors in a broad range of patients; avoid limiting the sample to those with more sleep-disruption in order to magnify the association and reduce risk of confounding

powered and rigorously designed studies which consider the time-dependency of sleep risk factors in the ICU, the inherent intra- and inter-patient variability, and covariates of risk depending on patient intrinsic, and/or non-modifiable risk factors. Although such research is extremely challenging, given the prevalence and significance of sleep disruption in the ICU, it behooves us to understand the factors contributing to sleep disruption and mitigate risk with personalized interventions tailored to our patients. Indeed, understanding risk factors and improving sleep in ICU may have dramatic impact on our patients' ICU experience, and potentially influence ICU and post-ICU outcomes.

References

1. Cooper AB, Thornley KS, Young GB, Slutsky AS, Stewart TE, Hanly PJ. Sleep in critically ill patients requiring mechanical ventilation. Chest. 2000;117(3):809–18.
2. Simini B. Patients' perceptions of intensive care. Lancet. 1999;354(9178):571–2.
3. Zhang L, Sha YS, Kong QQ, Woo JA, Miller AR, Li HW, et al. Factors that affect sleep quality: perceptions made by patients in the intensive care unit after thoracic surgery. Support Care Cancer. 2013;21(8):2091–6.
4. Drouot X, Quentin S. Sleep neurobiology and critical care illness. Sleep Med Clin. 2016;11(1):105–13.
5. Pulak LM, Jensen L. Sleep in the intensive care unit: a review. J Intensive Care Med. 2016;31(1):14–23.
6. Devlin JW, Skrobik Y, Gelinas C, Needham DM, Slooter AJC, Pandharipande PP, et al. Clinical practice guidelines for the prevention and management of pain, agitation/sedation, delirium, immobility, and sleep disruption in adult patients in the ICU. Crit Care Med. 2018;46(9):e825–e73.
7. Kamdar BB, King LM, Collop NA, Sakamuri S, Colantuoni E, Neufeld KJ, et al. The effect of a quality improvement intervention on perceived sleep quality and cognition in a medical ICU. Crit Care Med. 2013;41(3):800–9.
8. Skrobik Y, Duprey MS, Hill NS, Devlin JW. Low-dose nocturnal dexmedetomidine prevents ICU delirium. A randomized, placebo-controlled trial. Am J Respir Crit Care Med. 2018;197(9):1147–56.
9. Freedman NS, Gazendam J, Levan L, Pack AI, Schwab RJ. Abnormal sleep/wake cycles and the effect of environmental noise on sleep disruption in the intensive care unit. Am J Respir Crit Care Med. 2001;163(2):451–7.
10. World Health Organization. Environmental health: Estimations of attributable burden of disease due to a risk factor 2018. Available from: https://www.who.int/news-room/q-a-detail/environmental-health-estimations-of-attributable-burden-of-disease-due-to-a-risk-factor
11. Honarmand K, Rafay H, Le J, Mohan S, Rochwerg B, Devlin JW, et al. A systematic review of risk factors for sleep disruption in critically ill adults. Crit Care Med. 2020;48(7):1066–74.
12. Ehlers VJ, Watson H, Moleki MM. Factors contributing to sleep deprivation in a multidisciplinary intensive care unit in South Africa. Curationis. 2013;36(1):E1–8.
13. Frisk U, Nordstrom G. Patients' sleep in an intensive care unit—patients' and nurses' perception. Intensive Crit Care Nurs. 2003;19(6):342–9.
14. Little A, Ethier C, Ayas N, Thanachayanont T, Jiang D, Mehta S. A patient survey of sleep quality in the intensive care unit. Minerva Anestesiol. 2012;78(4):406–14.
15. Nicolas A, Aizpitarte E, Iruarrizaga A, Vazquez M, Margall A, Asiain C. Perception of nighttime sleep by surgical patients in an intensive care unit. Nurs Crit Care. 2008;13(1):25–33.
16. Simpson T, Lee ER, Cameron C. Patients' perceptions of environmental factors that disturb sleep after cardiac surgery. Am J Crit Care. 1996;5(3):173–81.
17. Storti LJ, Servantes DM, Borges M, Bittencourt L, Maroja FU, Poyares D, et al. Validation of a novel sleep-quality questionnaire to assess sleep in the coronary care unit: a polysomnography study. Sleep Med. 2015;16(8):971–5.
18. Hofhuis JG, Spronk PE, van Stel HF, Schrijvers AJ, Rommes JH, Bakker J. Experiences of critically ill patients in the ICU. Intensive Crit Care Nurs. 2008;24(5):300–13.

19. Ugras GA, Oztekin SD. Patient perception of environmental and nursing factors contributing to sleep disturbances in a neurosurgical intensive care unit. Tohoku J Exp Med. 2007;212(3):299–308.
20. Jones C, Dawson D. Eye masks and earplugs improve patient's perception of sleep. Nurs Crit Care. 2012;17(5):247–54.
21. Karaman Özlü Z, Özer N. The effect of enhancing environmental factors on the quality of patients' sleep in a cardiac surgical intensive care unit. Biol Rhythm Res. 2017;48(1):85–98.
22. Longley L, Simons T, Glanzer L, Du C, Trinks H, Letzkus L, et al. Evaluating sleep in a surgical trauma burn intensive care unit: an elusive dilemma. Dimens Crit Care Nurs. 2018;37(2):97–101.
23. Stewart JA, Green C, Stewart J, Tiruvoipati R. Factors influencing quality of sleep among non-mechanically ventilated patients in the intensive care unit. Aust Crit Care. 2017;30(2):85–90.
24. Dave K, Qureshi A, Lakshmanan G. Effects of earplugs and eye masks on perceived quality of sleep during night among patients in intensive care units. Asian J Nurs Educ Res. 2015;5:319.
25. Ugras GA, Babayigit S, Tosun K, Aksoy G, Turan Y. The effect of nocturnal patient care interventions on patient sleep and satisfaction with nursing care in neurosurgery intensive care unit. J Neurosci Nurs. 2015;47(2):104–12.
26. Yinnon AM, Ilan Y, Tadmor B, Altarescu G, Hershko C. Quality of sleep in the medical department. Br J Clin Pract. 1992;46(2):88–91.
27. Freedman NS, Kotzer N, Schwab RJ. Patient perception of sleep quality and etiology of sleep disruption in the intensive care unit. Am J Respir Crit Care Med. 1999;159(4 Pt 1):1155–62.
28. Bihari S, Doug McEvoy R, Matheson E, Kim S, Woodman RJ, Bersten AD. Factors affecting sleep quality of patients in intensive care unit. J Clin Sleep Med. 2012;8(3):301–7.
29. Chen CJ, Hsu LN, McHugh G, Campbell M, Tzeng YL. Predictors of sleep quality and successful weaning from mechanical ventilation among patients in respiratory care centers. J Nurs Res. 2015;23(1):65–74.
30. Diaz-Abad M, Verceles AC, Brown JE, Scharf SM. Sleep-disordered breathing may be under-recognized in patients who wean from prolonged mechanical ventilation. Respir Care. 2012;57(2):229–37.
31. Kamdar BB, Niessen T, Colantuoni E, King LM, Neufeld KJ, Bienvenu OJ, et al. Delirium transitions in the medical ICU: exploring the role of sleep quality and other factors. Crit Care Med. 2015;43(1):135–41.
32. Cicek H, Armutcu B, Dizer B, Yava A, Tosun N, editors. Sleep quality of patients hospitalized in the coron ary intensive care unit and the affecting factors; 2014.
33. Scotto CJ, McClusky C, Spillan S, Kimmel J. Earplugs improve patients' subjective experience of sleep in critical care. Nurs Crit Care. 2009;14(4):180–4.
34. Trompeo AC, Vidi Y, Locane MD, Braghiroli A, Mascia L, Bosma K, et al. Sleep disturbances in the critically ill patients: role of delirium and sedative agents. Minerva Anestesiol. 2011;77(6):604–12.
35. Drouot X, Roche-Campo F, Thille AW, Cabello B, Galia F, Margarit L, et al. A new classification for sleep analysis in critically ill patients. Sleep Med. 2012;13(1):7–14.
36. Hardin KA, Seyal M, Stewart T, Bonekat HW. Sleep in critically ill chemically paralyzed patients requiring mechanical ventilation. Chest. 2006;129(6):1468–77.
37. Litton E, Elliott R, Thompson K, Watts N, Seppelt I, Webb SAR, et al. Using clinically accessible tools to measure sound levels and sleep disruption in the ICU: a prospective multicenter observational study. Crit Care Med. 2017;45(6):966–71.
38. Roche Campo F, Drouot X, Thille AW, Galia F, Cabello B, d'Ortho MP, et al. Poor sleep quality is associated with late noninvasive ventilation failure in patients with acute hypercapnic respiratory failure. Crit Care Med. 2010;38(2):477–85.
39. Ersoy EO, Ocal S, Kara A, Ardic S, Topeli A. Sleep in mechanically ventilated patients in the intensive care unit. J Turk Sleep Med. 2016;3:10–3.
40. Chen JH, Chao YH, Lu SF, Shiung TF, Chao YF. The effectiveness of valerian acupressure on the sleep of ICU patients: a randomized clinical trial. Int J Nurs Stud. 2012;49(8):913–20.

41. Fanfulla F, Ceriana P. D'Artavilla Lupo N, Trentin R, Frigerio F, Nava S. Sleep disturbances in patients admitted to a step-down unit after ICU discharge: the role of mechanical ventilation. Sleep. 2011;34(3):355–62.
42. Friese RS, Diaz-Arrastia R, McBride D, Frankel H, Gentilello LM. Quantity and quality of sleep in the surgical intensive care unit: are our patients sleeping? J Trauma. 2007;63(6):1210–4.
43. Redeker NS, Mason DJ, Wykpisz E, Glica B. Sleep patterns in women after coronary artery bypass surgery. Appl Nurs Res. 1996;9(3):115–22.
44. Redeker NS, Wykpisz E. Gender differences in sleep and activity-rest after coronary bypass. Sleep. 1998:21–211.
45. Cheraghi M, Hazaryan M, Bahramnezhad F, Mirzaeipour F, Haghani H. Study of the relationship between sleep quality and prevalence of delirium in patients undergoing cardiac surgery. Int J Med Res Health Sci. 2016;5:38–43.
46. Zaal IJ, Slooter AJ. Delirium in critically ill patients: epidemiology, pathophysiology, diagnosis and management. Drugs. 2012;72(11):1457–71.
47. Pandharipande P, Ely EW. Sedative and analgesic medications: risk factors for delirium and sleep disturbances in the critically ill. Crit Care Clin. 2006;22(2):313–27, vii.
48. Lat I, McMillian W, Taylor S, Janzen JM, Papadopoulos S, Korth L, et al. The impact of delirium on clinical outcomes in mechanically ventilated surgical and trauma patients. Crit Care Med. 2009;37(6):1898–905.
49. Cabello B, Thille AW, Drouot X, Galia F, Mancebo J, d'Ortho MP, et al. Sleep quality in mechanically ventilated patients: comparison of three ventilatory modes. Crit Care Med. 2008;36(6):1749–55.
50. Elbaz M, Leger D, Sauvet F, Champigneulle B, Rio S, Strauss M, et al. Sound level intensity severely disrupts sleep in ventilated ICU patients throughout a 24-h period: a preliminary 24-h study of sleep stages and associated sound levels. Ann Intensive Care. 2017;7(1):25.
51. Elliott R, McKinley S, Cistulli P, Fien M. Characterisation of sleep in intensive care using 24-hour polysomnography: an observational study. Crit Care. 2013;17(2):R46.
52. Elliott R, Rai T, McKinley S. Factors affecting sleep in the critically ill: an observational study. J Crit Care. 2014;29(5):859–63.
53. Casida JM, Davis JE, Shpakoff L, Yarandi H. An exploratory study of the patients' sleep patterns and inflammatory response following cardiopulmonary bypass (CPB). J Clin Nurs. 2014;23(15–16):2332–42.
54. Navarro-Garcia MA, de Carlos AV, Martinez-Oroz A, Irigoyen-Aristorena MI, Elizondo-Sotro A, Indurain-Fernandez S, et al. Quality of sleep in patients undergoing cardiac surgery during the postoperative period in intensive care. Enferm Intensiva. 2017;28(3):114–24.
55. Lu W, Fu Q, Luo X, Fu S, Hu K. Effects of dexmedetomidine on sleep quality of patients after surgery without mechanical ventilation in ICU. Medicine (Baltimore). 2017;96(23):e7081.
56. Wu XH, Cui F, Zhang C, Meng ZT, Wang DX, Ma J, et al. Low-dose Dexmedetomidine improves sleep quality pattern in elderly patients after noncardiac surgery in the intensive care unit: a pilot randomized controlled trial. Anesthesiology. 2016;125(5):979–91.
57. Cordoba-Izquierdo A, Drouot X, Thille AW, Galia F, Roche-Campo F, Schortgen F, et al. Sleep in hypercapnic critical care patients under noninvasive ventilation: conventional versus dedicated ventilators. Crit Care Med. 2013;41(1):60–8.
58. Drouot X, Bridoux A, Thille AW, Roche-Campo F, Cordoba-Izquierdo A, Katsahian S, et al. Sleep continuity: a new metric to quantify disrupted hypnograms in non-sedated intensive care unit patients. Crit Care. 2014;18(6):628.
59. Andrejak C, Monconduit J, Rose D, Toublanc B, Mayeux I, Rodenstein D, et al. Does using pressure-controlled ventilation to rest respiratory muscles improve sleep in ICU patients? Respir Med. 2013;107(4):534–41.
60. Parthasarathy S, Tobin MJ. Effect of ventilator mode on sleep quality in critically ill patients. Am J Respir Crit Care Med. 2002;166(11):1423–9.

61. Toublanc B, Rose D, Glerant JC, Francois G, Mayeux I, Rodenstein D, et al. Assist-control ventilation vs. low levels of pressure support ventilation on sleep quality in intubated ICU patients. Intensive Care Med. 2007;33(7):1148–54.
62. Alexopoulou C, Kondili E, Vakouti E, Klimathianaki M, Prinianakis G, Georgopoulos D. Sleep during proportional-assist ventilation with load-adjustable gain factors in critically ill patients. Intensive Care Med. 2007;33(7):1139–47.
63. Bosma K, Ferreyra G, Ambrogio C, Pasero D, Mirabella L, Braghiroli A, et al. Patient-ventilator interaction and sleep in mechanically ventilated patients: pressure support versus proportional assist ventilation. Crit Care Med. 2007;35(4):1048–54.
64. Valente M, Placidi F, Oliveira AJ, Bigagli A, Morghen I, Proietti R, et al. Sleep organization pattern as a prognostic marker at the subacute stage of post-traumatic coma. Clin Neurophysiol. 2002;113(11):1798–805.
65. Hurley D. Sleep neurologists call it 'COVID-Somnia'—increased sleep disturbances linked to the pandemic. Neurol Today. 2020;20(13):1–31.
66. Lin LY, Wang J, Ou-Yang XY, Miao Q, Chen R, Liang FX, et al. The immediate impact of the 2019 novel coronavirus (COVID-19) outbreak on subjective sleep status. Sleep Med. 2021;77:348–54.
67. Meira ECM, Miyazawa M, Gozal D. Putative contributions of circadian clock and sleep in the context of SARS-CoV-2 infection. Eur Respir J. 2020;4;55(6):2001023.
68. Beck F, Leger D, Fressard L, Peretti-Watel P, Verger P, Coconel G. Covid-19 health crisis and lockdown associated with high level of sleep complaints and hypnotic uptake at the population level. J Sleep Res. 2021;30(1):e13119.
69. Farokhnezhad Afshar P, Bahramnezhad F, Asgari P, Shiri M. Effect of white noise on sleep in patients admitted to a coronary care. J Caring Sci. 2016;5(2):103–9.
70. Kim J, Choi D, Yeo MS, Yoo GE, Kim SJ, Na S. Effects of patient-directed interactive music therapy on sleep quality in postoperative elderly patients: a randomized-controlled trial. Nat Sci Sleep. 2020;12:791–800.

Effects of Common ICU Medications on Sleep

Patricia R. Louzon and Mojdeh S. Heavner

1 Introduction

Critically ill patients are usually prescribed many different medications during their ICU stay. Commonly administered medications can impact sleep through many distinct mechanisms. The purpose of this chapter is to review common pathways by which ICU medications can impact sleep, including administration-related sleep disruption, unintended physiologic effects, complication of underlying comorbid conditions, and withdrawal states.

As highlighted in chapter "Risk Factors for Disrupted Sleep in the ICU," medications are just one of the many factors known to disrupt sleep in the ICU. For example, medication administration during nighttime hours can induce care-related sleep disruption. Pharmacotherapy used in critical illness can also have unintended but important effects on sleep physiology, which includes direct effects on the central nervous system pathways that modulate sleep. As described in chapter "Normal Sleep Compared to Altered Consciousness During Sedation," the altered level of consciousness related to sedative agent administration differs both physiologically and clinically from normal, restful sleep. However, the sedative agents used to induce sedation in the ICU can have direct and distinct effects on stage 1 (N1), stage 2 (N2), stage 3 (N3)/slow wave sleep (SWS), and rapid eye movement (REM) sleep architecture when evaluated using electroencephalogram (EEG) approaches. Medications will also directly affect important parameters of sleep quality including

P. R. Louzon
Department of Pharmacy, AdventHealth Orlando, Orlando, FL, USA
e-mail: patricia.louzon@adventhealth.com

M. S. Heavner (✉)
Department of Pharmacy Practice and Science, School of Pharmacy, University of Maryland, Baltimore, MD, USA
e-mail: mheavner@rx.umaryland.edu

G. L. Weinhouse, J. W. Devlin (eds.), *Sleep in Critical Illness*,
https://doi.org/10.1007/978-3-031-06447-0_7

sleep efficiency (SE), sleep latency (SL), total sleep time (TST), and wakefulness (W).

Drugs associated with increased delirium can also deleteriously impact sleep quality; these mechanisms are described in depth in chapters "Sleep Disruption and Its Relationship with Delirium: Electroencephalographic Perspectives" and "Sleep Disruption and Its Relationship with Delirium: Clinical Perspectives." Common ICU medications can exacerbate underlying sleep disordered breathing (SDB) such as obstructive sleep apnea (OSA), periodic movement disorders (PMD), and parasomnias, all of which are known to impair sleep quality and quantity. Lastly, withdrawal states triggered by the abrupt cessation of chronic home therapies that have effects in the central nervous system (e.g., antidepressants, anxiolytics, stimulants) and drugs of abuse (e.g., alcohol, marijuana, and nicotine) can also complicate sleep in the ICU. The effects of commonly used medications in the ICU on sleep will be discussed in detail throughout the chapter, including strategies to reduce medication-associated sleep disruption in the ICU, current evidence gaps and opportunities for future research.

2 Medication Administration and Monitoring-Related Sleep Disruption

Medications may disrupt sleep beyond the effects of their known pharmacologic properties. Intermittent medication administration during the overnight hours may result in iatrogenic awakenings, particularly for medications with shorter half-lives that require every 4 to 6 h administration and drugs administered through the oral/enteral (vs. intravenous) route. The collection of serum drug concentrations for therapeutic drug monitoring (e.g., vancomycin) at night may also awaken patients. Consideration should be given to the timing of these medications to avoid overnight interruptions whenever possible. The administration times of medications scheduled every 8, 12 or 24 h should be revised to avoid administration between 10 pm and 5 am when possible. For example, a q8h medication scheduled for 6 pm, 2 am, and 10 am administration could be revised to 2 pm, 10 pm and 6 am. If this medication was vancomycin, serum trough concentrations could be drawn before any dose on this schedule without awakening the patient. Strategies to proactively optimize medication administration timing to promote sleep opportunity include standardization of order sets, intervention during the pharmacist order verification process, and protocols that permit retiming of medications by nurses and pharmacists after original order entry. Assessment and standardization of medication timing should be considered in sleep improvement bundles [1–3].

Table 1 Common ICU central nervous system medications known to effect sleep

Medication/Medication Class	Sleep Abnormalities							
	REM	SWS	SL	SE	TST	W	OSA	PMD
Gabaminergics								
Benzodiazepines	↓	↓	↓		↑	↓	↑	
Propofol	↓	↔	↓	↔	↔	↓		
Alpha-2 agonists								
Dexmedetomidine		↑	↓	↑	↑			
Clonidine	↑↓[a]	↑	↔	↔	↔			
Ketamine	↑↓[b]				↑↔[b]	↓↔[b]		
Antidepressants								
SSRIs/SNRIs	↓	↓		↓	↓	↑	↓	↑
Tricyclic—sedating	↓		↓	↑	↑	↓		
Tricyclic—non-sedating	↓		↑	↓				
Trazodone		↑	↓		↑	↓		
Mirtazapine	↑	↑	↓					
Antipsychotics								
Typical			↓	↑		↓		
Atypical		↑	↓	↑	↑	↓	↑	
Antihistamines						↓		
Anticonvulsants								
Gabapentin	↑	↑			↑	↓		
Phenobarbital	↓		↓		↑	↓	↑	
Phenytoin		↑	↓					
Opioids	↓↔[c]	↓			↓	↑↔[c]	↑	

[a]potential dose-related effects; [b]potential indication-related effects; [c]effect observed during initiation phase of methadone but not during maintenance

PMD = periodic movement disorders; REM = rapid eye movement; SE = sleep efficiency; SL = sleep latency; SSRI = selective serotonin reuptake inhibitor; SWS = slow wave sleep; TST = total sleep time; W = wakefulness

3 Medications that Physiologically Impact Sleep

Medications commonly utilized in the ICU and shown to physiologically impact sleep are discussed in detail by class. Table 1 summarizes current data on the effects of central nervous system (CNS) agents on sleep architecture and Table 2 summarizes sleep impact from other medication types and drug withdrawal. Figure 1 summarizes the pharmacodynamic mechanisms and pharmacokinetic properties that are involved in medication-related changes to sleep and the interplay of critical illness-related factors with these changes [4, 5]. These concepts are also discussed throughout as they pertain to specific drugs and drug classes.

Table 2 Sleep architecture impact of non-central nervous system medications and medication withdrawal

Medication/Medication Class	Sleep Abnormalities							
	REM	SWS	SL	SE	TST	W	OSA	PMD
Cardiovascular								
Beta-blockers	↓[a]		↑			↑		
Calcium-channel blockers				↓	↓			
Statins[a]			↓		↓			
Vasopressors Dopamine Epinephrine Norepinephrine	↓	↓						
Endocrine								
Corticosteroids[b] Dexamethasone Prednisone	↓	↑	↑	↓	↓	↑		
Estrogen/progestin							↓	
Testosterone						↑	↑	
Thyroid hormone							↓	
Pulmonary								
β-agonists					↑	↓		
Ipratropium	↑							
Nasal steroids							↓	
Theophylline[b,c]	↓		↓		↓	↑	↓	
Substance withdrawal								
Ethanol[d]	↓	↓			↓		↑	↑
Marijuana[c]	↑	↓	↑	↓	↓			
Nicotine			↑		↓			
Stimulants	↑			↓	↓	↑		↑

[a]impacted by lipid solubility of agent; [b]potential dose-related effects; [c]differs with acute versus chronic use; [d]differs between first and second half of night with consumption and withdrawal
PMD = periodic movement disorders; REM = rapid eye movement; SE = sleep efficiency; SL = sleep latency; SWS = slow wave sleep; TST = total sleep time; W = wakefulness

3.1 Central Nervous System Agents

Any medication that acts in the central nervous system (CNS) can impact sleep. However, the exact mechanisms for many of these effects are still not fully understood, given current gaps in our understanding of sleep physiology, the complex and dose-related pharmacologic response to many of these medications, the frequent administration of concomitant CNS-active drugs in the ICU, and the implications of critical illness disease-related effects on the brain in critical illness.

Although the clinical value of using CNS agents to improve sleep in the ICU will be discussed in chapter "Best Practices for Improving Sleep in the ICU. Part II: Pharmacologic", the potential implications of these agents on sleep physiology are important given that these drugs are commonly used for other indications in the ICU.

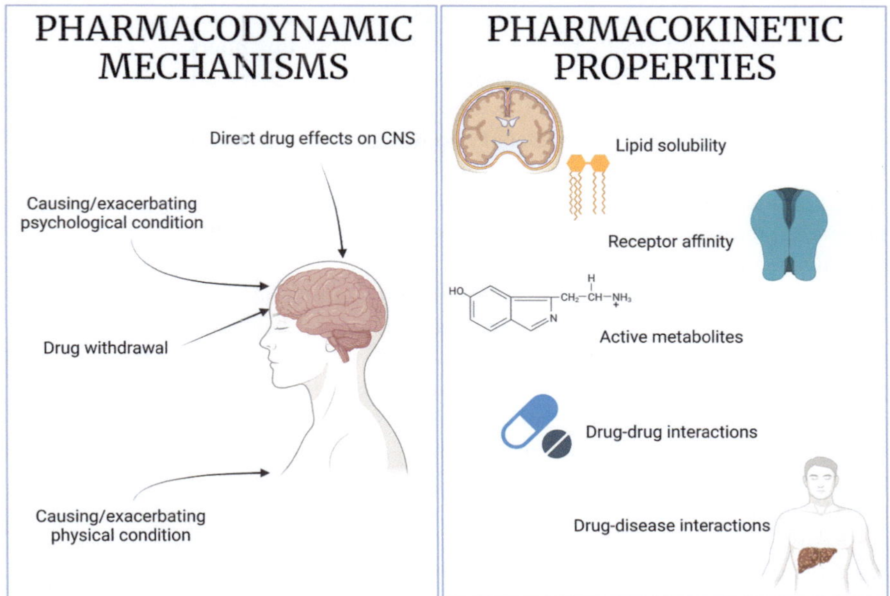

Fig. 1 Pharmacodynamic mechanisms and pharmacokinetic properties of commonly used drugs on sleep in the intensive care unit. Pharmacodynamic mechanisms affect the way by which medications affect sleep and include direct effects within the central nervous system, indirect effects causing or exacerbating a psychological or physical condition known to affect sleep pathway or inducing drug or substance withdrawal from the cessation of the agent after intensive care unit admission. Pharmacokinetic properties of drugs impacting the effects of medications on sleep include lipid solubility and the ability of the drug to enter the central nervous system to cause direct pharmacodynamic effects on sleep, affinity for receptors involved in sleep pathways (e.g., adrenergic, cholinergic, dopaminergic, noradrenergic, and serotonergic), interactions with other drugs prescribed in the ICU or from prior to admission, and interactions between drugs administered and either underlying comorbid disease states or changes related to critical illness. CNS = central nervous system

3.1.1 Gabaminergics

While benzodiazepines are not recommended as a first-line sedative in mechanically ventilation adults, they are still utilized in the ICU, especially for the management of alcohol withdrawal syndrome, seizures, procedural sedation, and to avoid withdrawal in chronic benzodiazepine users [6]. Patients requiring deep sedation (e.g., during neuromuscular blockade therapy) and not able to tolerate propofol may also be prescribed benzodiazepines. In general, benzodiazepine exposure increases TST, decreases wakefulness, increases stage N1 and N2 sleep and decreases stage N3 and REM sleep [7]. The data to support these effects in ICU patients are generally low quality but there are robust data across many studies evaluating the effects of sleep quality in healthy volunteers [8]. A practical consideration with benzodiazepines is that daytime (vs. nighttime) administration may cause daytime somnolence and disrupt circadian rhythms. Depending on the indication for use, daily benzodiaz-epine therapy should ideally be administered in the evening hours.

SDB may occur with benzodiazepine use in patients with obstructive sleep apnea (OSA) without an artificial airway, as benzodiazepines may aggravate upper airway obstruction and increase sleep-related hypoventilation. Patients with severe under-lying OSA, impaired respiratory function, chronic neuromuscular diseases, and the elderly are at the greatest risk for benzodiazepine-associated SDB. By increasing the arousal threshold, benzodiazepines may have a beneficial effect in patients with central sleep apneas [9].

Propofol is a gabaminergic sedative that is recommended for use in mechani-cally ventilated adults requiring continuous sedation. It is not recommended by clinical practice guidelines to improve sleep in the ICU [6]. The effects of pro-pofol and benzodiazepines on sleep would be expected to be similar given their shared gabaminergic mechanism of action. However, a systematic review and meta-analysis of four randomized controlled trials comparing the effects of pro-pofol to placebo on sleep in 149 critically ill adults reported that propofol does not affect TST, time spent in stage N1, N2, or N3 sleep, or SE. REM sleep was markedly diminished [10]. A trial comparing sleep architecture between criti-cally ill and normal sleeping, healthy adults found the administration of light sedation with either propofol or dexmedetomidine produced sleep that was close to normal in most patients. Propofol and dexmedetomidine produced sim-ilar effects on sleep, which is surprising given prior evidence suggesting the contrary [11].

3.1.2 Alpha-2 Agonists

Dexmedetomidine is an alpha-2-adrenoceptor agonist that is utilized in critically ill adults who require continuous sedation [6]. While dexmedetomidine has been preferred by many clinicians over propofol to better maintain light sedation and reduce delirium, a controlled trial found that time spent at light sedation and days without delirium or coma were similar between the dexmedetomidine and propofol groups [12]. Dexmedetomidine has been studied in the ICU for its potential sleep-promoting effects (see chapter "Best Practices for Improving Sleep in the ICU. Part II: Pharmacologic") [13–18]. Since dexmedetomidine is frequently used in the ICU for sedation, and not explicitly for sleep, its physiologic effects on sleep are impor-tant to consider when developing plans for sedation in the ICU. Dexmedetomidine produces a sleep-like state (phase N2 sleep) of sedation that can be readily reversed with external stimuli and does not cause respiratory depression [19–21]. The admin-istration of nighttime dexmedetomidine in non-intubated ICU patients is associated with increased state N2 (and possibly stage N3) sleep, longer TST, better SE, fewer arousals, and less stage N1 sleep [14]. Of note, whether dexmedetomidine improves patient-reported sleep quality is unclear, with only one study showing an improve-ment and at least two others reporting no change [13, 15, 22].

Clonidine, also an alpha-2-adrenoceptor agonist, does not penetrate the CNS as well as dexmedetomidine and thus has less potent sedative effects. It is more often used as an antihypertensive. When administered intravenously (not available in the USA), clonidine can effectively treat acute agitation, particularly in patients with delirium. The effects of clonidine on sleep in ICU patients have not been well-studied. When clonidine was administered as a 225 mcg dose to healthy adults, TST, SE, or SL remained unchanged, time in stage N3 sleep increased and time spent with REM sleep decreased [23]. These findings on REM sleep were confirmed in a study using a 100 mcg clonidine dose [24]. Notably, administration of clonidine at a very low dose (25 mcg) has been shown to increase REM sleep, suggesting the effects of clonidine on REM sleep may be dose-related [25]. An important consideration for alpha-2-agonists, like the gabaminergic sedatives, is the timing of medication administration and how that relates to timing of normal sleep. Daytime administration of clonidine, for example, and the potential implications of daytime sleepiness on circadian rhythmicity may be considerable and is worthy of future study.

3.1.3 Ketamine

Ketamine works primarily via N-methyl-D-aspartate receptor antagonist activity to produce sedative, hypnotic, analgesic, and amnestic properties. It may also directly influence CLOCK-BMAL1 complex function, leading to dose-related alterations in circadian gene expression [26]. Ketamine administration in rats has been shown to inhibit post-anesthetic W that is accompanied by increased stage N1/N2/N3 sleep on the first-post-anesthetic day at nighttime but no change in REM sleep [27]. The use of ketamine for treatment-resistant depression is associated with increased TST, stage N3, and REM sleep, although depression itself is also associated with disrupted sleep [28, 29]. This interplay between depression and sleep is further discussed in the next section. Pediatric burn patients receiving ketamine for procedural sedation were found to have reductions in REM sleep but no change in awakenings, W, or TST [30].

3.1.4 Antidepressants

Depression is common in critically ill adults and is associated with reduced REM latency, increased REM sleep, decreased stage N3 sleep, and increased awakenings [31]. Antidepressants may both be continued from home therapy and initiated in the ICU. Agents such as trazodone or mirtazapine are sometimes initiated to improve sleep and are discussed in more detail in chapter "Best Practices for Improving Sleep in the ICU. Part II: Pharmacologic". Trazodone increases TST and stage N3 sleep and decreases awakenings and SL. Whether it affects REM sleep remains unclear. Mirtazapine has been shown to increase both N3 and REM sleep and decrease awakenings and SL. Both drugs may cause significant daytime somnolence and therefore should be administered in the evening [32]. Sedating tricyclic antidepressants (e.g., amitriptyline) decrease SL, and increase SE; less sedating secondary amine tricyclics (e.g., desipramine, nortriptyline) have been shown to have the opposite sleep architecture effects [32]. Selective serotonin reuptake inhibitors (e.g., fluoxetine, citalopram) and selective norepinephrine reuptake inhibitors (e.g., venlafaxine, duloxetine) can be both activating and sedating. They can suppress REM, increase REM latency, and decrease SWS [31, 32]. Antidepressants decrease the risk for SDB by decreasing REM-associated apneas. Antidepressants also increase upper airway patency and act as a central respiratory stimulant [33].

3.1.5 Antipsychotics

In the ICU setting, antipsychotics may be continued for the chronic management of major psychiatric disorders and also acutely initiated for the treatment of agitation in patients with delirium [6]. Each antipsychotic has unique neurotransmitter effects; as a class they antagonize dopamine to varying degrees. Unwanted movement effects (e.g., haloperidol-associated extrapyramidal symptoms) may impact sleep quality. Typical antipsychotics (e.g., haloperidol) increase TST, SE, and REM latency, decrease stage N2 sleep but do not affect stage N3 sleep. The effects of atypical antipsychotics (e.g., olanzapine, quetiapine) on sleep architecture vary. Quetiapine is commonly associated with somnolence related to its strong antihistamine activity. When studied for insomnia, it improves both subjective (Pittsburgh Sleep Quality Index) and objective sleep quality measures (e.g., increased TST and SE; decreased SL) [31]. Olanzapine increases TST, SE, and SL, and N2 stage sleep and decreases N1 stage; its effect on N3 stage sleep remain unclear [31, 34]. Research regarding the effects of antipsychotics on sleep in the ICU is challenging as most patients have disrupted sleep because of an underlying psychiatric disorder (including delirium) before antipsychotic initiation. Sleep architecture changes with antipsychotics in healthy subjects are distinct from those with schizophrenia. As an example, REM sleep is generally not changed with atypical antipsychotics in healthy volunteers, but olanzapine and paliperidone have been shown to increase REM sleep, and quetiapine to decrease REM sleep in patients with schizophrenia [35].

Antipsychotics may exacerbate SDB (specifically OSA). Patients who are male, obese, and use antipsychotics chronically are at the greatest risk for experiencing these effects [33]. The cause for this independent risk is unclear, especially since the effects of these drugs on REM sleep are conflicting.

3.1.6 Antihistamines

Antihistamines are used in the ICU for a variety of indications and frequently self-administered by patients at home to initiate sleep. Histamine generally has an excitatory effect on target neurons but may also assist in the release of the inhibitory neurotransmitter gamma-aminobutyric acid (GABA). Histamine activity is vital at specific circadian phases; reducing neuronal histamine activity can produce sleep. Acute blockade of the H_1-receptor increases non-REM sleep. The relationship between histamine activity and circadian rhythms is implicated in worsening symptoms of asthma and allergic rhinitis at night. Neurons regulating histaminergic signaling are increased in the brains of patients with narcolepsy type 1 [36]. First-generation antihistamines (e.g., diphenhydramine) by being more lipophilic than second-generation antihistamines (e.g., cetirizine) have greater CNS penetration and are associated with larger sedating effects [36]. Antihistamine activity at the H_2-receptor is a target for gastric ulcer prophylaxis in the ICU. CNS-related adverse effects (e.g., agitation, delirium, confusion, and disturbing dreams) that may interrupt sleep are reported with H_2-receptor agonist (e.g., famotidine) use, particularly in older adults and patients with reduced renal clearance [37].

3.1.7 Anticonvulsants

Anticonvulsants are also commonly required in the ICU setting for new onset seizure management or prophylaxis. Sleep is often disrupted in patients with nocturnally predominant seizures; anticonvulsant therapy may positively impact sleep quality. Dose-related somnolence is common with the daytime initiation of the more sedating anticonvulsants (e.g., carbamazepine, phenytoin) and will disrupt circadian rhythm [38]. However, as therapy continues, these sedating effects, and their effect on sleep, will dissipate [7]. Barbiturates (e.g., phenobarbital), used in the ICU to treat seizures and acute agitation related to alcohol withdrawal and delirium are associated with reduced REM sleep and SL and increased REM latency and N2 stage sleep. Gabapentin is an anticonvulsant more recently used for management of alcohol withdrawal and neuropathic pain. It has not been shown to worsen sleep architecture, while increasing REM sleep and decreasing awakenings [7, 38].

3.1.8 Opioids

Opioids are mu-receptor agonists, and are a mainstay for pain management, sedation and ventilator optimization in the ICU [6]. Mu-receptor agonism is associated with REM sleep suppression [39]. The key opioid peptides (enkephalins, endorphins, and dynorphins) have a vital role in sleep onset and maintenance and influence the effect of vasopressin in circadian pacemaker activity and rhythms [39]. Although opioid-related activation of wake-promoting systems and inhibition of sleep-promoting systems in the brain have been observed, studies in healthy volunteers have reported conflicting data [40, 41]. Morphine and methadone have both been reported to increase stage N2 sleep and decrease stage N3 sleep. It is possible that duration of opioid therapy (i.e., acute vs. chronic therapy) or whether the opioid has been stopped and withdrawal is occurring, may affect sleep architecture differently [39]. For example, patients taking chronic methadone report poor sleep quality, reduced REM and N3, and increased W during the initiation phase. The N3 and REM effects tend to normalize during maintenance therapy [41].

Another important sleep-related concern with opioids is the ability to induce respiratory pauses, delays in expiration or prolonged expiratory time, irregular/periodic breathing and changes in tidal volume, and exacerbation of underlying SDB. [39] Patients at greatest risk for opioid-associated SDB include those with moderate-severe OSA, comorbid obesity, chronic lung diseases (e.g., COPD), and neuromuscular diseases [9].

3.2 Cardiovascular Agents

Changes in blood pressure and heart rate are a normal part of sleep-wake architecture, changing between each sleep stage. During non-REM sleep, parasympathetic tone predominates, leading to a decrease in heart rate, cardiac output, and a 5–15% decrease in systemic blood pressure. During REM sleep, fluctuations in sympathetic and parasympathetic tone cause greater variability in blood pressure with changes as much as 40 mm Hg [42].

Additionally, common underlying cardiac conditions (e.g., heart failure) increase the risk for SDB [42]. Any cardiovascular agent having the ability to alter a hemodynamic parameter(s) has the potential to disrupt sleep in the ICU by changing normal sleep associated fluctuations.

Beta-blockers
Beta-blockers have been shown to decrease REM sleep, induce nightmares and increase W [4, 43–45]. Those agents with the greatest lipid-solubility (and thus CNS penetration) (e.g., propranolol, labetalol, metoprolol) are most associated with sleep effects [4, 43]. Compared to placebo, metoprolol has been shown to increase awakenings and lead to greater wakefulness. [43, 46] ICU caregivers should be aware of these potential side effects and use a less lipophilic agent (e.g., atenolol) if their patients complain of disturbed sleep.

Statins
Statins, which are associated with potential anti-inflammatory effects, are often continued, or initiated in the ICU. Continuation of home statins is associated with reduced ICU delirium, an important risk factor for disrupted sleep [47]. Statin use has also specifically been associated with insomnia and impaired sleep initiation and maintenance, [48, 49] though statin-associated sleep effects may be dependent on the lipophilicity (and thus CNS penetration) of individual agents and the resulting neuroinflammatory effect that ensues. For example, use of simvastatin (high lipophilicity) is associated with decreased TST and increased awakenings, whereas pravastatin (low lipophilicity) has not been shown to affect sleep [50–52]. For a patient with potential statin-induced insomnia, a switch to pravastatin may be warranted.

Other

Limited evidence exists to suggest other cardiovascular medications commonly administered in the ICU have sleep effects. In the outpatient setting, calcium-channel blockers have been shown to decrease TST and lower SE in patients with OSA [53]. Diuretics and angiotensin converting enzyme inhibitors have not been shown to affect sleep. Amiodarone use is associated with insomnia and nightmares in up to 3% of outpatients [54, 55]. Vasopressors utilized to treat hypotension in the ICU have effects on alpha-1 (epinephrine, norepinephrine) or both alpha-1 and dopamine receptors (dopamine), as well as modulating melatonin secretion (norepinephrine) that help mediate the arousal state and result in insomnia and decreases in REM and SWS [45, 56, 57]. Animal studies demonstrate dopamine transmission helps control W and SWS and norepinephrine REM sleep regulation [58]. The clinical importance of any clinical effect adrenergic vasopressors may have on sleep remains unclear.

3.3   Endocrine

Steroids

Despite systemic steroid therapy being frequently utilized in the ICU to treat septic shock and acute inflammatory pulmonary disorders, the effects of steroids on sleep in critically ill adults has not been well researched. High-dose steroid therapy increases delirium, an important risk factor for sleep [59]. In chronic steroid users, patient reports of insomnia are common and are greater with higher daily doses [49, 60]. In outpatients, steroids increase REM latency, W, and the percent of time spent in SWS. These effects may be due to the effects of steroids on suprachiasmatic nucleus resulting in altered circadian rhythm and neuroinhibitory pathway alterations resulting in hyperarousal [49, 60, 61]. Most data is with dexamethasone, which decreases melatonin levels and augments tryptophan uptake [62, 63]. Healthy subjects on dexamethasone 3 mg every 8 h (compared to placebo) had increased W, longer REM SL, reduced number of REM periods, and decreased SE [61]. Limiting steroid duration and utilizing the lowest effective dose may help to mitigate steroid-related sleep disturbances in the ICU.

Hormonal Therapy

Hormonal therapy has been shown to impact sleep primarily through its effects on SDB [64]. OSA is less prevalent in females than males due to the SDB-lowering effects of estrogen and progestin [65]. In comparison, testosterone replacement, especially when administered at high doses, worsens OSA [66, 67]. As OSA is associated with hypothyroidism, it is possible that treatment with thyroid hormones such as levothyroxine may improve OSA, though study results vary from showing apnea improvement to no impact on sleep architecture with supraphysiologic doses of levothyroxine [33, 68].

3.4 Pulmonary

Patients with lung diseases (e.g., COPD, asthma) often have poor sleep; chronic dyspnea worsens sleep and contributes to OSA [69, 70]. When hypoxemia is treated with oxygen, increases in SE and all stages of sleep, including REM, increase [71, 72]. Medications used to treat lung disease may also affect sleep although it is difficult to distinguish the effects of medication use on sleep from those of the underlying disease-state, improvements of disease state symptoms that improve ability to sleep, or impact of individual agents since many are frequently utilized in combination.

Bronchodilators
Beta-agonist-related CNS stimulation may worsen sleep [70]. Salmeterol has been shown to improve objective sleep quality, time in deep sleep, and decrease W, [73] although at least one study has not shown any sleep architecture changes [69]. Clinical impact of beta-agonists on sleep may be related to symptom improvement that decreases sleep disruption. Ipratropium, an inhaled anticholinergic, improves perceived sleep quality (by visual analogue scale) and increases REM sleep in patients with COPD [74].

Other
Limited evidence suggests other pulmonary medications impact sleep architecture or SDB. Nasal steroids such as fluticasone and budesonide may decrease OSA by decreasing upper airway obstruction during sleep [33, 75, 76]. Theophylline is a central stimulating bronchodilator that is still occasionally used in asthma and COPD. Adenosine receptor antagonism increases alertness [77]. While reduced REM sleep and TST, increased awakenings, delayed SL, and improvements in OSA has been reported in some outpatient theophylline studies [33, 78–80], a lack of sleep effects have been reported in others [69, 81, 82]. Differences in study findings may depend on acute versus chronic use, underlying disease state, and the formulation and dose used. Acetazolamide is administered for altitude sickness due to inhibition of CO_2 to carbonic anhydrase. The resulting metabolic acidosis can help to stimulate respiration and has been shown to benefit OSA at regular and high altitudes [83–85].

3.5 Withdrawal from Chronic Therapies and Substances

When an ICU admission precludes use of a home medication that may positively affect sleep (e.g., inabilty to swallow a tablet), sleep may worsen. For example, when a medication that suppresses REM sleep (e.g., benzodiazepines, opioids, corticosteroids, illicit substances) is withdrawn, increased REM sleep, nightmares, and potential worsening of SDB such as OSA may be observed [4]. Acuity of illness or hospital formularies may lead ICU clinicians to stop chronic home medications known to improve sleep parameters, which can lead to both direct sleep impact and rebound effect. Medication reconciliation at the time of ICU admission is an important strategy to be able to predict potential withdrawal symptoms and rationalize the continuation of chronic home medications, including those focused on improving sleep. Introduction of agents such as opioids or benzodiazepine infusions in the ICU that are quickly withdrawn may also precipitate withdrawal symptoms that impact sleep during the later portion of an ICU stay.

Alcohol

Alcohol results in decreased SL and REM in the first half of the night, which may lead to a misconception of improved sleep, though increased REM sleep and nightmares in second half of night as alcohol is metabolized lead to overall poor sleep quality [86–88]. Alcohol use disorder (AUD) is a common cause of chronic insomnia. There are positive correlations between AUD scores and subjective association of sleep quality, duration, and disturbances [89, 90]. Alcohol ingestion may induce SDB even in those without pre-existing sleep apnea or worsen SDB in those with diagnosed SDB [33, 91]. Alcohol has been shown to increase periodic movement disorders (PMD) on a three-fold basis in women who consume two or more alcoholic drinks a day [92]. Alcohol withdrawal in the ICU is the most likely presentation of alcohol-related sleep disturbance, leading to decreased SWS and increased REM sleep and nightmares [93]. The impact of alcohol withdrawal on PMD is not known. Among AUD treatment medications, one systematic review demonstrated that naltrexone may negatively impact sleep by increasing insomnia, whereas acamprosate may be beneficial to improve sleep continuity. Both drugs decrease REM sleep [90].

Marijuana

Improved sleep may be a goal with marijuana use. While acute or intermittent use is associated with shorter SL and a longer sleep duration, chronic use is associated with poor sleep, including reduced REM sleep [94–96]. A study of withdrawal of marijuana in users with a history of heavy use demonstrated prolonged SL, worse SE, lower TST and less SWS, which may last as long as 45 days [97, 98]. These symptoms of poor sleep should be expected to occur in the ICU setting during marijuana withdrawal, especially in patients with a history of chronic use. Use of other formulations of cannabinoids such as cannabidiol (CBD) is increasing in the outpatient setting as a sleep aide, as early studies suggest potential efficacy to improve anxiety and increase TST in higher doses [98]. Impact of withdrawal is not known, but chronic use of CBD as a sleep aid could trigger healthcare professional awareness to expect potential sleep disturbances in the ICU resulting from discontinuation of a usual sleep aid.

Stimulants

Stimulants such as caffeine, nicotine, illicit drugs or medications for attention deficit hyperactivity disorder are rarely continued during hospitalization. While cocaine and 3,4-methylenedioxymethamphetamine (MDMA/ "Ecstasy") increase W, suppress REM sleep, decrease TST and SE, withdrawal can have an even more pronounced impact on sleep where REM rebound, decreased TST and nightmares are common [95]. The nightmares and delusions that occur during withdrawal may be confused with delirium.

Stimulant withdrawal has not been shown to impact SDB, though they may have long term improvements on SDB should their use lead to weight loss [33]. Nicotine replacement products may help mitigate withdrawal symptoms in appropriate patients. ICU patients and their families should be asked about use of stimulants prior to ICU admission to aid in recognizing potential impact on sleep and other symptoms of withdrawal.

4 Conclusions and Future Directions

Medications commonly used in the ICU can impact sleep through a variety of overlapping mechanisms including medication administration-related disruption, unintended physiologic effects, complication of underlying comorbid conditions or SDB, and withdrawal states. The complex interplay of these mechanisms and confounding by indication for the medications being prescribed are challenges to identifying direct impact of medications on sleep in this environment. Although commonly used ICU medications may have a rational physiologic basis to impact sleep, clinical data are often conflicting and generally sparse. This leads to limited knowledge of direct patient impact of medications used during ICU care on sleep. There are many practical challenges to measuring and reporting sleep characteristics in the ICU, including time and training difficulties with polysomnography measurements that provide the most detailed information on sleep architecture. As awareness of ICU sleep disturbances increase, and sleep improvement bundles are encouraged, [6] impact of medications on sleep should be considered as part of an overall medication evaluation strategy.

References

1. Andrews JL, Louzon PR, Torres X, et al. Impact of a pharmacist-led intensive care unit sleep improvement protocol on sleep duration and quality. Ann Pharmacother. 2021;55(7):863–9. https://doi.org/10.1177/1060028020973198.
2. Patel J, Baldwin J, Bunting P, Laha S. The effect of a multicomponent multidisciplinary bundle of interventions on sleep and delirium in medical and surgical intensive care patients. Anaesthesia. 2014;69(6):540–9. https://doi.org/10.1111/anae.12638.
3. Louzon PR, Heavner MS, Herod K, Wu T, Devlin JW. Sleep-promotion bundle development, implementation, and evaluation in critically ill adults: Roles for pharmacists. Ann Pharmacother. 2022;56(7):839–49. https://doi.org/10.1177/10600280211048494.
4. Novak M, Shapiro CM. Drug-induced sleep disturbances: focus on nonpsychotropic medications. Drug Saf. 1997;16(2):133–49. https://doi.org/10.2165/00002018-199716020-00005.
5. Boucher BA, Wood GC, Swanson JM. Pharmacokinetic changes in critical illness. Crit Care Clin. 2006;22(2):255–71., vi. https://doi.org/10.1016/j.ccc.2006.02.011.
6. Devlin JW, Skrobik Y, Gélinas C, Needham DM, Slooter AJC, Pandharipande PP, et al. Clinical practice guidelines for the prevention and management of pain, agitation/seda-

tion, delirium, immobility, and sleep disruption in adult patients in the ICU. Crit Care Med. 2018;46(9):e825–73. https://doi.org/10.1097/CCM.0000000000003299.

7. Geurkink EA, Sheth RD, Gidal BE, Hermann BP. Effects of anticonvulsant medication on EEG sleep architecture. Epilepsy Behav. 2000;1(6):378–83. https://doi.org/10.1006/ebeh.2000.0125.

8. de Mendonça FMR, de Mendonça GPRR, Souza LC, Galvão LP, Paiva HS, de Azevedo Marques Périco C, Torales J, Ventriglio A, Maurício Castaldelli-Maia J, Silva ASM. Benzodiazepines and sleep architecture: a systematic review. CNS Neurol Disord Drug Targets. 2021;17. https://doi.org/10.2174/1871527320666210618103344

9. Grote L. Drug-induced sleep-disordered breathing and ventilatory impairment. Sleep Med Clin. 2018;13(2):161–8. https://doi.org/10.1016/j.jsmc.2018.03.003.

10. Lewis SR, Schofield-Robinson OJ, Alderson P, Smith AF. Propofol for the promotion of sleep in adults in the intensive care unit. Cochrane Database Syst Rev. 2018;1(1):CD012454. https://doi.org/10.1002/14651858.CD012454.pub2.

11. Georgopoulos D, Kondili E, Alexopoulou C, Younes M. Effects of sedatives on sleep architecture measured with odds ratio product in critically ill patients. Crit Care Explor. 2021;3(8):e0503. https://doi.org/10.1097/CCE.0000000000000503.

12. Hughes CG, Mailloux PT, Devlin JW, Swan JT, Sanders RD, Anzueto A, Jackson JC, Hoskins AS, Pun BT, Orun OM, Raman R, Stollings JL, Kiehl AL, Duprey MS, Bui LN, O'Neal HR Jr, Snyder A, Gropper MA, Guntupalli KK, Stashenko GJ, Patel MB, Brummel NE, Girard TD, Dittus RS, Bernard GR, Ely EW, Pandharipande PP; MENDS2 Study Investigators. Dexmedetomidine or Propofol for Sedation in Mechanically Ventilated Adults with Sepsis. N Engl J Med. 2021;384(15):1424–36. https://doi.org/10.1056/NEJMoa2024922.

13. Skrobik Y, Duprey MS, Hill NS, Devlin JW. Low-dose nocturnal dexmedetomidine prevents ICU delirium. A randomized, placebo-controlled trial. Am J Respir Crit Care Med. 2018;197(9):1147–56. https://doi.org/10.1164/rccm.201710-1995OC.

14. Romagnoli S, Villa G, Fontanarosa L, Tofani L, Pinelli F, De Gaudio AR, Ricci Z. Sleep duration and architecture in non-intubated intensive care unit patients: an observational study. Sleep Med. 2020;70:79–87. https://doi.org/10.1016/j.sleep.2019.11.1265.

15. Wu XH, Cui F, Zhang C, Meng ZT, Wang DX, Ma J, Wang GF, Zhu SN, Ma D. Low-dose dexmedetomidine improves sleep quality pattern in elderly patients after noncardiac surgery in the intensive care unit: a pilot randomized controlled trial. Anesthesiology. 2016;125(5):979–91. https://doi.org/10.1097/ALN.0000000000001325.

16. Alexopoulou C, Kondili E, Diamantaki E, Psarologakis C, Kokkini S, Bolaki M, Georgopoulos D. Effects of dexmedetomidine on sleep quality in critically ill patients: a pilot study. Anesthesiology. 2014;121(4):801–7. https://doi.org/10.1097/ALN.0000000000000361.

17. Oto J, Yamamoto K, Koike S, Onodera M, Imanaka H, Nishimura M. Sleep quality of mechanically ventilated patients sedated with dexmedetomidine. Intensive Care Med. 2012;38(12):1982–9. https://doi.org/10.1007/s00134-012-2685-y.

18. Lu W, Fu Q, Luo X, Fu S, Hu K. Effects of dexmedetomidine on sleep quality of patients after surgery without mechanical ventilation in ICU. Medicine (Baltimore). 2017;96(23):e7081. https://doi.org/10.1097/MD.0000000000007081.

19. Huupponen E, Maksimow A, Lapinlampi P, Särkelä M, Saastamoinen A, Snapir A, Scheinin H, Scheinin M, Meriläinen P, Himanen SL, Jääskeläinen S. Electroencephalogram spindle activity during dexmedetomidine sedation and physiological sleep. Acta Anaesthesiol Scand. 2008;52(2):289–94. https://doi.org/10.1111/j.1399-6576.2007.01537.x.

20. Guldenmund P, Vanhaudenhuyse A, Sanders RD, Sleigh J, Bruno MA, Demertzi A, Bahri MA, Jaquet O, Sanfilippo J, Baquero K, Boly M, Brichant JF, Laureys S, Bonhomme V. Brain functional connectivity differentiates dexmedetomidine from propofol and natural sleep. Br J Anaesth. 2017;119(4):674–84. https://doi.org/10.1093/bja/aex257.

21. Hsu YW, Cortinez LI, Robertson KM, Keifer JC, Sum-Ping ST, Moretti EW, Young CC, Wright DR, Macleod DB, Somma J. Dexmedetomidine pharmacodynamics: part I: crossover comparison of the respiratory effects of dexmedetomidine and remifentanil in healthy volunteers. Anesthesiology. 2004;101(5):1066–76. https://doi.org/10.1097/00000542-200411000-00005.

22. Corbett SM, Rebuck JA, Greene CM, Callas PW, Neale BW, Healey MA, Leavitt BJ. Dexmedetomidine does not improve patient satisfaction when compared with propofol during mechanical ventilation. Crit Care Med. 2005;33(5):940–5. https://doi.org/10.1097/01. ccm.0000162565.18193.e5.

23. Kanno O, Clarenbach P. Effect of clonidine and yohimbine on sleep in man: polygraphic study and EEG analysis by normalized slope descriptors. Electroencephalogr Clin Neurophysiol. 1985;60(6):478–84. https://doi.org/10.1016/0013-4694(85)91107-1.

24. Gentili A, Godschalk MF, Gheorghiu D, Nelson K, Julius DA, Mulligan T. Effect of clonidine and yohimbine on sleep in healthy men: a double-blind, randomized, controlled trial. Eur J Clin Pharmacol. 1996;50(6):463–5. https://doi.org/10.1007/s002280050141.

25. Miyazaki S, Uchida S, Mukai J, Nishihara K. Clonidine effects on all-night human sleep: opposite action of low- and medium-dose clonidine on human NREM-REM sleep proportion. Psychiatry Clin Neurosci. 2004;58(2):138–44. https://doi.org/10.1111/j.1440-1819.2003.01207.x.

26. Bellet MM, Vawter MP, Bunney BG, Bunney WE, Sassone-Corsi P. Ketamine influences CLOCK:BMAL1 function leading to altered circadian gene expression. PLoS One. 2011;6(8):e23982. https://doi.org/10.1371/journal.pone.0023982.

27. Kushikata T, Sawada M, Niwa H, Kudo T, Kudo M, Tonosaki M, Hirota K. Ketamine and propofol have opposite effects on postanesthetic sleep architecture in rats: relevance to the endogenous sleep-wakefulness substances orexin and melanin-concentrating hormone. J Anesth. 2016;30(3):437–43. https://doi.org/10.1007/s00540-016-2161-x.

28. Duncan WC Jr, Zarate CA Jr. Ketamine, sleep, and depression: current status and new questions. Curr Psychiatry Rep. 2013;15(9):394. https://doi.org/10.1007/s11920-013-0394-z.

29. Kohtala S, Alitalo O, Rosenholm M, Rozov S, Rantamäki T. Time is of the essence: coupling sleep-wake and circadian neurobiology to the antidepressant effects of ketamine. Pharmacol Ther. 2021;221:107741. https://doi.org/10.1016/j.pharmthera.2020.107741.

30. Gottschlich MM, Mayes T, Khoury J, McCall J, Simakajornboon N, Kagan RJ. The effect of ketamine administration on nocturnal sleep architecture. J Burn Care Res. 2011;32(5):535–40. https://doi.org/10.1097/BCR.0b013e31822ac7d1.

31. Doghramji K, Jangro WC. Adverse effects of psychotropic medications on sleep. Sleep Med Clin. 2016;11(4):503–14. https://doi.org/10.1016/j.jsmc.2016.08.001.

32. Riemann D, Krone LB, Wulff K, Nissen C. Sleep, insomnia, and depression. Neuropsychopharmacology. 2020;45(1):74–89. https://doi.org/10.1038/s41386-019-0411-y. Epub 2019 May 9

33. Seda G, Tsai S, Lee-Chiong T, et al. Medication effects on sleep and breathing. Clin Chest Med. 2014;35:557–69. https://doi.org/10.1016/j.ccm.2014.06.011.

34. Lazowski LK, Townsend B, Hawken ER, Jokic R, du Toit R, Milev R. Sleep architecture and cognitive changes in olanzapine-treated patients with depression: a double blind randomized placebo controlled trial. BMC Psychiatry. 2014;14:202. https://doi.org/10.1186/1471-244X-14-202.

35. Monti JM, Torterolo P, Pandi Perumal SR. The effects of second generation antipsychotic drugs on sleep variables in healthy subjects and patients with schizophrenia. Sleep Med Rev. 2017;33:51–7. https://doi.org/10.1016/j.smrv.2016.05.002.

36. Scammell TE, Jackson AC, Franks NP, Wisden W, Dauvilliers Y. Histamine: neural circuits and new medications. Sleep. 2019;42(1):zsy183. https://doi.org/10.1093/sleep/zsy183.

37. Werbel T, Cohen PR. Ranitidine-associated sleep disturbance: case report and review of H2 antihistamine-related central nervous system adverse effects. Cureus. 2018;10(4):e2414. https://doi.org/10.7759/cureus.2414.

38. Moore JL, Carvalho DZ, St Louis EK, Bazil C. Sleep and epilepsy: a focused review of pathophysiology, clinical syndromes, co-morbidities, and therapy. Neurotherapeutics. 2021;18(1):170–80. https://doi.org/10.1007/s13311-021-01021-w.

39. Wang D, Teichtahl H. Opioids, sleep architecture and sleep-disordered breathing. Sleep Med Rev. 2007;11(1):35–46. https://doi.org/10.1016/j.smrv.2006.03.006.

40. Eacret D, Veasey SC, Blendy JA. Bidirectional relationship between opioids and disrupted sleep: putative mechanisms. Mol Pharmacol. 2020;98(4):445–53. https://doi.org/10.1124/mol.119.119107.

41. Cutrufello NJ, Ianus VD, Rowley JA. Opioids and sleep. Curr Opin Pulm Med. 2020;26(6):634–41. https://doi.org/10.1097/MCP.0000000000000733.
42. Mehra R. Sleep apnea and the heart. Cleve Clin J Med. 2019;86(9 Suppl 1):10–8. https://doi.org/10.3949/ccjm.86.s1.03.
43. McAnish J, Cruickshank JM. Beta-blockers and central nervous system side effects. Pharmacol Ther. 1990;46:163–97. https://doi.org/10.1016/0163-7258(90)90092-g.
44. Betts TA, Alford C. Beta-blockers and sleep: a controlled trial. Eur J Clin Pharmacol. 1985;28:65–8. https://doi.org/10.1007/BF00543712.
45. Bourne RS, Mills GH. Sleep disruption in critically ill patients-pharmacological considerations. Anaesthesia. 2004;59:374–84. https://doi.org/10.1111/j.1365-2044.2004.03664.x.
46. Kostis JB, Raymond RC. Central nervous system effects of Beta-adrenergic-blocking drugs: the role of ancillary properties. Circulation. 1987;75(1):204–12. https://doi.org/10.1161/01.cir.75.1.204.
47. Page VJ, Davis D, Zhao XB, et al. Statin use and risk of delirium in the critically ill. Am J Respir Crit Care Med. 2014;189(6):666–73. https://doi.org/10.1164/rccm.201306-1150CC.
48. Takada M, Fujimoto M, Yamazaki K, Takamoto M, Hosomi K. Association of statin use with sleep disturbances: data mining of a spontaneous reporting database and a prescription database. Drug Saf. 2014;37:421–61. https://doi.org/10.1007/s40264-014-0163-x.
49. Szmyd B, Rogut M, Bialasiewicz, Gabryelska A. The impact of glucocorticoids and statins on sleep quality. Sleep Med Rev. 2021;55:101380. https://doi.org/10.1016/j.smrv.2020.101380.
50. Schaefer EJ. HMG-CoA reductase inhibitors for hypercholesterolemia. N Engl J Med. 1988;319:1222–3. https://doi.org/10.1056/NEJM198811033191811.
51. Barth JD, Kruisbrink OAE, Van Dijk AL. Inhibitors of hydroxymethylglutaryl coenzyme a reductase for treating hypercholesterolemia. Br Med J. 1990;301:669. https://doi.org/10.1136/bmj.301.6753.669-a.
52. Vgontzas AN, Kales A, Bixler ER, Manfredi RL, Tyson KL. Effects of lovastatin and pravastatin on sleep efficiency and sleep stages. Clin Pharmacol Ther. 1991;50:730–7. https://doi.org/10.1038/clpt.1991.213.
53. Nerbass FB, Pedrosa RP, Genta PR, Drager LF, Lorenzi-Filho G. Calcium channel blockers are independently associated with short sleep duration in hypertensive patients with obstructive sleep apnea. J Hypertens. 2011;29:1236–41. https://doi.org/10.1097/HJH.0b013e3283462e8b.
54. Amiodarone hydrochloride [package insert]. Philadelphia, Pennsylvania: Wyeth pharmaceuticals; 2004.
55. Hilleman D, Miller MA, Parker R, Doering P, Pieper JA. Optimal management of amiodarone therapy: efficacy and side effects. Pharmacotherapy. 1998;18(6 Pt 2):138S–45S.
56. Olendorf WH. Brain uptake of radiolabeled amino acids, amines, and hexoses after arterial injection. Am J Phys. 1971;221:1629–39. https://doi.org/10.1152/ajplegacy.1971.221.6.1629.
57. Mitchell HA, Weinshenker D. Good night and good luck: norepinephrine in sleep pharmacology. Biochem Pharmacol. 2010;79(6):801–9. https://doi.org/10.1016/j.bcp.2009.10.004.
58. Nishino S, Mao J, Sampathkumaran R, Shelton J. Increased dopaminergic transmission mediates the wake-promoting effects of CNS stimulants. Sleep Res Online. 1998;1(1):49–61.
59. Cole JL. Steroid-induced sleep disturbance and delirium: a focused review for critically ill patients. Fed Pract. 2020;37(6):260–7.
60. Curtis J, Westfall A, Allison J, et al. Population-based assessment of adverse effects associated with long-term glucocorticoid use. Arthritis Rheum. 2006;55(3):420–6. https://doi.org/10.1002/art.21984.
61. Moser NJ, Phillips BA, Guthrie G, Barnett G. Effects of dexamethasone on sleep. Pharmcol Toxicol. 1996;79:100–2. https://doi.org/10.1111/j.1600-0773.1996.tb00249.x.
62. Demish L, Demish K, Neckelsen T. Influence of dexamethasone on nocturnal melatonin production in healthy adult subjects. J Pineal Res. 1988;5(3):317–21. https://doi.org/10.1111/j.1600-079x.1988.tb00657.x.
63. McEwen BS, Davis PG, Parsons B, Pfaff DW. The brain as a target for steroid hormone secretion. Ann Rev Neurosci. 1979;2:65–112. https://doi.org/10.1146/annurev.ne.02.030179.000433.

64. Young T, Palta M, Dempsey J, et al. The occurrence of sleep-disordered breathing among middle-aged adults. N Engl J Med. 1993;328(17):1230–5. https://doi.org/10.1056/NEJM199304293281704.
65. Shahar E, Redline S, Young T, et al. Hormone replacement therapy and sleep disordered breathing. Am J Respir Crit Cre Med. 2003;167(9):1186–92. https://doi.org/10.1164/rccm.200210-1238OC.
66. Hanafy HM. Testosterone therapy and obstructive sleep apnea: is there a real connection? J Sex Med. 2007;4(5):1241–6. https://doi.org/10.1111/j.1743-6109.2007.00553.x.
67. Cistulli PA, Grunstein RR, Sullivan CE. Effect of testosterone administration on upper airway collapsibility during sleep. Am J Respir Crit Care Med. 1994;149(2 Pt 1):530–2. https://doi.org/10.1164/ajrccm.149.2.8306057.
68. Kraemer S, Danker-Hopfe H, Pilhatsch M, et al. Effects of supraphysiological doses of levothyroxine on sleep in healthy subjects: a prospective polysomnography study. J Thyroid Res. 2011;2011:420580. https://doi.org/10.4061/2011/420580.
69. Man GW, Chapman KR, Habib A, Darke A. Sleep quality and nocturnal respiratory function with once-daily theophylline and inhaled salbutamol in patients with COPD. Chest. 1996;110:648–53. https://doi.org/10.1378/chest.110.3.648.
70. Janson C, Gislason T, Bowman G, Hetta J, Roos BE. Sleep disturbances in patients with asthma. Respir Med. 1990;84:37–42. https://doi.org/10.1016/s0954-6111(08)80092-3.
71. Kearley R, Wynne JW, et al. The effect of low-flow oxygen on sleep-disordered breathing and oxygen desaturation: a study of patients with chronic obstructive lung disease. Chest. 1980;78:682–5. https://doi.org/10.1378/chest.78.5.682.
72. Calverley PMA, Brezinova V, Douglas NJ, et al. The effect of oxygenation on sleep quality in chronic bronchitis and emphysema. Am Rev Respir Dis. 1982;126:206–10. https://doi.org/10.1164/arrd.1982.126.2.206.
73. Fitzpatrick MF, Mackay T, Driver H, et al. Salmeterol in nocturnal asthma: a double-blind, placebo controlled trial of a long acting inhaled beta-2 agonist. BMJ. 1990;301:1365–8. https://doi.org/10.1136/bmj.301.6765.1365.
74. Martin RM, Bucher Bartelson BL, Smith P, et al. Effect of ipratropium bromide treatment on oxygen saturation and sleep quality in COPD. Chest. 1999;115:1338–45. https://doi.org/10.1378/chest.115.5.1338.
75. Kiely JL, Nolan P, McNichols WT. Intranasal corticosteroid therapy for obstructive sleep apnoea in patients with co-existing rhinitis. Thorax. 2004;59(1):50–5.
76. Kheirandish-Gozal L, Gozal D. Intranasal budesonide treatment for children with mild obstructive sleep apnea syndrome. Pediatrics. 2008;122(1):e149–55. https://doi.org/10.1542/peds.2007-3398.
77. Roux FJ, Kryger MH. Medication effects on sleep. Clin Chest Med. 2010;31(2):397–405. https://doi.org/10.1016/j.ccm.2010.02.008.
78. Roehrs T, Merlotti L, Halpin D, et al. Effects of theophylline on nocturnal sleep and daytime sleepiness/alertness. Chest. 1995;108(2):382–7. https://doi.org/10.1378/chest.108.2.382.
79. Fleetham JA, Fera T, Edgell G, et al. The effect of theophylline therapy on sleep disorders in COPD patients. Am Rev Respir Dis. 1983;127(suppl):A85. https://doi.org/10.1164/arrd.1983.127.1.125.
80. Mulloy E, McNicholas WT. Theophylline improves gas exchange during rest, exercise and sleep in severe chronic obstructive pulmonary disease. Am Rev Respir Dis. 1993;148:1030–6. https://doi.org/10.1164/ajrccm/148.4_Pt_1.1030.
81. Berry RB, Desa MM, Branum JP, et al. Effect of theophylline on sleep and sleep disordered breathing in patients with chronic obstructive pulmonary disease. Am Rev Respir Dis. 1991;143:245–50. https://doi.org/10.1164/ajrccm/143.2.245.
82. Fitzpatrick MF, Engleman HM, Boellert F, et al. Effect of therapeutic theophylline levels on sleep quality and daytime cognitive performance of normal subjects. Am Rev Respir Dis. 1992;145:540–4. https://doi.org/10.1164/ajrccm/145.6.1355.
83. DeBacker WA, Vorbraecken J, Willemen M, et al. Central apnea index decreases after prolonged treatment with acetazolamide. Am J Respir Crit Care Med. 1995;151:87–91. https://doi.org/10.1164/ajrccm.151.1.7812578.

84. Nussbaumer-Ochsner Y, Latshang TF, Ulrich S, et al. Patients with obstructive sleep apnea syndrome benefit from acetazolamide during an altitude sojourn: a randomized, placebo-controlled, double blind trial. Chest. 2012;141(1):131–8. https://doi.org/10.1378/chest.11-0375.
85. Latshang TD, Nussbaumer-Ochsner Y, Henn RM, et al. Effect of acetazolamide and sutoCPAP therapy on breathing disturbances among patients with obstructive sleep apnea syndrome who travel to altitude: a randomized controlled trial. JAMA. 2012;308(22):2390–8. https://doi.org/10.1001/jama.2012.94847.
86. Yules RB, Lippman ME, Freedman DX. Alcohol administration prior to sleep: the effect of EEG sleep stages. Arch Gen Phychiatry. 1967;16:94–7. https://doi.org/10.1001/archpsyc.1967.01730190096012.
87. Lobo LL, Tufik S. Effects of alcohol on sleep parameters of sleep-deprived healthy volunteers. Sleep. 1997;20:52–9. https://doi.org/10.1093/sleep/20.1.52.
88. Madsen BW, Rossi L. Sleep and Michael-Menten elimination of ethanol. Clin Pharmaol Therap. 1980;27:114–9. https://doi.org/10.1038/clpt.1980.17.
89. Park S, Oh M, Lee B, et al. The effects of alcohol on quality of sleep. Korean J Fam Med. 2015;36:294–9. https://doi.org/10.4082/kjfm.2015.36.6.294.
90. Panin F, Peana AT. Sleep and the pharmacotherapy of alcohol use disorder: unfortunate bed-fellows. A systematic review with meta-analysis. Front Pharmacol. 2019;10:1164. https://doi.org/10.3389/fphar.2019.01164.
91. Taasan VC, Block AJ, Boysen PG, et al. Alcohol increases sleep apnea and oxygen desaturation in asymptomatic men. Am J Med. 1981;71(2):240–5. https://doi.org/10.1016/0002-9343(81)90124-8.
92. Aldrich MS, Shipley JE. Alcohol use and periodic limb movements of sleep. Alcohol Clin Exp Res. 1993;17:192–6. https://doi.org/10.1111/j.1530-0277.1993.tb00747.x.
93. Koob GF, Colrain IM. Alcohol use disorder and sleep disturbances: a feed-forward allostatic framework. Neuropsychopharmacology. 2020;45:141–65. https://doi.org/10.1038/s41386-019-0446-0.
94. Winiger EA, Hitchcock LN, Bryan AD, Bidwell LC. Cannabis use and sleep: expectations, outcomes and the role of age. Addict Behav. 2021;112:106642. https://doi.org/10.1016/j.addbeh.2020.106642.
95. Schierenbeck T, Riemann D, Berger M, Hornyak M. Effect of illicit recreational drugs upon sleep: cocaine, ecstasy and marijuana. Sleep Med Rev. 2008;12:381–9. https://doi.org/10.1016/j.smrv.2007.12.004.
96. Conroy DA, Kurth ME, Strong DR, Brower KJ, Stein MD. Marijuana use patterns and sleep among community-based young adults. J Addict Dis. 2015;35(2):135–43. https://doi.org/10.1080/10550887.2015.1132986.
97. Bolia KL, Lesage SR, Gamaldo CE, et al. Sleep disturbance in heavy marijuana users. Sleep. 2008;31(6):901–8. https://doi.org/10.1093/sleep/31.6.901.
98. Babson KA, Sottile J, Morabito D. Cannabis, cannabinoids, and sleep: a review of the literature. Curr Psychiatry Rep. 2017;19(4):23. https://doi.org/10.1007/s11920-017-0775-9.

Sleep Disruption and Its Relationship with Delirium: Electroencephalographic Perspectives

Isabel Okinedo, Patricia S. Andrews, E. Wesley Ely, and Shawniqua Williams Roberson

1 Introduction

The cognitive benefits of sleep are most evident when normal sleep is disrupted. The neurophysiologic processes underlying these benefits have been the subject of investigation for nearly a century. An important tool in this line of investigation is electroencephalography (EEG), the recording and interpretation of patterns of electrical signals from the brain. Unique patterns have been identified in EEG signals that indicate specific stages of sleep and signify particular interactions among neuronal populations within the brain. Sleep disruption is associated with altered EEG dynamics both during wakefulness and in subsequent sleep. Significant sleep disruption can precipitate delirium, a syndrome of brain dysfunction characterized by altered mental status, fluctuating levels of arousal, inattention and disordered

I. Okinedo
Department of Neuroscience, Vanderbilt University, Nashville, TN, USA

P. S. Andrews
Department of Psychiatry and Behavioral Sciences, Critical Illness, Brain dysfunction and Survivorship (CIBS) Center, Vanderbilt University Medical Center, Nashville, TN, USA
e-mail: patricia.andrews@vumc.org

E. W. Ely
Critical Illness, Brain dysfunction and Survivorship (CIBS) Center, Division of Allergy, Pulmonary, and Critical Care Medicine, Vanderbilt University Medical Center, and Geriatric Research Education and Clinical Center (GRECC), VA Tennessee Valley Healthcare System, Nashville, TN, USA
e-mail: wes.ely@vumc.org

S. Williams Roberson (✉)
Critical Illness, Brain dysfunction and Survivorship (CIBS) Center,
Departments of Neurology and Biomedical Engineering, Vanderbilt University,
Nashville, TN, USA
e-mail: shawniqua.w.roberson@vumc.org

© The Author(s), under exclusive license to Springer Nature Switzerland AG 2022
G. L. Weinhouse, J. W. Devlin (eds.), *Sleep in Critical Illness*,
https://doi.org/10.1007/978-3-031-06447-0_8

thinking. Given that delirium is also characterized by altered physiologic patterns on EEG, this modality may provide clues to the mechanistic processes underlying the relationship between sleep disruption and delirium. In the present chapter we explore this relationship through the lens of EEG. The clinical relationship between sleep disruption and delirium is covered in chapter "Sleep Disruption and Its Relationship with Delirium: Clinical Perspectives".

2   The Restorative Neurophysiology of Sleep

Building on the chapter "Characteristics of Sleep in Critically Ill Patients. Part I: Sleep Fragmentation and Sleep Stage Disruption", electroencephalography (EEG) consists of the recording and interpretation of time-varying patterns of electrical signals from the brain. Identification of these patterns in the brain's electrical activity allows one to distinguish sleep states from wakefulness and other states of consciousness (e.g. coma or delirium). Neurophysiologists examine, either by visual inspection or by quantitative analysis, the relative contributions to the EEG signal of oscillations in specific frequency ranges. The ranges most commonly identifiable on scalp EEG in adults are slow oscillations (less than 1 Hz), delta (1–4 Hz), theta (4–7 Hz), alpha (7–13 Hz), and beta (13–35 Hz) frequencies. In healthy individuals the EEG typically demonstrates alpha activity during wakefulness, theta activity during drowsiness, slow oscillations and delta activity during non-rapid eye movement (NREM) sleep and beta activity during rapid eye movement (REM) sleep (Fig. 1). Sleep spindles are a defining feature of stage II sleep. These sporadic 12–15 Hz oscillations have an outline that resembles an old-fashioned sewing spindle (broad in the middle and tapered at either end). They frequently occur in association with K-complexes - brief, high amplitude deflections of about 1 s in duration. K-complexes can often be elicited by sudden acoustic stimuli during sleep (K stands for "knock") and likely reflect the integrity of the brain's ability to 'filter' sensory stimuli [1, 2].

The oscillatory patterns recorded during sleep EEG are associated with specific neurophysiologic activities that support healthy cerebral function. Theta oscillations in sleep are associated with replaying memories acquired during wakefulness. Delta waves drive clearance of the brain's waste products and may facilitate synaptic homeostasis, a mechanism by which the brain is theorized to "reorganize" itself to allow for more efficient processing. Sleep spindles are associated with memory consolidation and thus likely facilitate learning and cognitive processing. These patterns are postulated to result from interactions between the brain cortex and the thalamus, an egg-shaped structure near the center of the brain that largely serves as a relay between the brainstem and the cortex. Coordinated oscillations across disparate brain regions (also known as "functional connectivity") allow for these regions to communicate in support of processes such as memory replay. In the remainder of this section we discuss recent work to elucidate the functions supported by these

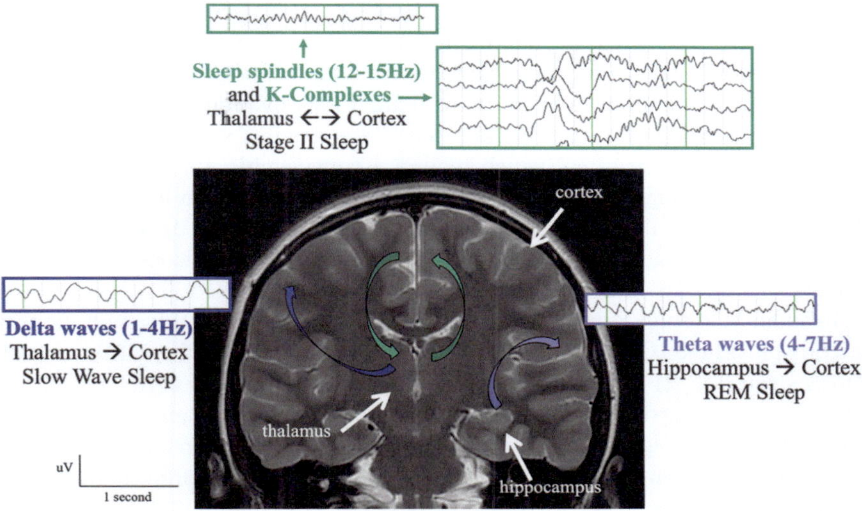

Fig. 1 Selected EEG patterns related to sleep and brain structures involved in their generation. Sleep spindles and K complexes [green] indicate stage II sleep and are generated through bidirectional interactions between the thalamus and the cortex. Delta (1–4 Hz) waves [blue] predominate in slow-wave sleep and are largely driven by thalamocortical cells, though local cortical regions can generate their own intrinsic delta activity. Hippocampal theta (4–7 Hz) activity [purple] is characteristically present during REM sleep but may also appear during stages I and II

patterns of electrical activity during sleep. Though much of our knowledge to date is informed by animal studies, we focus primarily on oscillatory activity that can be measured by scalp EEG in vivo in humans.

2.1　Slow Oscillations and Delta Waves

Slow oscillations reflect neuronal firing patterns that typically fluctuate at less than 1 Hz and occur synchronously throughout the brain. They are generated by bidirectional interactions between neurons in the thalamus and the brain cortex during NREM sleep. Slow oscillations are characterized by alternating UP states (periods of increased activity of neurons in the thalamus and primary sensorimotor areas of the cortex) and DOWN states (periods of relative quiescence). These rhythms are postulated to modulate the brain's delta wave activity during sleep [3]. They are important for sleep-dependent learning and memory processing [4], especially that of declarative (fact-based or explicit) and recognition memories [5, 6]. Delta waves, also characteristically present in NREM sleep, fluctuate between 1 Hz and 4 Hz in regional populations of neurons. Delta waves appear to be generated by intrinsic activity in the cortex that is augmented by input from the thalamus [7, 8]. Kim et al. [4] used optogenetic silencing of neurons to disrupt delta waves and observed an increase in performance gains on a skill learned prior to sleep. These observations suggest that delta waves are important for homeostatic *forgetting* of memories acquired prior to sleep, a function that may support effective memory consolidation [9]. Since encoding of information in the brain occurs by sequential replay of neuronal firing patterns [10, 11], memory formation requires strengthening synaptic connections among neurons (which require a considerable amount of energy to maintain). According to the synaptic homeostasis hypothesis, an important role of sleep is to "prune" these connections to allow efficient energy expenditure while integrating newly acquired information into the lived experience of the individual [9].

In addition to supporting memory consolidation, delta waves drive pulsations of cerebrospinal fluid (CSF) in and out of the skull cavity through the fourth ventricle during sleep (Fig. 2) [12]. In anesthetized animals, delta activity correlates with an influx of CSF alongside perivascular spaces through the glymphatic system [13], a paravascular pathway that facilitates clearance of interstitial solutes in the brain [14]. Delta waves thus play a role in the homeostatic evacuation of the brain's waste products. This may explain why delta activity reduces buildup of tau protein [15] and why suppression of slow-wave activity results in buildup of amyloid beta protein [16], both markers of age-related dementia. It also may explain why suppression of delta waves is associated with age-related memory impairment [17].

The improved efficiencies in memory resulting from slow oscillations and delta waves may facilitate cognitive performance after sleep. A computational model of sleep spindles and slow oscillations with delta waves showed that the latter allow competition between memories such that memories with more reinforcement take precedence over weaker memories in the memory replay and consolidation process [18]. A separate model of sleep-like slow oscillations generated by interactions between the thalamus and the cortex showed that these oscillations are beneficial to cognitive task performance [19].

2.2 Sleep Spindles and K Complexes

Sleep spindles and K complexes result from a complex interplay among the thalamus, the hippocampus and the brain's cortex [20, 21]. Maingret and colleagues [22] examined this phenomenon using intracranial electrodes implanted in a series of male Long-Evans rats. The authors used timed electrical stimulation to modulate the electrical patterns underlying spindles and the associated delta waves that together form K complexes during sleep. Using a spatial memory task before and after sleep, they observed that tighter coupling between cortical spindles and hippocampal fast ripples was associated with improvements in memory consolidation. Van Schalkwijk and colleagues [23] recorded sleep before and after a procedural

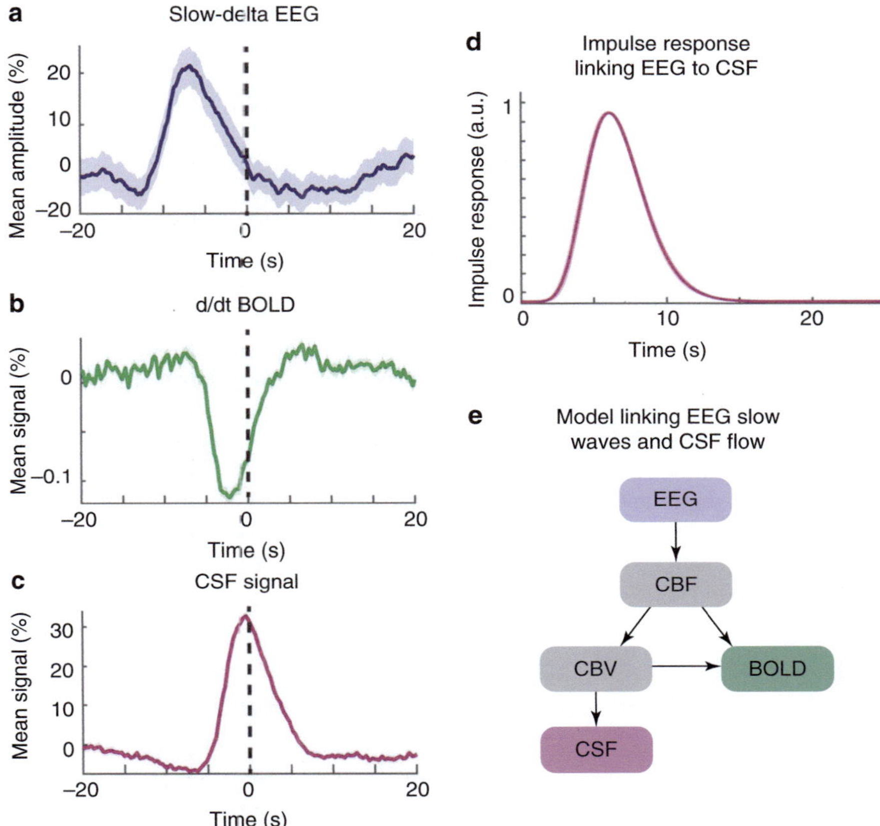

Fig. 2 EEG slow-delta waves are coupled to CSF oscillations. (**a**) Mean amplitude envelope of slow-delta EEG, (**b**) mean derivative of BOLD signals, and (**c**) mean CSF signal, all locked to the peaks of CSF waves during sleep in 13 humans undergoing simultaneous EEG and fMRI during NREM sleep. The shaded region represents the standard error across peak-locked trials (n = 123 peaks). (**d**) Calculated impulse response of the CSF signal to the EEG envelope shows a time course similar to that of previously established hemodynamic models. Shading indicates standard deviation across model folds. (**e**) Diagram of model linking the time course of neural activity to CSF flow. Variables include CBF and cerebral blood volume (CBV). *With permission from The American Association for the Advancement of Science* © 2019

memory task in humans and found improved task performance (fewer errors) the following day in those whose sleep spindle activity increased after learning the task. The authors concluded that spindle activity was important for memory consolidation in this sample. On the other hand, deficits in sleep spindles correlate with impaired memory consolidation among patients with schizophrenia [24]. These findings support the theory that sleep spindles are a key mechanism by which sleep supports memory consolidation.

2.3 Theta Waves

The hippocampi are a pair of horn-shaped structures in the medial regions of the brain bilaterally. The hippocampi are important for memory encoding and retrieval, and are postulated to be the primary source of theta (4–7 Hz) activity during NREM and REM sleep [25–27]. The hippocampus uses theta oscillations to encode memories of specific sequences of locations, such as the path an animal might take to find food [28] and reactivate when planning to repeat the same sequence [29]. REM theta oscillations are also proposed to mediate processing of emotional memories by way of coordinated activity between the hippocampus and the cortex [30]. Coordinated theta activity between the hippocampus and the ventral striatum, a brain structure important to salience, facilitates replay of memories during sleep [27, 31]. This 'memory replay' phenomenon has been observed in humans and rodents, and is postulated to be the first step in the process of sleep-dependent memory consolidation [32].

2.4 Functional Connectivity Patterns in Normal Sleep

Functional connectivity refers to the degree of covariance between two physiologic signals recorded from distinct regions of the brain. Commonly recorded signals include electrical fluctuations, as recorded using EEG, and hemodynamic fluctuations, as measured using blood oxygen level dependent (BOLD) fMRI. An observed correlation between two signals suggests some form of communication between the neuronal populations that generate them, either by causal influence of one population over the other, or by virtue of a third party generator that exerts a synchronizing influence over both populations simultaneously [33]. The synchronizing population may or may not represent part of a "rich club"—a group of highly interconnected brain regions that play a key role in global integration of information across the entire brain [34]. Measures of instantaneous connectivity across the cerebral cortex are lower in slow-wave sleep compared to wakefulness [35, 36]. This phenomenon may reflect the corresponding decrease in sensory integration that occurs with diminished conscious awareness during sleep [37].

The functional utility of altered connectivity patterns during sleep has been under much speculation. During slow wave sleep, sequences of neuronal firing patterns observed during wakefulness are spontaneously replayed at an accelerated timescale [38]. Berkers et al. trained volunteers on 50 visual stimuli paired with 50 auditory stimuli during wakefulness and monitored the same individuals using EEG and fMRI during sleep. When the participants reached slow-wave sleep, the investigators prompted reactivation of memories by replaying the auditory stimuli at low volume. They then tested the participants' memory of the audio-visual pairings after awakening. They found that greater connectivity between stimulus-relevant areas of the cortex and the hippocampus during memory reactivation correlated with better performance on the post-sleep memory task [39]. This finding suggests dynamic changes in brain connectivity patterns during sleep may support memory replay, a key step in sleep-related memory consolidation [5]. Computational models suggest the observed changes in connectivity may in turn be driven by theta oscillations [40], and this is supported by a study of post-sleep recall of vocabulary learned prior to sleep [27].

Functional connectivity may also play a role in determining when sleep may be disrupted by external sensory stimuli. Bastuji and colleagues [41] used lasers to deliver stimuli during slow-wave sleep to 14 individuals undergoing intracranial EEG monitoring for epilepsy. They observed a significant increase in the probability of awakening when there was enhanced connectivity among areas of the brain responsible for sensory processing. This association was maintained independent of sleep stage and may explain, in part, the observation that ICU patients exhibit very little slow-wave sleep. If the brain's intrinsic response to sepsis or sedation, for example, results in greater connectivity among sensory regions, this may result in higher sensitivity to the variety of stimuli in the ICU environment.

3   Neural Dynamics in Sleep Disruption

During and after sleep disruption, there are observable changes in EEG activity patterns. Sleep deprivation disrupts functional connectivity, primarily in the prefrontal cortex and related regions. Sleep deprivation was associated with decreased connectivity between left central and right frontocentral regions during wakefulness in a series of 18 healthy, right-handed young men [42]. Vermeij and colleagues [43] compared high-density resting state EEGs in a series of eight healthy participants during a day following normal sleep versus a day following sleep disruption. Using a graph theoretical analysis approach, the authors found sleep deprivation to affect the EEG in a manner that was topographically specific: a significant decrease in prefrontal interconnectedness in the alpha frequency band (typically associated with normal wakefulness), and a significant increase in global functional connectivity in the theta frequency range. The fact that the prefrontal region was the most strongly affected, may explain why functions mediated by this region may be most impacted by sleep deprivation [43]. Such functions include the process of initiating or sustaining any non-reflex response (energization), developing and implementing a plan (task setting), periodically checking that one remains on task (monitoring), behavioral/emotional regulation, understanding of one's own thoughts (metacognition), vigilant attention, working memory, and learning that is dependent on the hippocampus [44, 45]. Deficits in functional connectivity of the prefrontal cortex due to sleep deprivation may be expected to result in deficits in any or all of these executive functions which are some of the defining clinical features of delirium (see chapter "Sleep Disruption and Its Relationship with Delirium: Clinical Perspectives").

Aberrant functional connectivity may also be the mechanism by which sleep deprivation leads to neuropsychological dysfunction and impairment of fine motor control. Decreased connectivity between the prefrontal cortex and the amygdala, an almond-shaped region important for processing of fear and other emotions, results in impaired emotional regulation in sleep-deprived individuals. In a study of 30 healthy adult males undergoing 36 h of complete sleep deprivation, alterations in connectivity among regions involved in motor regulatory control were associated with impaired somatic fine motor function [46]. The same study revealed aberrant communication of sensory information in areas responsible for sensory processing. Altogether these findings suggest that changes in functional connectivity among specific brain networks underlie cognitive and motor deficits after sleep deprivation [46].

EEG activity patterns can be quantified to measure the brain's response to sleep deprivation. Skorucak and colleagues [47] conducted a cross-over study to investigate the response to 7 days of sleep restriction (6 h in bed) versus sleep extension (10 h in bed) followed by 40 h of sleep deprivation and 12 h of recovery sleep in healthy participants. The investigators used polysomnographic recordings during the sleep sessions to examine sleep architecture and slow-wave activity. Sleep deprivation resulted in less REM sleep during sleep restriction and greater frontal and central slow wave activity during recovery sleep [47, 48].

The recovery period that follows sleep deprivation is more intense than normal sleep. Characteristics of this increased intensity include decreased responsiveness to the environment, altered EEG properties (specifically increased delta power and decreased sleep spindle activity), and increased sleep time. In a study by Mander and colleagues [49], 9 healthy adults underwent functional magnetic resonance imaging (fMRI) on two occasions: once after 9 h of normal sleep following 38 h of being awake, and once after 10 h of recovery sleep, also following 38 hours of being awake. It was found that recovery sleep was an average of 111 min longer than normal sleep. Recovery sleep also altered markers of prefrontal activation the following day. The increase in delta power during recovery sleep was most prominent in the frontal cortex, and task performance increased with recovery sleep. These findings reinforce the claim that slow-wave sleep is important for the recovery of prefrontal functions (including task performance) that may be lost or diminished during sleep deprivation.

4 Neural Dynamics in Delirium

The electrophysiologic characteristics of delirium were first described by Engel and Romano in the 1940s [50]. They placed electrodes at the frontal, central and posterior areas of the scalp in 53 patients and grouped recordings into five stages of delirium based on their observations of the patients' degree of disturbance in awareness. Delirium severity progressively worsened from stage I to stage V. In stages I and II (mild to moderate delirium) the authors observed normal waking EEG patterns with increased theta (5–7 Hz) activity. In stages II and III there was a predominance of low voltage fast (beta) activity. Stages III and IV were characterized by prominent delta and theta activity (2–7 Hz oscillations) with very little of the alpha (8–13 Hz) activity typically seen in normal wakefulness. In stage IV there were periods of regular (monomorphic), high amplitude delta (0.5–3 Hz) waves, at times with superimposed low voltage fast beta activity. In the most severe stage of delirium (stage V), the EEG was almost entirely composed of fairly regular, moderately high amplitude delta activity (3–7 Hz). Little to no normal alpha or beta activity was apparent at this stage.

In the decades since this original investigation, the patterns of activity described by Romano and Engel have been observed in groups of patients with specific etiologies of delirium. Increased irregular theta and delta activity is typically present in delirium due to endocrine or metabolic disorders [51]. Repetitive, frontally predominant delta waves with a characteristic triphasic morphology are historically associated with hepatic encephalopathy but have also been observed in renal failure, respiratory failure, severe sepsis and medication toxicity [52–54]. Intoxication with benzodiazepines or other substances that activate gamma aminobutyric acid (GABA) receptors in the brain is associated with increased beta activity, particularly in frontal regions [55]. Monomorphic delta waves with overriding beta activity can be observed in patients with autoimmune encephalitis [56]. Yet for the most part, attempts to obtain diagnostic specificity in regard to delirium etiology have been disappointing using conventional analysis techniques [53].

Some investigators have attempted to characterize electroencephalographic patterns in delirium using more computational techniques. Numan and colleagues [57] recorded EEGs in 18 patients with postoperative hypoactive delirium and 40 age- and sex-matched controls (20 recovering from anesthesia and 20 non-delirious control patients). In general, EEGs in the delirious patients were similar to those in the sedated patients, demonstrating increased delta activity and decreased global functional connectivity in the alpha range compared to non-delirious controls. Compared to patients recovering from anesthesia, the EEG in delirious patients exhibited less activity in the alpha (8–13 Hz) frequency range. Betweenness centrality, a measure of global integration, was also decreased in the alpha range in delirium compared with controls and with sedated patients [57].

Importantly, EEG recordings change dynamically. The features we have described thus far may fluctuate over time in terms of their relative contributions to the overall EEG signal. These fluctuations can reasonably be expected to be even more prominent in the case of delirium, which is commonly characterized by changes in level of arousal and alertness, and transient phenomena such as hallucinations. Van der Kooi and Slooter [58] captured these fluctuations elegantly by measuring the coefficient of variation (CV) of the canonical frequency ranges among 26 delirious and 28 non-delirious patients after cardiac surgery. Delirium was associated with increased CV in the alpha (8–13 Hz) range globally, and increased CV in the beta (13–20 Hz) range in the frontal region. Contrary to other frequency ranges, CV in the delta (0.5–4 Hz) range was decreased in the delirium group. The mechanisms for this difference are incompletely understood but may relate to post-anesthetic sleep intrusions among non-delirious participants that are suppressed in delirium. Importantly, alterations in the variability of delta activity not only may occur in acute delirium but may give hints to patterns of cognitive impairment long after critical illness [59]. Further exploration of these phenomena may provide clues to the distinction between the pathological delta activity associated with delirium and 'normal' delta oscillations contributing to healthy brain activity during sleep.

The EEG patterns classically associated with mild to moderate stages of delirium have also been described in mechanically ventilated patients, who commonly experience severe sleep disruption [60, 61]. Clinical evidence of delirium (as determined by Glasgow Coma Scale [62] score less than 15 or a Richmond Agitation-Sedation Scale [63] score less than −1 and positive Confusion Assessment Method for the ICU) was an exclusion criterion for this study. Yet 16 (28%) of 57 patients demonstrated periods of high amplitude irregular (polymorphic) delta activity without sleep spindles or K complexes, which the authors termed "atypical sleep". During wakefulness, these patients exhibited excessive theta (6 Hz and below) activity, which the authors described as "pathologic wakefulness". The striking similarity between these patterns and those classically described by Romano and Engel [50], along with the observation that sleep deprived patients are at higher risk of delirium [64], raises the possibility that delirium and atypical sleep/pathologic wakefulness may reflect two sides of the same coin. Chapter "Atypical Sleep and Pathologic Wakefulness" describes these findings in greater detail.

5 Sleep Deprivation: Toward a Hypothesis of Deliriogenesis

The electrophysiologic changes observed in sleep deprivation give a window into possible mechanisms by which sleep disruption may precipitate delirium in compromised individuals (Table 1). When wakefulness persists and normal NREM sleep is not permitted to take place, a lack of slow oscillations and delta waves lead to disrupted CSF flow dynamics [12]. This may result in a buildup of the brain's waste products, a consequence that may have effects akin to hepatic or renal compromise, wherein systemic toxins are allowed to build up in the bloodstream. In such cases patients often experience fluctuations in level of arousal and impaired judgment. Decreased waste clearance might be expected to have more pronounced acute effects in the context of neurodegenerative diseases, such that this may preferentially affect people already vulnerable because of an underlying condition such as dementia [65]. Indeed, accumulation of toxic protein aggregates is a pathological hallmark of Alzheimer's Disease (AD) [66], and patients with AD experience worse cognitive decline after an episode of delirium [67].

A lack of coordinated theta waves, delta waves and spindles due to sleep disruption likely impairs the brain's ability to process and consolidate memories [3].

Table 1 Summary of EEG features and potentially deliriogenic effects of disruption

Characteristic	Condition	Function	Potential effect of loss
Theta waves	REM sleep	Memory replay	Impaired memory consolidation
Slow oscillations	Slow wave sleep	Coordinate delta waves	Impaired memory consolidation
Delta waves	Slow wave sleep	Drive CSF pulsations Facilitate memory pruning	Waste accumulation Impaired memory consolidation
Spindles	NREM sleep	Memory reorganization	Network disorganization Impaired learning
Prefrontal connectivity	Wakefulness	Executive function (e.g. planning) Emotional regulation	Behavioral disturbances
Sensorimotor connectivity	REM sleep	Memory replay Memory pruning	Impaired retention of information Perceptual disturbances

Absent or diminished memory consolidation hinders retention of past information and, according to prevailing theory of memory consolidation mechanisms, may result in a progressively disorganized cortical network. This disorganization is characterized by worsening metabolic inefficiencies, i.e. higher energy requirements resulting from un-pruned synapses coupled with inefficient acquisition and storage of new information [9, 68]. Deficits in processing of recently acquired information and impaired ability to integrate new information may combine to produce an acute state of confusion. Thus, although the diagnostic criteria of delirium pivot primarily on inattention, when we focus on the genesis of delirium from sleep disruption, what we find is a problem that is precipitated by impairments in memory processing [69, 70].

As described above, sleep disruption is also associated with diminished connectivity within the prefrontal region and between prefrontal and emotion processing centers. These physiologic changes can further exacerbate symptoms of inattention and result in impaired emotional control [71] and perceptual distortions [72], effects that may underlie the behavioral dysregulation observed in patients with hyperactive delirium.

Disruptions in the brain's metabolic waste processing, impaired memory processing and acquisition, perceptual distortions and executive disinhibition may combine to create a syndrome akin to delirium in sleep-deprived individuals (Fig. 3). Yet delirium itself may also worsen sleep disruption and exacerbate impairments in the associated cognitive processes. In a convenience sample of 12 postoperative patients recovering from orthopedic surgery, delirium severity (as measured by the revised Delirium Rating Scale [73]) was associated with shorter total sleep time on night 1 and increased waking delta power on postoperative day 1, but decreased delta power on night 2 after surgery [74]. While delirium is classically associated with increased theta and delta activity during wakefulness, there is a lack of the organized sleep architecture defining various sleep stages. This may be due to

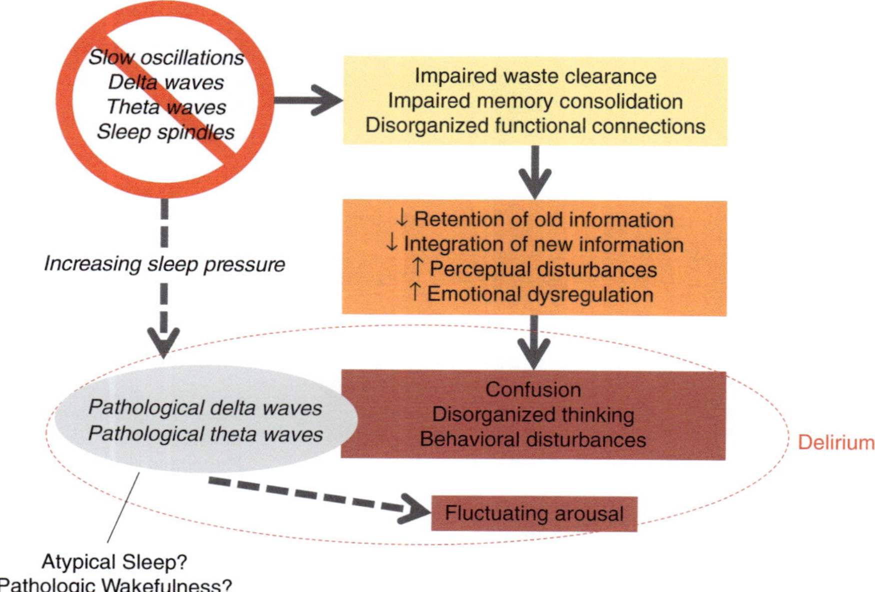

Fig. 3 Deliriogenic Potential of Sleep Disruption (A Neurophysiologic Perspective): Lack of the normal physiologic activity characterizing sleep leads to 1) disruptions in CSF flow dynamics and impaired clearance of the brain's metabolic waste products, 2) reductions in the normal memory consolidation processes that allow for efficient memory processing and efficient acquisition of new information, and 3) disorganized connectivity among brain regions responsible for memory processing, perception, emotional control and other cognitive functions. These deficits cause a cascade of symptoms that are characterized by pathological neuronal firing patterns (manifest on EEG recordings as pathological delta and theta waves) and ultimately, due to increasing sleep pressure, lead to characteristic signs of delirium. Atypical sleep and pathological wakefulness, though present in non-delirious patients, may represent subsyndromal delirium or EEG harbingers of impending delirium onset

absence of coordinated slow oscillations modulating cerebral function as observed by Dash and Colleagues [3]. Whether the delta and theta waves thus observed is the brain's attempt to 'catch up' on homeostatic sleep functions versus an entirely disparate pattern (i.e. driven by unique generators unrelated to sleep homeostasis and decoupled from CSF pulse flow dynamics) remains to be elucidated. Nonetheless, the bidirectional effect of sleep disruption and delirium may result in a self-propelling cycle, with escalating impairments in memory, cognition and metabolic waste clearance that become difficult for the brain to regulate without external interventions (Fig. 3). Such interventions may include reorientation to familiar faces and voices, modulation of sensory stimuli and promotion of regular sleep-wake cycles. These effects underscore the importance of preserving quality sleep, particularly among individuals at higher risk of delirium, and motivate adherence to systematic protocols that include optimizing sleep quality to minimize risk of delirium in inpatient settings [75, 76].

6　Clinical Implications: Sleep in the ICU and Beyond

The propensity for sleep disruption to precipitate or contribute to delirium in at-risk patients raises the question of how best to ensure optimal sleep quality in the ICU. Though polysomnography (PSG) is the gold standard for monitoring and assessing sleep quality, PSG is often impractical in the ICU environment and traditional scoring criteria do not translate well to this setting [61]. Sleep questionnaires are limited by subjectivity and are not suitable for patients with impaired communication. Accelerometry devices may be hindered by restrictions in spontaneous movement due to indwelling catheters or physical injuries. A role can be envisioned for limited-montage EEG as a standardized measurement of sleep in the ICU. Attempts have been made to use bispectral index to stage sleep in critically ill patients [77], and emerging wearable EEG devices may find utility in this setting [78, 79]. Importantly, these will require careful study for optimal implementation given the ICU-specific conditions (e.g. sedation, hepatic or renal failure, mechanical ventilation) that frequently influence EEG signals [80, 81]. Chapter "Methods for Routine Sleep Assessment and Monitoring" reviews sleep assessment in more detail.

While delirium in the ICU confers a dose-dependent increase in the risk of long-term cognitive impairment [82] and sleep deprivation is associated with worse cognitive trajectory among the general population [83], little is known about sleep disruption and cognitive impairment in the post-ICU period. Between 10 and 61% of ICU survivors experience persistent sleep disturbances up to 6 months after critical illness [84]. Wilcox et al. followed 102 ICU survivors to estimate sleep using actigraphy and assess cognition using the Repeatable Battery for the Assessment of Neuropsychological Status (RBANS). They found an association between sleep fragmentation and cognitive impairment at 7 days after ICU discharge but not at 6- or 12-month follow-up [85]. Though EEG features of sleep and wakefulness improve simultaneously with improvements in cognitive function during critical illness, the timing and trajectory of these changes in the post-ICU period is yet to be elucidated [86].

7　Summary and Conclusions

Normal sleep is characterized by a series of neurophysiologic processes that are identifiable in EEG activity patterns. Slow oscillations, delta and theta waves, and sleep spindles indicate particular types of activity within and between specialized structures in the brain. The hippocampus, thalamus, and cerebral cortex play integral parts in the processes of waste clearance, memory consolidation and cortical reorganization during sleep. These functions are important for maintenance of cerebral function and their disruption leads to symptoms and signs consistent with delirium, particularly among at-risk individuals. These patterns give insight to possible neurophysiologic mechanisms underlying the relationship between sleep disruption and delirium. We propose that sleep disruption may be characterized by specific alterations in EEG activity patterns that result in inefficient clearance of cerebral metabolic waste, impaired memory consolidation and disrupted brain connectivity, leading to memory loss, inattention, and difficulty processing new information. The physiologic processes underlying delirium may further exacerbate sleep disruption, fueling a self-propelling cycle and motivating interventions to maintain appropriate sleep hygiene in at-risk populations.

Yet several gaps exist in our understanding of this relationship. Are the delta waves of delirium and those of slow-wave sleep borne of the same neural generators? What of the theta activity that is typically observed in earlier stages of delirium? Does the modulatory effect of slow oscillations remain intact in delirium? And fundamentally: does impaired memory consolidation increase risk of delirium independent of other functions of sleep? Both sleep disruption and delirium are associated with long-term cognitive decline and increased risk of dementia [82, 87]. Are the neurophysiologic processes linking these conditions also responsible for cognitive aging? Investigations to elucidate these questions will inform development of therapeutic interventions and motivate approaches to optimizing the restorative functions of sleep.

References

1. Loomis AL, Harvey EN, Hobart G. Potential rhythms of the cerebral cortex during sleep. Science 1935;81(0036-8075 (Print)):597–8.
2. Caporro M, Zulfi H, Yeh HJ, Lenartowicz A, Buttinelli C, Parvizi J, et al. Functional MRI of sleep spindles and K-complexes. Clin Neurophysiol. 2012;123(2):303–9. https://doi.org/10.1016/j.clinph.2011.06.018.
3. Dash MB. Infraslow coordination of slow wave activity through altered neuronal synchrony. Sleep. 2019;42(12):1–13. https://doi.org/10.1093/sleep/zsz170.
4. Kim J, Gulati T, Ganguly K. Competing roles of slow oscillations and Delta waves in memory consolidation versus forgetting. Cell. 2019;179(2):514–26.e13. https://doi.org/10.1016/j.cell.2019.08.040.
5. Diekelmann S, Born J. The memory function of sleep. Nat Rev Neurosci. 2010;11(2):114–26. https://doi.org/10.1038/nrn2762.
6. Daurat A, Terrier P, Foret J, Tiberge M. Slow wave sleep and recollection in recognition memory. Conscious Cogn. 2007;16(2):445–55. https://doi.org/10.1016/j.concog.2006.06.011.
7. Gent TC, Bandarabadi M, Herrera CG, Adamantidis AR. Thalamic dual control of sleep and wakefulness. Nat Neurosci. 2018;21(7):974–84. https://doi.org/10.1038/s41593-018-0164-7.
8. Steriade M, Nunez A, Amzica F. Intracellular analysis of relations between the slow (<I Hz) neocortical oscillation and other sleep rhythms of the electroencephalogram. J Neurosci. 1993;13(8):3266–83. https://doi.org/10.1016/S0040-4039(97)01107-6.
9. Tononi G, Cirelli C. Sleep and the price of plasticity: from synaptic and cellular homeostasis to memory consolidation and integration. Neuron. 2014;81(1):12–34. https://doi.org/10.1016/j.neuron.2013.12.025.

10. Peters AJ, Chen SX, Komiyama T. Emergence of reproducible spatiotemporal activity during motor learning. Nature. 2014;510(7504):263–7. https://doi.org/10.1038/nature13235.
11. Okubo TS, Mackevicius EL, Payne HL, Lynch GF, Fee MS. Growth and splitting of neural sequences in songbird vocal development. Nature. 2015;528(7582):352–7. https://doi.org/10.1038/nature15741.
12. Fultz NE, Bonmassar G, Setsompop K, Stickgold RA, Rosen BR, Polimeni JR, et al. Coupled electrophysiological, hemodynamic, and cerebrospinal fluid oscillations in human sleep. Science. 2019;366(6465):628–31. https://doi.org/10.1126/science.aax5440.
13. Hablitz LM, Vinitsky HS, Sun Q, Staeger FF, Sigurdsson B, Mortensen KN, et al. Increased glymphatic influx is correlated with high EEG delta power and low heart rate in mice under anesthesia. Sci Adv. 2019;5(2):eaav5447. https://doi.org/10.1126/sciadv.aav5447.
14. Iliff JJ, Wang M, Liao Y, Plogg BA, Peng W, Gundersen GA, et al. A paravascular pathway facilitates CSF flow through the brain parenchyma and the clearance of interstitial solutes, including amyloid beta. Sci Transl Med. 2012;4(147):147ra11. https://doi.org/10.1126/scitranslmed.3003748.
15. Iaccarino HF, Singer AC, Martorell AJ, Rudenko A, Gao F, Gillingham TZ, et al. Gamma frequency entrainment attenuates amyloid load and modifies microglia. Nature. 2016;540(7632):230–5. https://doi.org/10.1038/nature20587.
16. Ju YS, Ooms SJ, Sutphen C, Macauley SL, Zangrilli MA, Jerome G, et al. Slow wave sleep disruption increases cerebrospinal fluid amyloid-beta levels. Brain. 2017;140(8):2104–11. https://doi.org/10.1093/brain/awx148.
17. Mander BA, Rao V, Lu B, Saletin JM, Lindquist JR, Ancoli-Israel S, et al. Prefrontal atrophy, disrupted NREM slow waves and impaired hippocampal-dependent memory in aging. Nat Neurosci. 2013;16(3):357–64. https://doi.org/10.1038/nn.3324.
18. Wei Y, Krishnan GP, Komarov M, Bazhenov M. Differential roles of sleep spindles and sleep slow oscillations in memory consolidation. 2018.
19. Capone C, Pastorelli E, Golosio B, Paolucci PS. Sleep-like slow oscillations improve visual classification through synaptic homeostasis and memory association in a thalamo-cortical model. Sci Rep. 2019;9(1):1–11. https://doi.org/10.1038/s41598-019-45525-0.
20. Schabus M, Dang-Vu TT, Albouy G, Balteau E, Boly M, Carrier J, et al. Hemodynamic cerebral correlates of sleep spindles during human non-rapid eye movement sleep. Proc Natl Acad Sci U S A. 2007;104(32):13164–9. https://doi.org/10.1073/pnas.0703084104.
21. Andrillon T, Nir Y, Staba RJ, Ferrarelli F, Cirelli C, Tononi G, et al. Sleep spindles in humans: insights from intracranial EEG and unit recordings. J Neurosci. 2011;31(49):17821. https://doi.org/10.1523/JNEUROSCI.2604-11.2011.
22. Maingret N, Girardeau G, Todorova R, Goutierre M, Zugaro M. Hippocampo-cortical coupling mediates memory consolidation during sleep. Nat Neurosci. 2016;19(7):959–64. https://doi.org/10.1038/nn.4304.
23. van Schalkwijk FJ, Hauser T, Hoedlmoser K, Ameen MS, Wilhelm FH, Sauter C, et al. Procedural memory consolidation is associated with heart rate variability and sleep spindles. J Sleep Res. 2020;29(3):1–8. https://doi.org/10.1111/jsr.12910.
24. Manoach DS, Stickgold R. Abnormal sleep spindles, memory consolidation, and schizophrenia. Annu Rev Clin Psychol. 2017;2019(15):451–79. https://doi.org/10.1146/annurev-clinpsy-050718-095754.
25. Sirota A, Montgomery S, Fujisawa S, Isomura Y, Zugaro M, Buzsáki G. Entrainment of neocortical neurons and gamma oscillations by the hippocampal theta rhythm. Neuron. 2008;60(4):683–97. https://doi.org/10.1016/j.neuron.2008.09.014.
26. Goutagny R, Jackson J, Williams S. Self-generated theta oscillations in the hippocampus. Nat Neurosci. 2009;12(12):1491–3. https://doi.org/10.1038/nn.2440.
27. Schreiner T, Doeller CF, Jensen O, Rasch B, Staudigl T. Theta phase-coordinated memory reactivation reoccurs in a slow-oscillatory rhythm during NREM sleep. Cell Rep. 2018;25(2):296–301. https://doi.org/10.1016/j.celrep.2018.09.037.

28. Dragoi G, Buzsáki G. Temporal encoding of place sequences by hippocampal cell assemblies. Neuron. 2006;50(1):145–57. https://doi.org/10.1016/j.neuron.2006.02.023.

29. Wikenheiser AM, Redish AD. Hippocampal theta sequences reflect current goals. Nat Neurosci. 2015;18(2):289–94. https://doi.org/10.1038/nn.3909.

30. Hutchison IC, Rathore S. The role of REM sleep theta activity in emotional memory. Front Psychol. 2015;6:1439.

31. Lansink CS, Goltstein PM, Lankelma JV, McNaughton BL, Pennartz CMA. Hippocampus leads ventral striatum in replay of place-reward information. PLoS Biol. 2009;7(8) https://doi.org/10.1371/journal.pbio.1000173.

32. Klinzing JG, Niethard N, Born J. Mechanisms of systems memory consolidation during sleep. Nat Neurosci. 2019;22(October) https://doi.org/10.1038/s41593-019-0467-3.

33. Buzsaki G, Draguhn A. Neuronal oscillations in cortical networks. Science. 2004;304(5679):1926–9. https://doi.org/10.1126/science.1099745.

34. van den Heuvel MP, Sporns O. Rich-club organization of the human connectome. J Neurosci. 2011;31(44):15775–86. https://doi.org/10.1523/JNEUROSCI.3539-11.2011.

35. Imperatori LS, Betta M, Cecchetti L, Canales-Johnson A, Ricciardi E, Siclari F, et al. EEG functional connectivity metrics wPLI and wSMI account for distinct types of brain functional interactions. Sci Rep. 2019;9(1):1–15. https://doi.org/10.1038/s41598-019-45289-7.

36. Massimini M, Ferrarelli F, Huber R, Esser SK, Singh H, Tononi G. Breakdown of cortical effective connectivity during sleep. Science. 2005;309(5744):2228–32. https://doi.org/10.1126/science.1117256.

37. Tononi G. Consciousness as integrated information: a provisional manifesto. Biol Bull. 2008;215(3):216–42. https://doi.org/10.2307/25470707.

38. Lee AK, Wilson MA. Memory of sequential experience in the hippocampus during slow wave sleep. Neuron. 2002;36(6):1183–94. https://doi.org/10.1016/s0896-6273(02)01096-6.

39. Berkers RMWJ, Ekman M, van Dongen EV, Takashima A, Barth M, Paller KA, et al. Cued reactivation during slow-wave sleep induces brain connectivity changes related to memory stabilization. Sci Rep. 2018;8(1):1–12. https://doi.org/10.1038/s41598-018-35287-6.

40. Theodoni P, Rovira B, Wang Y, Roxin A. Theta-modulation drives the emergence of connectivity patterns underlying replay in a network model of place cells. elife. 2018;7:1–33. https://doi.org/10.7554/eLife.37388.

41. Bastuji H, Cadic-Melchior A, Magnin M, Garcia-Larrea L. Intracortical functional connectivity predicts arousal to noxious stimuli during sleep in humans. J Neurosci. 2021;41(23):5115–23. https://doi.org/10.1523/JNEUROSCI.2935-20.2021.

42. Na SH, Jin SH, Kim SY. The effects of total sleep deprivation on brain functional organization: mutual information analysis of waking human EEG. Int J Psychophysiol. 2006;62(2):238–42. https://doi.org/10.1016/j.ijpsycho.2006.03.006.

43. Verweij IM, Romeijn N, Smit DJA, Piantoni G, Van Someren EJW, van der Werf YD. Sleep deprivation leads to a loss of functional connectivity in frontal brain regions. BMC Neurosci. 2014;15:1–10. https://doi.org/10.1186/1471-2202-15-88.

44. Henri-Bhargava A, Stuss DT, Freedman M. Clinical assessment of prefrontal lobe functions. CONTINUUM lifelong learning in Neurology. 2018;24(3, BEHAVIORAL NEUROLOGY AND PSYCHIATRY):704–26. https://doi.org/10.1212/CON.0000000000000609.

45. Qi J, Li BZ, Zhang Y, Pan B, Gao YH, Zhan H, et al. Disrupted small-world networks are associated with decreased vigilant attention after total sleep deprivation. Neuroscience. 2021;471:51–60. https://doi.org/10.1016/j.neuroscience.2021.07.010.

46. Wang H, Yu K, Yang T, Zeng L, Li J, Dai C, et al. Altered functional connectivity in the resting state neostriatum after complete sleep deprivation: impairment of motor control and regulatory network. Front Neurosci. 2021;15(August):1–11. https://doi.org/10.3389/fnins.2021.665687.

47. Skorucak J, Arbon EL, Dijk DJ, Achermann P. Response to chronic sleep restriction, extension, and subsequent total sleep deprivation in humans: adaptation or preserved sleep homeostasis? Sleep. 2018;41(7):1–17. https://doi.org/10.1093/sleep/zsy078.

48. Vyazovskiy VV, Delogu A. NREM and REM sleep: complementary roles in recovery after wakefulness. Neuroscientist. 2014;20(3):203–19. https://doi.org/10.1177/1073858413518152.

49. Mander BA, Reid KJ, Baron KG, Tjoa T, Parrish TB, Paller KA, et al. EEG measures index neural and cognitive recovery from sleep deprivation. J Neurosci. 2010;30(7):2686–93. https://doi.org/10.1523/JNEUROSCI.4010-09.2010.

50. Romano J, Engel GL. Delirium: Electroencephalographic data. Arch Neurol Psychiatr. 1944;51:356–77.

51. Faigle R, Sutter R, Kaplan PW. Electroencephalography of encephalopathy in patients with endocrine and metabolic disorders. J Clin Neurophysiol. 2013;30(5):505–16. https://doi.org/10.1097/WNP.0b013e3182a73db9.

52. Kaplan PW. The EEG in metabolic encephalopathy and coma. J Clin Neurophysiol. 2004;21(5):307–18.

53. Sutter R, Kaplan PW. Clinical and electroencephalographic correlates of acute encephalopathy. J Clin Neurophysiol. 2013;30(5):443–53. https://doi.org/10.1097/WNP.0b013e3182a73bc2.

54. Payne LE, Gagnon DJ, Riker RR, Seder DB, Glisic EK, Morris JG, et al. Cefepime-induced neurotoxicity: a systematic review. Crit Care. 2017;21(1):276. https://doi.org/10.1186/s13054-017-1856-1.

55. Akeju O, Pavone KJ, Westover MB, Vazquez R, Prerau MJ, Harrell PG, et al. A comparison of propofol- and dexmedetomidine-induced electroencephalogram dynamics using spectral and coherence analysis. Anesthesiology. 2014;121(5):978–89. https://doi.org/10.1097/ALN.0000000000000419.

56. Schmitt SE, Pargeon K, Frechette ES, Hirsch LJ, Dalmau J, Friedman D. Extreme delta brush. Neurology. 2012;79(11):1094. https://doi.org/10.1212/WNL.0b013e3182698cd8.

57. Numan T, Slooter AJC, van der Kooi AW, Hoekman AML, Suyker WJL, Stam CJ, et al. Functional connectivity and network analysis during hypoactive delirium and recovery from anesthesia. Clin Neurophysiol. 2017;128(6):914–24. https://doi.org/10.1016/j.clinph.2017.02.022.

58. van der Kooi AW, Slooter AJ, van Het Klooster MA, Leijten FS. EEG in delirium: increased spectral variability and decreased complexity. Clin Neurophysiol. 2014;125(10):2137–9. https://doi.org/10.1016/j.clinph.2014.02.010.

59. Williams Roberson S, Azeez N, Taneja R, Pun BT, Pandharipande P, Jackson JC, et al. The relationship between EEG characteristics during critical illness and long-term cognitive impairment. Neurology. 2020;94(15 Supp)

60. Drouot X, Roche-Campo F, Thille AW, Cabello B, Galia F, Margarit L, et al. A new classification for sleep analysis in critically ill patients. Sleep Med. 2012;13(1):7–14. https://doi.org/10.1016/j.sleep.2011.07.012.

61. Watson PL, Pandharipande P, Gehlbach BK, Thompson JL, Shintani AK, Dittus BS, et al. Atypical sleep in ventilated patients: empirical electroencephalography findings and the path toward revised ICU sleep scoring criteria. Crit Care Med. 2013;41(8):1958–67. https://doi.org/10.1097/CCM.0b013e31828a3f75.

62. Teasdale G, Jennett B. Assessment of coma and impaired consciousness. A practical scale. Lancet. 1974;2(7872):81–4. https://doi.org/10.1016/s0140-6736(74)91639-0.

63. Sessler CN, Gosnell MS, Grap MJ, Brophy GM, O'Neal PV, Keane KA, et al. The Richmond agitation-sedation scale: validity and reliability in adult intensive care unit patients. Am J Respir Crit Care Med. 2002;166(10):1338–44. https://doi.org/10.1164/rccm.2107138.

64. Weinhouse GL, Schwab RJ, Watson PL, Patil N, Vaccaro B, Pandharipande P, et al. Bench-to-bedside review: delirium in ICU patients – importance of sleep deprivation. Crit Care. 2009;13(6) https://doi.org/10.1186/cc8131.

65. Da Mesquita S, Papadopoulos Z, Dykstra T, Brase L, Farias FG, Wall M, et al. Meningeal lymphatics affect microglia responses and anti-Aβ immunotherapy. Nature. 2021;593(7858):255–60. https://doi.org/10.1038/s41586-021-03489-0.

66. Tarasoff-Conway JM, Carare RO, Osorio RS, Glodzik L, Butler T, Fieremans E, et al. Clearance systems in the brain-implications for Alzheimer disease. Nat Rev Neurol. 2015;11(8):457–70. https://doi.org/10.1038/nrneurol.2015.119.

67. Fong TG, Jones RN, Marcantonio ER, Tommet D, Gross AL, Habtemariam D, et al. Adverse outcomes after hospitalization and delirium in persons with Alzheimer disease. Ann Intern Med. 2012;156(12):848–56, W296. https://doi.org/10.7326/0003-4819-156-12-201206190-00005

68. Vyazovskiy VV, Olcese U, Lazimy YM, Faraguna U, Esser SK, Williams JC, et al. Cortical firing and sleep homeostasis. Neuron. 2009;63(6):865–78. https://doi.org/10.1016/j.neuron.2009.08.024.

69. Sanders RD. Hypothesis for the pathophysiology of delirium: role of baseline brain network connectivity and changes in inhibitory tone. Med Hypotheses. 2011;77(1):140–3. https://doi.org/10.1016/j.mehy.2011.03.048.

70. Maldonado JR. Delirium pathophysiology: an updated hypothesis of the etiology of acute brain failure. Int J Geriatr Psychiatry. 2018;33(11):1428–57. https://doi.org/10.1002/gps.4823.

71. Simon EB, Oren N, Sharon H, Kirschner A, Goldway N, Okon-Singer H, et al. Losing neutrality: the neural basis of impaired emotional control without sleep. J Neurosci. 2015;35(38):13194–205. https://doi.org/10.1523/JNEUROSCI.1314-15.2015.

72. Petrovsky N, Ettinger U, Hill A, Frenzel L, Meyhöfer I, Wagner M, et al. Sleep deprivation disrupts prepulse inhibition and induces psychosis-like symptoms in healthy humans. J Neurosci. 2014;34(27):9134. https://doi.org/10.1523/JNEUROSCI.0904-14.2014.

73. Trzepacz PT, Mittal D, Torres R, Kanary K, Norton J, Jimerson N. Validation of the delirium rating scale-revised-98: comparison with the delirium rating scale and the cognitive test for delirium. J Neuropsychiatry Clin Neurosci. 2001;13(2):229–42. https://doi.org/10.1176/jnp.13.2.229.

74. Evans JL, Nadler JW, Preud'homme XA, Fang E, Daughtry RL, Chapman JB, et al. Pilot prospective study of post-surgery sleep and EEG predictors of post-operative delirium. Clin Neurophysiol. 2017;128(8):1421–5. https://doi.org/10.1016/j.clinph.2017.05.004.

75. Pun BT, Balas MC, Barnes-Daly MA, Thompson JL, Aldrich JM, Barr J, et al. Caring for critically ill patients with the ABCDEF bundle: results of the ICU liberation collaborative in over 15,000 adults. Crit Care Med. 2019;47(1):3–14. https://doi.org/10.1097/CCM.0000000000003482.

76. Devlin JW, Skrobik Y, Gelinas C, Needham DM, Slooter AJC, Pandharipande PP, et al. Clinical practice guidelines for the prevention and Management of Pain, agitation/sedation, delirium, immobility, and sleep disruption in adult patients in the ICU. Crit Care Med. 2018;46(9):e825–e73. https://doi.org/10.1097/CCM.0000000000003299.

77. Nicholson T, Patel J, Sleigh JW. Sleep patterns in intensive care unit patients: a study using the bispectral index. Crit Care Resusc. 2001;3(2):86–91.

78. Arnal PJ, Thorey V, Debellemaniere E, Ballard ME, Bou Hernandez A, Guillot A, et al. The Dreem headband compared to polysomnography for electroencephalographic signal acquisition and sleep staging. Sleep. 2020;43(11) https://doi.org/10.1093/sleep/zsaa097.

79. Mikkelsen KB, Tabar YR, Kappel SL, Christensen CB, Toft HO, Hemmsen MC, et al. Accurate whole-night sleep monitoring with dry-contact ear-EEG. Sci Rep. 2019;9(1):16824. https://doi.org/10.1038/s41598-019-53115-3.

80. Watson PL. Measuring sleep in critically ill patients: beware the pitfalls. Crit Care. 2007;11(4):159. https://doi.org/10.1186/cc6094.

81. Pisani MA, Friese RS, Gehlbach BK, Schwab RJ, Weinhouse GL, Jones SF. Sleep in the intensive care unit. Am J Respir Crit Care Med. 2015;191(7):731–8. https://doi.org/10.1164/rccm.201411-2099CI.

82. Pandharipande PP, Girard TD, Jackson JC, Morandi A, Thompson JL, Pun BT, et al. Long-term cognitive impairment after critical illness. N Engl J Med. 2013;369(14):1306–16. https://doi.org/10.1056/NEJMoa1301372.

83. Ma Y, Liang L, Zheng F, Shi L, Zhong B, Xie W. Association between sleep duration and cognitive decline. JAMA Netw Open. 2020;3(9):e2013573. https://doi.org/10.1001/jamanetworkopen.2020.13573.
84. Altman MT, Knauert MP, Pisani MA. Sleep disturbance after hospitalization and critical illness: a systematic review. Ann Am Thorac Soc. 2017;14(9):1457–68. https://doi.org/10.1513/AnnalsATS.201702-148SR.
85. Wilcox ME, McAndrews MP, Van J, Jackson JC, Pinto R, Black SE, et al. Sleep fragmentation and cognitive trajectories after critical illness. Chest. 2021;159(1):366–81. https://doi.org/10.1016/j.chest.2020.07.036.
86. Wilcox ME, Lim AS, McAndrews MP, Wennberg RA, Pinto RL, Black SE, et al. A study protocol for an observational cohort investigating COGnitive outcomes and WELLness in survivors of critical illness: the COGWELL study. BMJ Open. 2017;7(7):e015600. https://doi.org/10.1136/bmjopen-2016-015600.
87. Waser M, Lauritzen MJ, Fagerlund B, Osler M, Mortensen EL, Sørensen HBD, et al. Sleep efficiency and neurophysiological patterns in middle-aged men are associated with cognitive change over their adult life course. J Sleep Res. 2019;28(4):e12793. https://doi.org/10.1111/jsr.12793.

Sleep Disruption and Its Relationship with Delirium: Clinical Perspectives

Yoanna Skrobik and John W. Devlin

1 Introduction

Delirium, a syndrome characterized by acute alteration in mental status, occurs in up to 50% of mechanically ventilated critically ill adults [1, 2] and is an independent risk factor for poor ICU and post-ICU outcomes [3]. Delirium reduction has become a priority in the care of the critically ill. As detailed in chapters "Characteristics of Sleep in Critically Ill Patients. Part I: Sleep Fragmentation and Sleep Stage Disruption" and "Characteristics of Sleep in Critically Ill Patients. Part II: Circadian Rhythm Disruption" sleep disruption and abnormal sleep architecture are common in the ICU. Sleep in patients who are critically ill demonstrates prolonged sleep latency, sleep fragmentation, and numerous arousals. These abnormalities are associated with important effects on ICU (chapter "ICU Sleep Disruption and Its Relationship with ICU Outcomes") and post-ICU (chapter "Long-Term Outcomes: Sleep in Survivors of Critical Illness") outcomes. While several non-pharmacological sleep promotion efforts have been shown to reduce delirium, they have not been demonstrated to improve sleep, regardless of whether it is evaluated by objective or subjective means (chapter "Best Practices for Improving Sleep in the ICU. Part I: Non-pharmacologic"). As outlined in chapter "Best Practices for Improving Sleep in the ICU. Part II: Pharmacologic", evidence that pharmacologic interventions improve sleep is sparse.

Although many clinicians assume poor sleep provokes delirium and delirium provokes poor sleep [4], any association between delirium and disrupted sleep in the

Y. Skrobik
Department of Medicine, McGill University, Quebec, Canada

J. W. Devlin (✉)
Bouve College of Health Sciences, Northeastern University and Division of Pulmonary and Critical Care Medicine, Brigham and Women's Hospital, Boston, MA, USA
e-mail: jwdevlin@bwh.harvard.edu

G. L. Weinhouse, J. W. Devlin (eds.), *Sleep in Critical Illness*,
https://doi.org/10.1007/978-3-031-06447-0_9

149

complex ICU environment remains unclear. Abnormal sleep is present in more than one quarter of patients hospitalized in critical care units [5, 6]. Further, since severe sleep deprivation in critically ill adults can lead to symptoms of inattention, emotional lability (and thus inappropriateness), and delusional thoughts or hallucinations, the value of psychometric evaluations in the ICU setting remains unclear where confounders abound and links between clinical features of sleep deprivation and relevant outcomes remain challenging to align [7–9]. Moreover, the mechanical ventilator settings known to affect sleep in critically ill adults have not been evaluated for their effect on delirium symptoms (chapter "Mechanical Ventilation and Sleep") [10].

Consideration of the impact of pre-morbid status on outcomes pertinent to ICU sleep and delirium remains challenging as the presence of chronic disease, cognitive decline and frailty are usually not systematically screened for at the time of ICU admission. Baseline frailty increases the delirium risk and is frequent among older adults [11–13]. In one recent non-pharmacological delirium prevention interventional RCT, 75% of patients aged 70 or more presented with at least mild baseline cognitive deficits despite living autonomously and seemingly without overt cognitive abnormalities prior to hospitalization [14]. The physiologic relationship between sleep and delirium in the ICU is reviewed in chapter "Sleep Disruption and Its Relationship with Delirium: Electroencephalographic Perspectives". The objective of this chapter is to review the clinical relationship between sleep and delirium in critically ill adults.

2   Risk Factors

Risk factors for delirium and disrupted sleep before the ICU, at the time of ICU admission and during the ICU stay (see also chapter "Risk Factors for Disrupted Sleep in the ICU") are compared in Table 1 [11, 12, 15]. Important challenges exist in comparing risk factors for delirium and disrupted sleep given a lack of published studies comparing delirium and sleep risk factors in the same cohort of patients, the presence of delirium has not been controlled for in ICU sleep risk factor studies, and the multiple ways an ICU patient can be deemed to have 'disrupted sleep". Moreover, the pathophysiologic mechanisms for some risk factors common to both delirium and sleep (e.g., sedative-induced coma) may be different (see chapter "Normal Sleep Compared to Altered Consciousness During Sedation").

Several studies have found a relationship between preexisting sleep disorder syndromes and postoperative delirium [16, 17]. Following cardiac surgery, for example, sleep disordered breathing risk has been associated with a six-fold increase in delirium risk [17]. Circadian misalignment is a known risk factor for delirium [18–20]. In healthy patients, release of melatonin is highly influenced by sleep-wake

Table 1 Comparison of risk factors for delirium and disrupted sleep in critically ill adults

	Delirium	Disrupted sleep
Before ICU admission		
Male gender	X	X
Older age	X	X
Reduced cognitive function	X	
Psychiatric co-morbidity	X	X
Frailty	X	
Insomnia		X
Obstructive sleep apnea		X
Hearing/visual loss	X	
≥ Moderate alcohol use	X	X
Functional impairment	X	
ICU admission		
Severity of illness	X	X
Infection/sepsis	X	
Sedative-induced coma	X	X
Urgent ICU admission	X	X
Pain	X	X
During ICU admission		
Severity of illness	X	X
Infection/sepsis	X	X
Sedative-induced coma	X	X
Medication use/withdrawal	X	X
Mechanical ventilation/ hypoxia	X	X
Immobility	X	X
Blood transfusion	X	
Lack of family presence	X	X
Noise		X
Pain	X	X
Light		X

rhythms and zeitbegers such as ambient light, the feeding schedule and social interactions. However, in the ICU setting, lighting is often kept low throughout the day, continuous (vs. scheduled) enteral feedings are common and the ability of patients to interact with their environment is reduced, particularly when sedatives are used. In the face of these reduced zeitgebers, circadian misalignment is common in critically ill adults (chapter "Characteristics of Sleep in Critically Ill Patients. Part II: Circadian Rhythm Disruption").

3 Epidemiology and Outcomes

Disrupted sleep and delirium each are associated with negative ICU and post-ICU outcomes, many of which are of high concern to patients and their families [1, 3–5, 15, 21].

3.1 Disrupted Sleep

Sleep is a periodic, reversible state of cognitive and sensory disengagement from the external environment. As outlined in chapters "Characteristics of Sleep in Critically Ill Patients. Part I: Sleep Fragmentation and Sleep Stage Disruption" and "Sleep Disruption and Its Relationship with delirium: Electroencephalographic Perspectives", sleep can be staged using EEG criteria into non-rapid eye movement (NREM) [stage 1, stage 2 (light sleep), stage 3 (deep sleep)] and rapid eye movement (REM) phases that are associated with distinct physiologic changes, neuroanatomic substrates, and neurochemical correlates.

As reviewed in chapter "Characteristics of Sleep in Critically Ill Patients. Part II: Circadian Rhythm Disruption", sleep and wakefulness are controlled by the circadian regulatory system and by the sleep homeostatic process [19, 20]. The circadian timing system is responsible for multiple biologic processes including endocrine regulation of hormones including cortisol. Although establishing a circadian rhythm pattern of care in the ICU has been proposed as one non-pharmacological approach to diminish sleep disruption in the noisy, busy, caregiver-focused critical care environment, it may be difficult to operationalize given the 50% of individuals who are 'night owls' rather than 'morning people' [22], while most ICUs function with a rigid schedule where sleep is expected to start in the evening and care activities early in the morning. Beyond physiology, clinical context-dependent symptoms including pain and anxiety drive sleep disruption.

3.2 Delirium

Delirium, the phenotypic expression of acute encephalopathy [23], has four cardinal features: (1) a disturbed level of consciousness (i.e., a reduced clarity of awareness of the environment), with a reduced ability to focus, sustain, or shift attention; and (2) either a change in cognition (i.e., memory deficit, disorientation, language disturbance), or the development of a perceptual disturbance (i.e., hallucinations, delusions) [24]. A common misconception is that delirious patients are either hallucinating or delusional, but neither of these symptoms is required to make the diagnosis.

Whether the long-term cognitive impairment [25] attributable to ICU delirium is related in part to pre-ICU cognitive frailty and severity of illness is challenging to analyze. These confounders were not considered in most ICU trials other than those permitting cognitive assessments prior to ICU admission [14]. Moreover, although frailty is increasingly becoming recognized as the single most important driver of overall prognosis beyond severity of illness in the critically ill [13, 26], none of its metrics consider functionality beyond autonomy and physical strength. Cognitive 'frailty', therefore' has not been well- established or linked to delirium. Whether frailty in the context of sleep disruption even exists or is linked to predisposition to delirium or frailty in other dimensions remains unclear. Even though sleep patterns and cognitive patterns change over time, particularly after age 60 for sleep and 45 for cognition, these observations and studies have not, to our knowledge, been duplicated in a critically ill population.

4   Sleep Deprivation and Delirium Symptoms

Sleep deprivation and delirium share many common symptoms (Table 2). Patients who experience acute sleep deprivation demonstrate many of the same sequelae of delirium including diminished psychomotor performance, short-term memory impairment and difficulty with executive functioning [1]. In addition, sleep deprivation leads to mood disturbances including irritability, inattention, disorientation, anxiety, depression, and paranoia [21, 26]. One study of young healthy adults demonstrated severe sleep deprivation to be associated with symptoms within 24 h of its occurrence including perceptual distortions, visual hallucinations, and changes in mood ranging from apathy to disordered thoughts with impairment in attention [27]. The marked similarity in symptoms between sleep disruption and delirium have prompted experts to draw links between the two and question both the relationship and the directionality of this relationship.

The Diagnostic and Statistical Manual of Mental Disorders, fifth edition [24], reorganized sleep disorders into three major categories: insomnia, hypersomnia and arousal disorders that incorporate 11 different diagnostic groups. Growing evidence has shown that sleep disorders coexist with other medical and psychiatric disorders and may not be mutually exclusive. DSM-5 underscores the need for independent clinical attention of sleep disorder(s) regardless of other mental or medical problems that may be present. DSM-5 also recognizes that coexisting medical conditions, mental disorders, and sleep disorders are interactive and bidirectional. Two previous diagnoses have been eliminated: sleep disorder related to another mental disorder and sleep disorder related to another medical condition. The DSM-5 criteria for delirium shares many of the symptoms of these DSM-5 sleep disorders.

Table 2 Common symptoms of sleep deprivation and delirium

Anxiety
Agitation/restlessness
Confusion
Circadian dysregulation: Nighttime wakefulness
Emotional lability
Irritability
Lethargy
Reduced short-term memory
Reduced executive function
Reduced responsiveness
Sympathetic stimulation: Increased heart rate/blood pressure

5 Assessment of Sleep and Delirium

5.1 Sleep

Although a number of different objective and subjective methods to evaluate sleep in the ICU exist (chapter "Best Practice for Improving Sleep in the ICU. Part I: Non-pharmacologic"), limitations exist with each assessment method and thus sleep is usually not routinely evaluated in the ICU setting [28]. Patient self-reported sleep poses challenges in sedated patients and those who experience moderate to severe delirium or have delirium symptoms during the assessment. Beyond scales and physiologic measurements, patients report a significant proportion of sleep disruption as originating from psychological distress, anxiety, fear, and pain. Yet, other than pain, these symptoms are not routinely evaluated by bedside clinicians and their potential relationship with sleep deprivation may not be considered.

Standard sleep quality assessment from patients and family members at the time of ICU admission will identify the 25% of patients who have baseline disrupted sleep. Routinely making the patient comfortable, in a familiar sleep position and asking about fears and worries may mitigate patient fears and diminish the need for sedatives and restraints. Making a more concentrated effort to understand patient preferences for comfort and stress reduction to facilitate natural sleep intuitively should lead to better quality sleep.

5.2 Delirium

Practice guidelines [12] and care improvement bundles [29] advocate critically ill adults be routinely assessed for delirium using validated assessment tools like the Confusion Assessment Method for the ICU (CAM-ICU) [30] or the Intensive Care Delirium Screening Checklist [31] in an effort to facilitate delirium risk factor recognition (and modulation) and non-pharmacologic interventions to reduce its duration. However, the potential benefit from this process assumes ICU clinicians are well-trained to evaluate delirium, will document assessment results, are motivated to engage with the rest of the ICU interprofessional team when delirium is recognized, and do the hard work in reducing risk factors and implementing non-pharmacologic improvement strategies [11, 12]. Regular evaluation of patient symptoms in critically ill adults is clearly important. One controlled trial found the time from ICU delirium recognition to the initiation of treatment was similar between clinicians using the CAM-ICU compared to clinicians who were educated on the symptoms of delirium and the importance of delirium-related outcomes [32].

Even twice per day routine screening may miss delirium (and its symptoms) when one considers 40% of delirium symptoms occur between midnight and 6 am, a period when ICU clinicians are infrequently at patients' bedsides [33]. Whether routine screening is necessary if clinicians are interested and engaged in evaluating delirium is not clear. Regardless, the recognition and mitigation of fear, through patient reassurance, remains an important component of bedside care at night in patients unable to sleep. Both authors have witnessed narratives from ICU survivors describing how comforting such reassurance can be in fostering hope and stabilizing anxiety. This simple approach has not been studied either for its impact in de-escalating anxiety, minimizing sedative use or improving outcomes.

6 Patient-Centered Evaluations Linked to Both Sleep and Delirium

Below, we wish to highlight the importance of considering such metrics in a broader context of humanizing care, both from the patient perspective and from the point of view of the caregiver.

Patients report that their loss of a sense of agency was among the most distressful parts of their critical illness. Realizing ICUs may be one of the last frontiers of autocratic care, and patients may be positioned in ways deemed 'safe' and convenient for staff to deliver interventions, patient's sleep preferences and habits should be determined and applied when possible. Unfortunately, no matter how assiduously nursing staff record delirium or sleep assessments in the health record, if physicians and other ICU caregivers disregard these reports, the value of conducting these monitoring efforts becomes diminished to bedside nurses.

Sedation and restraints are administered in the name of safety [34]. Neither approach has been shown to reduce risk of invasive ICU-care related instrument (endotracheal tube, central line) removal. Both approaches add risk and significant disadvantages in terms of patient outcome in association with delirium; the impact of sedatives is discussed in detail in the chapter "Effects of Common ICU Medications on Sleep." The impact of restraints on sleep quality has not, to our knowledge, been evaluated. Patients remember being restrained as an unpleasant and distressful component of their critical care stay [35].

The rate of clinician burnout was about 50% before the COVID-19 pandemic; it is now much higher [36]. Any suggestion of improving care at the bedside that incorporates additional measures is likely to be met with the resistance of already overstretched or tired staff [37, 38]. Three elements should be considered: (1) it should be simple to do and document; (2) the change should make the caregiver feel good so they keep doing it beyond 'data' supporting it is good for patients, and this work should be recognized by other team members; (3) for any sustainability there has to be ongoing benchmarking and preferably comparators with other units or hospitals to ensure ongoing friendly competition to perform.

7 The Relationship Between Sleep and Delirium Reported in ICU Clinical Studies

A number of ICU clinical studies evaluating interventions focused on improving sleep in the ICU have reported reduced delirium but no improvement in sleep [39–42]. For example, one randomized controlled trial (RCT) comparing low-dose nocturnal dexmedetomidine to placebo in non-delirious ICU patients reported dexmedetomidine significantly reduces delirium occurrence (relative risk 0.44; 95% CI 0.23 to 0.82) but patient-reported sleep quality was similar between groups (mean difference, 0.02; 95% CI 0.42 to 1.92) [42]. In a follow up study, the association between morning Leeds Sleep Evaluation Questionnaire (LSEQ) score and delirium occurrence in the prior 24 h (retrospective analysis) and the association between morning LSEQ score and delirium occurrence in the following 24 h (predictive analysis) was measured for all 24 h periods where the patient had both a delirium and LSEQ assessment and remained free of coma [43]. Using a model that accounted for age, severity of illness and dexmedetomidine (vs. placebo) use, the LSEQ score had no relationship to subsequent delirium. Similarly, the implementation of multi-component sleep improvement protocols in critically ill adults have reported a reduction in delirium but no change in sleep improvement [44]. For example, in one cohort of 300 medical ICU patients [40], implementation of a stepped protocol increased ICU days free of delirium and coma by more than half but had little effect on patient-perceived sleep.

8 Areas for Future Investigation

The relationship between subjective sleep quality and delirium remains poorly explored; multiple investigative challenges exist in critically ill adults. Any study addressing whether a link between subjective sleep quality and delirium exists should pair delirium and sleep assessments in individual patients and consider them over short time periods given the natural fluctuation of both of these outcomes over the course of the ICU stay. In any ICU sleep-delirium cohort study, established baseline and daily ICU risk factors know to disrupt sleep (see chapter "Risk Factors for Disrupted Sleep in the ICU"), increase delirium, or both must be considered.

9 Conclusions

Delirium and sleep disruption, and the symptoms associated with both, should be rigorously evaluated in critically ill adults. Non pharmacologic interventions focused on improving sleep should be optimized given their use will reduce delirium. A number of important avenues of research are required to better understand the inter-relationship between delirium and sleep in the ICU and those interventions best suited to improve both.

References

1. Wilson JE, Mart MF, Cunningham C, et al. Nat Rev Dis Primers. 2020; 6(1):90.
2. Rood P, Huisman-de Waal G, Vermeulen H, Schoonhoven L, Pickkers P, van den Boogaard M. Effect of organizational factors on the variation in incidence of delirium in intensive care unit patients: a systematic review and meta-regression analysis. Aust Crit Care. 2018;31(3):180–7.
3. Salluh JI, Wang H, Schneider EB, Nagaraja N, Yenokyan G, Damluji A, et al. Outcome of delirium in critically ill patients: systematic review and meta-analysis. BMJ. 2015;350:2538.
4. Kamdar BB, Knauert MP, Jones SF, Parsons EC, Parthasarathy S, Pisani MA, et al. Perceptions and practices regarding sleep in the intensive care unit. A survey of 1,223 critical care providers. Ann Am Thorac Soc. 2016;13:1370–7.
5. Weinhouse GL, Schwab RJ, Watson PL, Patil N, Vaccaro B, Pandharipande P, et al. Bench-to-bedside review: delirium in ICU patients – importance of sleep deprivation. Crit Care. 2009;13:234.
6. Telias I, Wilcox ME. Sleep and circadian rhythm in critical illness. Crit Care. 2019;23:82.
7. Fisher S. The microstructure of dual-task interaction. 4. Sleep deprivation and the control of attention. Perception. 1980;9(3):327–37.
8. Boesen HC, Andersen JH, Bendtsen AO, Jennum PJ. Sleep and delirium in unsedated patients in the intensive care unit. Acta Anaesthiol Scand. 2016;60(1):59–68.
9. Waters F, Chiu V, Atkinson A, Blon JD. Severe sleep deprivation causes hallucinations and a gradual progression towards psychosis with increasing time awake. Front Psych. 2018;9:303.
10. Cooper AB, Thornley KS, Young GB, Slutsky AS, Stewart TE, Hanly PJ. Sleep in critically ill patients requiring mechanical ventilation. Chest. 2000;117(3):809–18.
11. Zaal IJ, Devlin JW, Peelen LM, Slooter AJ. A systematic review of risk factors for delirium in the ICU. Crit Care Med. 2015;43:40–7.
12. Devlin JW, Skrobik Y, Gélinas C, et al. Clinical practice guidelines for the prevention and management of pain, agitation/sedation, delirium, immobility, and sleep disruption in adult patients in the ICU. Crit Care Med. 2018;46(9):e825–73.
13. Muscedere J, Waters B, Varambally A, et al. The impact of frailty on intensive care unit outcomes: a systematic review and meta-analysis. Intensive Care Med. 2017;43(8):1105–22.

14. Deeken F, Sanchez A, Rapp MA, et al. Outcomes of a delirium prevention program in older persons after elective surgery: a stepped-wedge, cluster randomized clinical trial. JAMA Surg. 2022;157:e216370.
15. Honarmond K, Rafay H, Le J, et al. A systematic review of risk factors for sleep disruption in critically ill adults. Crit Care Med. 2020;48(7):1066–74.
16. Roggenbach J, Klamman M, von Haken R, Bruckner T, Karck M, Hofer S. Sleep-disordered breathing is a risk factor for delirium after cardiac surgery: a prospective cohort study. Crit Care. 2014;18(5):477.
17. Fadayomi AB, Ibala R, Bilotta F, Westover MB, Akeju O. A systematic review and meta-analysis examining the impact of sleep disturbances on postoperative delirium. Crit Care Med. 2018;46(12):e1204–12.
18. Balan S, Leibovitz A, Zila SO, Ruth M, ChanaW YB, et al. The relation between the clinical subtypes of delirium and the urinary level of 6-SMT. J Neuropsychiatry Clin Neurosci. 2003:15:363–6. https://doi.org/10.1176/jnp.15.3.363.
19. Li CX, Liang DD, Xie GH, et al. Altered melatonin secretion and circadian gene expression with increased proinflammatory cytokine expression in early-stage sepsis patients. Mol Med Rep. 2013;7:1117–22.
20. Gehlbach BK, Chapotot F, Leproult R, et al. Temporal disorganization of circadian rhythmicity and sleep-wake regulation in mechanically ventilated patients receiving continuous intravenous sedation. Sleep. 2012;35(8):1105–14.
21. Altman MT, Knauert MP, Pisani MA. Sleep disturbance after hospitalization and critical illness: a systematic review. Ann Am Thorac Soc. 2017;14(9):1457–68.
22. https://www.sleepfoundation.org/how-sleep-works/chronotypes. Accessed March 5, 2022.
23. Slooter AJC, Otte WM, Devlin JW, et al. Updated nomenclature of delirium and acute encephalopathy: statement of ten societies. Intensive Care Med. 2020;46(5):1020–2.
24. American Psychiatric Association. Diagnostic and statistical manual of mental disorders. 5th ed. Arlington, VA: American Psychiatric Association; 2013.
25. Pandharipande PP, Girard TD, Jackson JC, et al. Long-term cognitive impairment after critical illness. N Engl J Med. 2013;1(14):1306–16.
26. Wilcox ME, McAndrews MP, Van J, et al. Sleep fragmentation and cognitive trajectories after critical illness. Chest. 2020;56:112–9.
27. Bishir M, Bhat A, Essa MM, et al. Sleep deprivation and neurological disorders. Biomed Res Int. 2020;5764017
28. Weinhouse GL, Kimchi E, Watson P, Devlin JW. Sleep assessment in critically ill adults: established methods and emerging strategies. Crit Care Explor. 2022;4(2):E0628.
29. Pun BT, Balas MC, Barnes-Daly MA, et al. Caring for critically ill patients with the ABCDEF bundle: results of the ICU liberation collaborative in over 15,000 adults. Crit Care Med. 2019;47(1):3–14.
30. Ely EW, Margolin R, Francis J, et al. Evaluation of delirium in critically ill patients: validation of the Confusion Assessment Method for the Intensive Care Unit (CAM-ICU). Crit Care Med. 2001;29(7):1370–9.
31. Bergeron N, Dubois MJ, Dumont M, et al. Intensive care delirium screening checklist: evaluation of a new screening tool. Intensive Care Med. 2001;27:859–64.
32. Bigatello LM, Amirfarzan H, Haghighi AK, et al. Effects of routine monitoring of delirium in a surgical/trauma intensive care unit. Trauma Acute Care Surg. 2013;74(3):876–83.
33. Devlin JW, Fraser GF, Joffe A, Riker RR, Skrobik Y. The accurate recognition of delirium in the ICU: more new clothes for the emperor. Intensive Care Med. 2013;39(12):2196–9.
34. Guidelines FS, Hallett C, McHugh G. Physical restraint: experiences, attitudes and opinions of adult intensive care unit nurses. Nurs Crit Care. 2016;21(2):78–87.
35. Simini B. Patients' perceptions of intensive care. Lancet. 1999;354(9178):571–2.
36. Krause AJ, Simon EB, Mander BA, et al. The sleep-deprived human brain. Nat Rev Neurosci. 2017;18(7):404–18.

37. Ben Simon E, Vallat R, Barnes CM, Walker MP. Sleep loss and the socio-emotional brain. Trends Cogn Sci. 2020;24(6):435–50.
38. Moll V, Meissen H, Pappas S, et al. The coronavirus disease 2019 pandemic impacts burnout syndrome differently among multi professional critical care clinicians – a longitudinal survey study. Crit Care Med. 2022;50(3):440–8.
39. Ibrahim MG, Bellomo R, Hart GK, et al. A double-blind placebo-controlled randomised pilot study of nocturnal melatonin in tracheostomised patients. Crit Care Resusc. 2006;8(3):187–91.
40. Kamdar BB, King LM, Collop NA, et al. The effect of a quality improvement intervention on perceived sleep quality and cognition in a medical ICU. Crit Care Med. 2013;41:800–9.
41. Litton E, Carnegie V, Elliott R, Webb SA. The efficacy of earplugs as a sleep hygiene strategy reducing delirium in the ICU: a systematic review and meta-analysis. Crit Care Med. 2016;44(5):992–9.
42. Skrobik Y, Duprey MS, Hill NS, Devlin JW. Low-dose nocturnal dexmedetomidine prevents ICU delirium. A randomized, placebo-controlled trial. Am J Respir Crit Care Med. 2018;197:1147–56.
43. Duprey MS, Devlin JW, Skrobik Y. Association between subjective sleep quality and daily delirium occurrence in critically ill adults: a post-hoc evaluation of a randomized controlled trial. BMJ Open Respir Res. 2020;7(1):e000576.
44. Louzon PR, Heavner MS, Herod K, Wu TT, Devlin JW. Sleep-promotion bundle development, implementation, and evaluation in critically ill adults: roles for pharmacists. Ann Pharmacotherapy. 2022;56(7):839–49.

Mechanical Ventilation and Sleep

Lauren E. Estep and Sairam Parthasarathy

1 Introduction

The objective of this chapter is to synthesize the current literature regarding the inter-relationship between mechanical ventilation and sleep to help the reader apply such knowledge at the bedside and identify future knowledge gaps. Researchers have studied the impact of mechanical ventilation on sleep and, conversely, they have also studied the potential effects of sleep disturbances on aspects of mechanical ventilation in the critical care setting. Considering the paucity of studies evaluating the effect of sleep on mechanical ventilation in the critical care setting, we will also draw upon robust findings from experimental physiology, where appropriate. Such experiments may have involved healthy subjects or participants with respiratory disease who are not critically ill, and we will identify the associated caveats and cautions pertaining to such extrapolation.

L. E. Estep
Division of Pulmonary, Allergy, Critical Care and Sleep Medicine, University of Arizona, Tucson, AZ, USA
e-mail: lestep@arizona edu

S. Parthasarathy (✉)
Division of Pulmonary, Allergy, Critical Care & Sleep Medicine, University of Arizona College of Medicine, Tucson, AZ, USA
e-mail: spartha1@arizona.edu

G. L. Weinhouse, J. W. Devlin (eds.), *Sleep in Critical Illness*,
https://doi.org/10.1007/978-3-031-06447-0_10

2 Conceptual Framework

A conceptual framework with the need for mechanical ventilatory assistance as being central (Fig. 1; red box) presents the reader with the length and breadth of the complexity of the study of sleep and mechanical ventilation. By nature, invasive mechanical ventilation through an endotracheal tube is very uncomfortable and the attendant noxious stimuli can disturb sleep (Fig. 1; blue box). Other required invasive devices (e.g., nasogastric or urinary catheters, arterial lines, etc.), or the application of physical restraints that are placed by virtue of initiating invasive mechanical ventilation, can similarly produce discomfort and thereby disrupt sleep. (see chapter "Risk Factors for Disrupted Sleep in the ICU"). Moreover, intravenous sedation and analgesia that are administered to reduce the discomfort of invasive mechanical ventilation, may, in turn, inadvertently alter the very nature of sleep (see chapter "Effects of Common ICU Medications on Sleep"). It should be noted here that non-invasive ventilation approaches such as high flow nasal cannula (HFNC), noninvasive intermittent positive pressure ventilation (NIPPV), or nasal continuous positive airway pressure (NCPAP) do not necessarily require escalation in administering sedatives or analgesics. The lower use of sedative/analgesia during noninvasive versus invasive ventilation suggests noninvasive ventilation approaches are less noxious than invasive mechanical ventilation, and thus less likely to disrupt sleep, despite a lack of empirical evidence directly evaluating the relationship between pain/discomfort and sleep in these individuals. Lastly, the administration of supplemental oxygen through a face mask or traditional nasal cannula could be used as another comparator in being the least intrusive to sleep. However, in the absence of

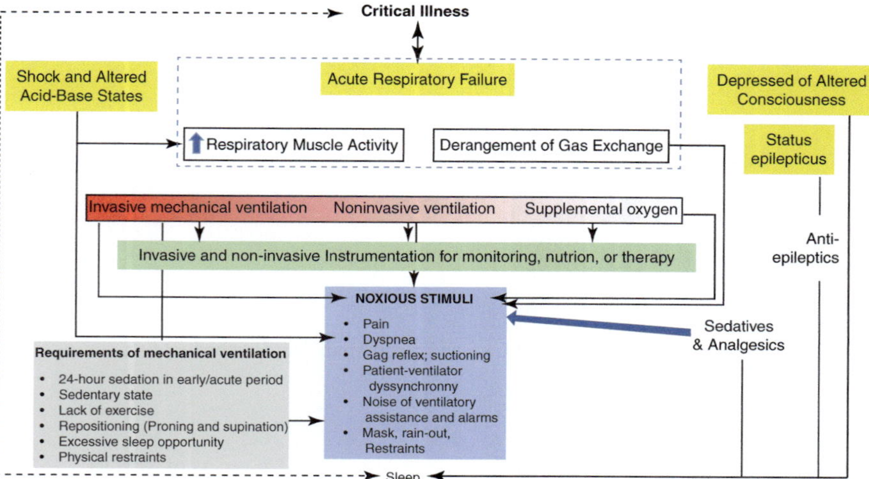

Fig. 1 A schematic review of variables both directly and indirectly related to mechanical ventilation which can have affects on patients' ability to sleep. The highlighted yellow boxes represent the indications for mechanical ventilation

randomized controlled trial (RCTs) data, direct comparisons of sleep across the spectrum of patients needing invasive mechanical ventilation, noninvasive ventilation, or supplemental oxygen, cannot be made given the confounding influence of acuity of underlying illness on sleep quality.

Besides acute respiratory failure, there are other indications for mechanical ventilation that can independently—or together with concomitant medications and therapies—adversely affect sleep (Fig. 1; yellow boxes). Altered gas-exchange, increased respiratory muscle activity, and other noxious stimuli secondary to mismatch of ventilator settings and patient demands (patient-ventilator desynchrony) may be disruptive to sleep. Such respiratory stimuli incurred by increased respiratory muscle activity are more potent in causing arousals than derangements in gas exchange (hypoxia or hypercapnia) [1–3]. More directly, the noise of the respiratory assistance and associated ventilator alarms in addition to other noise emanating in an ICU can adversely impact sleep [4, 5] (see chapter "Risk Factors for Disrupted Sleep in the ICU"). Also, suctioning of endotracheal or tracheostomy tubes, noninvasive mask interface, nasal fluids due to the "rain out" from high humidity systems used in high flow systems of oxygen delivery are noxious stimuli that disturb sleep [6–8].

There are certain requirements that are peculiar to patients receiving mechanical ventilation that by virtue of their *prima facie* nature do not deserve the needed attention for scientific inquiry. There is an unhealthy level of opportunity for sleep when a critically ill patient is recumbent for 24-h a day that inherently works against 7–8 h of good and well-timed sleep, i.e. good sleep hygiene [9, 10] (see chapter "Characteristics of Sleep in Critically Ill Patients. Part II: Circadian Rhythm Disruption"). This creates a conundrum for the field of study of sleep during mechanical ventilation considering that there are 16 h of the day when the patient is being exposed to the afore-mentioned noxious setting without the "cover" of unconsciousness if the goal is to get 8 h of continuous, good quality sleep (Fig. 1; grey box). The sedentary nature, at least early in the acute state, combined with the lack of exercise can disrupt sleep or is at least not conducive for facilitating sleep onset [11]. Moreover, after prolonged periods of mechanical ventilation or in individuals who are uncooperative or delirious, the need to apply physical restraints to prevent accidental extubation or disconnection from ventilator causes greater distress and anxiety that are not conducive for sleep [12, 13] (see chapter "Sleep Disruption and Its Relationship with Delirium: Clinical Perspectives").

3 Epidemiology and Scope of the Problem

The birth of the intensive care unit (ICU) revolved around invasive mechanical ventilation for acute respiratory failure and is therefore highly relevant to the discussions regarding sleep in critically ill patients [14]. Today, treatment of acute respiratory failure accounts for more than one-third of ICU admissions globally [15]. Among these patients only 35% received invasive mechanical ventilation (as compared with almost all patients two decades ago); two-thirds received other forms of respiratory support including noninvasive mechanical ventilation [16]. Conceivably, the burden posed by mechanical ventilation on sleep in critically ill patients could be posited to have decreased with the sea shift from invasive to non-invasive mechanical ventilation. Over the past 2 decades, there has also been a reduction in the administration of sedatives effected by daily sedation interruptions and lighter sedation targets [17]. During the early Coronavirus disease 2019 (COVID-19) pandemic, however, there was a shift towards early intubation and heavier sedation [18], Now, however, the pendulum has swung back with cautionary notes against early intubation [19, 20]. With such seesawing trends, with regards to invasive versus noninvasive mechanical ventilation, similar swings on the impact to sleep in critically ill patients receiving ventilatory assist should be anticipated and used to contextualize the findings of a given observational or intervention-based study.

Through the remainder of this chapter, we highlight intervention-based studies over observational approaches considering the number and complexity of confounding variables and the possibility of residual confounding, reverse causation, or confounding by indication in observational studies. In the absence of intervention-based or experimental data derived from participants who are not critically ill, we will highlight the observational studies and the knowledge gaps that needs addressing.

4　Modes of Mechanical Ventilation

Mechanical ventilation allows manipulation of various respiratory parameters which may affect the quality and continuity of sleep by their effects on patient comfort, synchrony with the mechanical breaths, and potentially by their effectiveness at managing gas exchange. It is, therefore, not just the mode of ventilation but also the skill with which it is adjusted that can relieve dyspnea, dyssynchrony, and hypercarbia for example. Investigators have performed RCTs that studied various modes of mechanical ventilation with cross over design intended to reduce the effects of inter-individual variability [21–28].

4.1　Assist Control Versus Pressure Support

In an early study comparing assist control ventilation (ACV) against pressure support ventilation (PSV) in patients receiving mechanical ventilation, patients supported on ACV developed less sleep fragmentation (measured as arousals and awakenings per hour of sleep) when compared to when they were receiving PSV [21] (see also chapter "Characteristics of Sleep in Critically Ill Patients. Part I: Sleep Fragmentation and Sleep Stage Disruption"). The absence of a back-up rate during pressure support combined with an unstable respiratory controller associated with congestive heart failure played a mechanistic role in creating central apneas and hyperpneas that associated with arousal from sleep. A third arm consisting of pressure support with added dead space elevated the operating partial pressure of CO_2 ($PaCO_2$) above the apnea threshold and reduced the respiratory instability and thereby improved sleep when compared to pressure support alone. While there were concerns that the presence of central apneas signified excessive support, it should be noted that the level of pressure assist was determined during calm wakefulness to ensure comparable tidal volume to that set during assist control ventilation. Conceivably, the reduction in apnea threshold with sleep onset combined with a high loop gain due to underlying heart failure may have played a role in the development of respiratory instability and consequent sleep disruption [29].

To address the issue of excessive levels of pressure assist, Toublanc and colleagues undertook a study comparing low levels of pressure support versus assist control ventilation in patients who were soon to be extubated [22]. In a single night RCT with cross over design, they performed polysomnography and found that both measured sleep quality (as indicated by greater slow wave sleep) and perceived sleep quality was better while receiving assist control ventilation when compared to pressure support [22]. In contrast, Cabello and colleagues did not notice differences between assist control ventilation, manually adjusted pressure support, and automatically adjusted pressure support ventilation in a 3-arm RCT with cross over design [24]. While on average the level of pressure assist delivered in this study was lower than that in the study by Parthasarathy and Tobin, they had included conscious patients who were free of sedative medications and had been ventilated for prolonged periods with only one of the 15 patients having a diagnosis of heart failure. Conceivably, the concomitant presence of sedative-analgesics and underlying heart failure can pose interactive effects by which the mode of ventilation (pressure support ventilation) played a deterministic role in sleep and breathing in the critically ill patients that were studied.

4.2 Proportional Assist Versus Pressure Support

Bosma and colleagues compared proportional assist ventilation versus pressure support in an RCT with cross-over design. They found that overall sleep quality was better during proportional assist ventilation as measured by less sleep fragmentation (arousals and awakenings), and greater proportion of time in slow wave and rapid eye movement (REM) sleep. Moreover, during pressure support there was greater tidal volume and minute ventilation and lower $PaCO_2$ than during proportional assist ventilation suggesting that respiratory controller instability may have played a role. In keeping with such rationale, patient-ventilator asynchronies per hour were greater with pressure support ventilation than during proportional assist ventilation and correlated with the number of arousals per hour. Despite ventilator settings being set to reduce the inspiratory work (measured as pressure time product per minute) by 50%, these ventilator-related sleep alterations were observed. Such findings suggest that even during modest levels of pressure support ventilation, the aforementioned patient-related factors (heart failure or opiate analgesics) or other ventilator-related factors can propagate ventilatory instability and consequent sleep disruption. One such ventilator-related factor could be the inherent oscillatory behavior of pressure support algorithms that are evident in mathematical modeling and bench experiments and that may result in substantial variations in tidal volume even when patient effort is constant [30, 31]. Another ventilator-related factor may be the absence of a back-up rate during pressure support ventilation administered by many commercial ventilators that could lead to the development of central apneas and consequent apnea ventilation and attendant alarms.

4.3 Pressure Control, Neurally Adjusted Ventilator Assistance, or Proportional Assist Plus Versus Pressure Support

Other studies include a RCT comparing pressure control ventilation (with a backup rate) versus low-levels of pressure support ventilation (without a backup rate) performed by Andrejak and colleagues in 13 critically ill patients receiving mechanical ventilation [27]. In this study, pressure control ventilation was associated with significantly better sleep quality and quantity compared to low-levels of pressure support: sleep efficiency, proportion of time in stage 2 non-REM sleep, slow wave sleep, and REM sleep were greater during pressure control ventilation than pressure support [3]. In another study performed by Delisle and colleagues, neurally adjusted ventilatory assistance (NAVA) was superior to pressure support in a RCT of patients undergoing weaning from mechanical ventilation. During the NAVA condition the patients were found to spend a greater proportion of time in REM sleep and suffer less sleep fragmentation and ineffective breathing efforts [25]. In yet another study, Alexopoulou and colleagues compared pressure support versus proportional assist ventilation plus (PAV+) using polysomnography [26]. They concluded that even though patient-ventilator synchrony was improved on PAV+ (similar to the study by Bosma and colleagues), sleep quality was not different between the two modes of mechanical ventilation [23, 26].

4.4 Summary

A synthesis of all the studies involving modes of mechanical ventilation that qualified as level I according to US Preventive Services Task Force hierarchy of study design was performed by Poongkunran and colleagues. In this meta-analysis of 8 RCTs

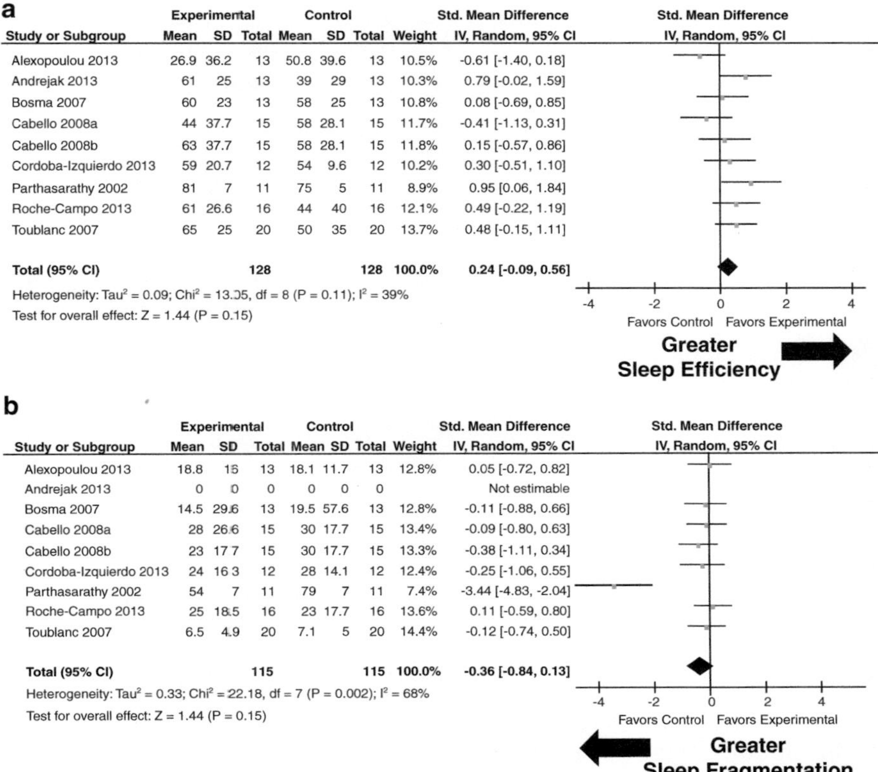

Fig. 2 (**a**) Forrest plot of studies overall demonstrating that adjusting ventilator mode can improve sleep quantity by increasing sleep efficiency [32]. (**b**) Forrest plot of studies overall demonstrating that adjusting ventilator mode can improve sleep quantity by decreasing sleep fragmentation [32]

involving 115 patients, the authors found that changes to modes of mechanical ventilation tended to improve sleep quantity by increasing sleep efficiency (Fig. 2a) and tended to improve sleep quality by decreasing sleep fragmentation (Fig. 2b) [32]. There was significant heterogeneity among these studies [32]. Sensitivity analysis of a subgroup of four RCTs revealed that, when compared to spontaneous modes of ventilation, timed modes of mechanical ventilation improved sleep quantity (Fig. 3a) [32]. However, timed modes of mechanical ventilation did not improve sleep quality measured as sleep fragmentation when compared to spontaneous modes of ventilation (Fig. 3b) [32]. Such a pooled analysis of the literature suggests that while a back-up rate is advantageous to preserving breathing stability and sleep, more adequately powered RCTs are needed to study the inter-relationship between sleep, modes of ventilation, medications, and patient-related factors (such as loop gain).

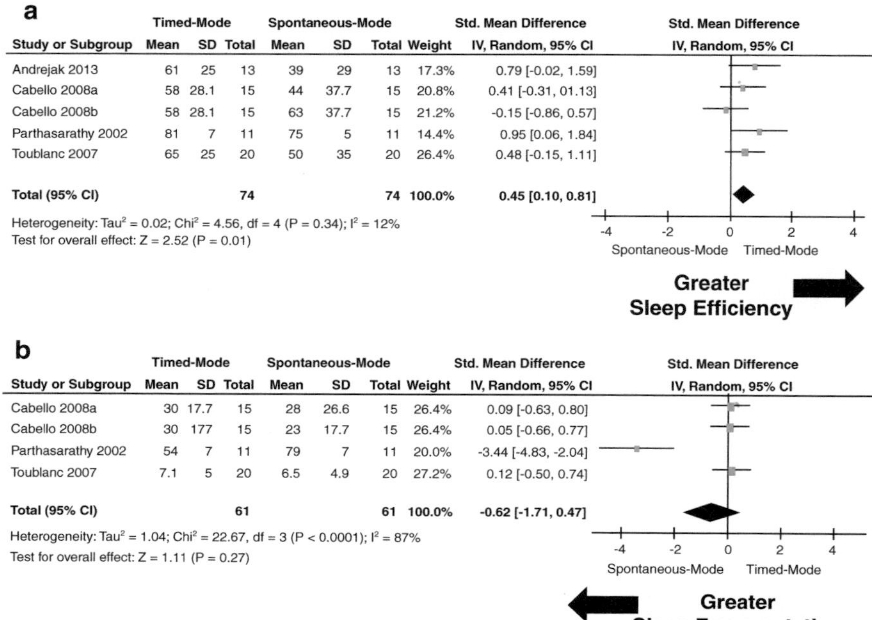

Fig. 3 (a) Forrest plot of subgroup of studies demonstrating that compared with spontaneous modes of ventilation, timed modes of ventilation improved sleep efficiency [32]. (b) Forrest plot of subgroup of studies demonstrating that timed modes did not improve sleep quality as measured by sleep fragmentation when compared with spontaneous modes [32]

5 Effect of Ventilator Management Strategies on Sleep; Low Tidal Volume Ventilation

Low tidal volume ventilation (4–6 ml/kg predicted body weight) is advocated for patients with acute respiratory distress syndrome (ARDS) and even in patients without ARDS by clinical practice guidelines [33]. Tidal volumes that are too high can lead to harm manifesting as alveolar overdistention, ventilator-induced lung injury, ventilator non-triggering, and eccentric respiratory muscle injury [34–38]. However, when tidal volumes are too low they can cause hypercarbic acidosis, increased work of breathing, and patient-ventilator dyssynchrony that create noxious stimuli, which, in turn, can disrupt sleep (Fig. 1) [39–41]. Patient-ventilator dyssynchrony can manifest as strenuous inspiratory efforts and double-triggering, either of which can paradoxically lead to alveolar overdistention [41–44]. Insufficient tidal volume can also cause atelectrauma, increased respiratory rate (stress frequency) and increased sedation requirements [45]. Such increased sedation requirements may be in response to the mismatch between the respiratory demand of the patient versus the ventilatory assistance delivered by the ventilator and cause discomfort manifesting as dyspnea. Reduced flow, tidal volume, or greater trigger sensitivity can lead to significant increases in the patients' inspiratory work of breathing and thereby contribute to dyspnea and consequent sleep disruption [46]. As such the greater sedation requirements given to combat the perception of increased respiratory (elastic and resistive) load due to low tidal volume and inspiratory flow rate has been associated with greater mortality in recent observational studies and reanalysis of prior RCTs [47–50]. Although sleep measurements were not performed in any of these studies, such a pathobiological state would not be conducive for restorative sleep but warrants artificial drug-induced deep sedation that may not mimic the restorative nature of true sleep [51] (see chapter "Normal Sleep Compared to Altered Consciousness During Sedation") and may increase the risk for delirium besides increasing length of ICU stay and mortality [52].

6 Effect of Sleep on Noninvasive Mechanical Ventilation and Monitoring

Sleep deprivation has systemic effects that may prolong the need for mechanical ventilation and length of stay in critical care and result in worse outcomes [53] (see also chapter "ICU Sleep Disruption and Its Relationship with ICU Outcomes"). However, objective studies that measure the effect of sleep disruption or deprivation on length of mechanical ventilation or ICU stay have not been performed. Moreover, physiological studies are equivocal with regards to whether sleep deprivation can reduce load response measured as hypercapnic ventilatory response [54].

6.1 Monitoring

Sleep disturbances and respiratory instability associated with sleep perturbations can impact monitoring in the ICU. For example, the coefficient of variation of end-tidal CO_2 was ~9% during pressure support and ~5% during assist-control ventilation in one of the studies that measured sleep fragmentation and respiratory variables [21]. The end-tidal CO_2 can vary by as much as 7 mmHg during sleep versus wakefulness, and such a magnitude of difference may impact the ventilator settings adopted by healthcare providers. Moreover, in most cases, adjustments to ventilator settings are done in the morning rounds during daily sedation interruptions, and the provider may not be aware of the impact of such changes on gas exchange and patient-ventilator interactions at nighttime especially if the patient were on a spontaneous mode of ventilation without a back-up rate. A practical consideration would be to adopt a mode of ventilation with a back-up rate when patients are asleep.

6.2 Noninvasive Ventilation

In a study of 27 hypercapnic patients who required noninvasive ventilation in a medical intensive care unit, Roche Campo and colleagues found that patients who failed noninvasive ventilation suffered worse sleep with greater disruption of diurnal sleep-wake cycles and less nocturnal REM sleep than patients who were successfully treated with noninvasive ventilation [55]. Such findings suggest that sleep in critically ill patients may be a reflection of the underlying brain dysfunction associated with critical illness and may be a prognosticator. In the same study, they found that failure of noninvasive ventilation was associated with a greater risk for delirium during the ICU stay. There is very little known about the relationship between various types of noninvasive ventilation such as NIPPV, HFNC, or CPAP and sleep quality in critically ill patients. Despite such noninvasive modalities being the most common modes of ventilatory assistance, this area is largely unexplored and ripe for future investigation.

7 Conclusion

In sum, sleep in critically ill patients is influenced by mode of mechanical ventilation in critically ill patients. However, this area of study suffers from lack of large level 1 adequately powered studies that can address important questions regarding whether such modes of mechanical ventilation can affect long- or short-term outcomes such as sedation requirements, neurocognitive function, ICU length of stay, duration of mechanical ventilation, and health-related quality of life upon survivorship. Moreover, there is a paucity of studies in critically ill patients receiving noninvasive ventilation. Nevertheless, practical implications for the ICU provider are that there are sleep-related instabilities in breathing control that may be facilitated by certain modes of ventilation such as pressure support ventilation without a back-up rate and the clinician should be cautious in interpreting respiratory gas exchange and setting the ventilator in the context of sleep-wakefulness state of the patient.

Acknowledgements S.P. was funded by NIH (HL138377; HL126140; HL151254; OT2-HL156812; OT2-HL161847-01; AG065346, MD011600), DoD (PT130770; W81XWH-21-1-0025, W81XWH20C0051), PCORI (DI-2018C2-13161; CER-2018C2-13262; PCS-1504-30430), U.S. Dept. of HHS (CT-HD-22-089); Sergey Brin Family Foundation; Philips-Respironics, Inc., WHOOP, Inc., Regeneron, Inc. The funders had no role in study design, data collection and analysis, decision to publish, or preparation of the manuscript. S.P. is a consultant for Jazz Pharmaceuticals, Inc. and holds a US patent (US20160213879A1) that is licensed to SaiOx, Inc. and receives royalty from UpToDate, Inc (Wolters Kluwer, Inc.).

References

1. Phillipson EA, Sullivan CE. Arousal: the forgotten response to respiratory stimuli. Am Rev Respir Dis. 1978;118:807–9.
2. Douglas NJ, White DP, Weil JV, Pickett CK, Zwillich CW. Hypercapnic ventilatory response in sleeping adults. Am Rev Respir Dis. 1982;126:758–62.
3. Douglas NJ, White DP, Weil JV, Pickett CK, Martin RJ, Hudgel DW, Zwillich CW. Hypoxic ventilatory response decreases during sleep in normal men. Am Rev Respir Dis. 1982;125:286–9.
4. Topf M. Effects of personal control over hospital noise on sleep. Res Nurs Health. 1992;15:19–28.
5. Parthasarathy S, Tobin MJ. Sleep in the intensive care unit. Intensive Care Med. 2004;30:197–206.
6. Borel JC, Tamisier R, Dias-Domingos S, Sapene M, Martin F, Stach B, Grillet Y, Muir JF, Levy P, Series F, Pepin JL. Type of mask may impact on continuous positive airway pressure adherence in apneic patients. PLoS One. 2013;8:e64382.
7. Kamdar BB, Knauert MP, Jones SF, Parsons EC, Parthasarathy S, Pisani MA. Perceptions and practices regarding sleep in the ICU: a survey of 1,223 critical care providers. Ann Am Thorac Soc. 2016.
8. Andrade RG, Piccin VS, Nascimento JA, Viana FM, Genta PR, Lorenzi-Filho G. Impact of the type of mask on the effectiveness of and adherence to continuous positive airway pressure treatment for obstructive sleep apnea. J Bras Pneumol. 2014;40:658–68.
9. Morin CM, Hauri PJ, Espie CA, Spielman AJ, Buysse DJ, Bootzin RR. Nonpharmacologic treatment of chronic insomnia. An American Academy of Sleep Medicine review. Sleep. 1999;22:1134–56.
10. Klerman EB, Dijk D-J. Age-related reduction in the maximal capacity for sleep—implications for insomnia. Curr Biol. 2008;18:1118–23.
11. Fan E, Cheek F, Chlan L, Gosselink R, Hart N, Herridge MS, Hopkins RO, Hough CL, Kress JP, Latronico N, Moss M, Needham DM, Rich MM, Stevens RD, Wilson KC, Winkelman C, Zochodne DW, Ali NA. An official American Thoracic Society Clinical Practice guideline: the diagnosis of intensive care unit-acquired weakness in adults. Am J Respir Crit Care Med. 2014;190:1437–46.
12. Franks ZM, Alcock JA, Lam T, Haines KJ, Arora N, Ramanan M. Physical restraints and post-traumatic stress disorder in survivors of critical illness. A systematic review and meta-analysis. Ann Am Thorac Soc. 2021;18:689–97.
13. Pun BT, Balas MC, Barnes-Daly MA, Thompson JL, Aldrich JM, Barr J, Byrum D, Carson SS, Devlin JW, Engel HJ, Esbrook CL, Hargett KD, Harmon L, Hielsberg C, Jackson JC, Kelly TL, Kumar V, Millner L, Morse A, Perme CS, Posa PJ, Puntillo KA, Schweickert WD, Stollings JL, Tan A, D'Agostino McGowan L, Ely EW. Caring for critically ill patients with the ABCDEF bundle: results of the ICU liberation collaborative in over 15,000 adults. Crit Care Med. 2019;47:3–14.
14. Reisner-Sénélar L. The birth of intensive care medicine: Björn Ibsen's records. Intensive Care Med. 2011;37:1084–6.
15. Laffey JG, Madotto F, Bellani G, Pham T, Fan E, Brochard L, Amin P, Arabi Y, Bajwa EK, Bruhn A, Cerny V, Clarkson K, Heunks L, Kurahashi K, Laake JH, Lorente JA, McNamee L, Nin N, Palo JE, Piquilloud L, Qiu H, Jiménez JIS, Esteban A, McAuley DF, van Haren F, Ranieri M, Rubenfeld G, Wrigge H, Slutsky AS, Pesenti A. Geo-economic variations in epidemiology, patterns of care, and outcomes in patients with acute respiratory distress syndrome: insights from the LUNG SAFE prospective cohort study. Lancet Respir Med. 2017;5:627–38.
16. Esteban A, Anzueto A, Alia I, Gordo F, Apezteguia C, Palizas F, Cide D, Goldwaser R, Soto L, Bugedo G, Rodrigo C, Pimentel J, Raimondi G, Tobin MJ. How is mechanical ventilation employed in the intensive care unit? An international utilization review. Am J Respir Crit Care Med. 2000;161:1450–8.

17. Barr J, Fraser GL, Puntillo K, Ely EW, Gélinas C, Dasta JF, Davidson JE, Devlin JW, Kress JP, Joffe AM, Coursin DB, Herr DL, Tung A, Robinson BR, Fontaine DK, Ramsay MA, Riker RR, Sessler CN, Pun B, Skrobik Y, Jaeschke R. Clinical practice guidelines for the management of pain, agitation, and delirium in adult patients in the intensive care unit. Crit Care Med. 2013;41:263–306.
18. Radovanovic D, Santus P, Coppola S, Saad M, Pini S, Giuliani F, Mondoni M, Chiumello DA. Characteristics, outcomes and global trends of respiratory support in patients hospitalized with COVID-19 pneumonia: a scoping review. Minerva Anestesiol. 2021;87:915–26.
19. Garg S, Patel K, Pham H, Whitaker M, O'Halloran A, Milucky J, Anglin O, Kirley PD, Reingold A, Kawasaki B, Herlihy R, Yousey-Hindes K, Maslar A, Anderson EJ, Openo KP, Weigel A, Teno K, Ryan PA, Monroe ML, Reeg L, Kim S, Como-Sabetti K, Bye E, Shrum Davis S, Eisenberg N, Muse A, Barney G, Bennett NM, Felsen CB, Billing L, Shiltz J, Sutton M, Abdullah N, Talbot HK, Schaffner W, Hill M, Chatelain R, Wortham J, Taylor C, Hall A, Fry AM, Kim L, Havers FP. Clinical trends among U.S. Adults hospitalized with COVID-19, March to December 2020: a cross-sectional study. Ann Intern Med. 2021(174):1409–19.
20. Tobin MJ, Laghi F, Jubran A. Caution about early intubation and mechanical ventilation in COVID-19. Ann Intensive Care. 2020;10:78.
21. Parthasarathy S, Tobin MJ. Effect of ventilator mode on sleep quality in critically ill patients. Am J Respir Crit Care Med. 2002;166:1423–9.
22. Toublanc B, Rose D, Glerant JC, Francois G, Mayeux I, Rodenstein D, Jounieaux V. Assist-control ventilation vs. low levels of pressure support ventilation on sleep quality in intubated ICU patients. Intensive Care Med. 2007;33:1148–54.
23. Bosma K, Ferreyra G, Ambrogio C, Pasero D, Mirabella L, Braghiroli A, Appendini L, Mascia L, Ranieri VM. Patient-ventilator interaction and sleep in mechanically ventilated patients: pressure support versus proportional assist ventilation. Crit Care Med. 2007;35:1048–54.
24. Cabello B, Thille AW, Drouot X, Galia F, Mancebo J, d'Ortho MP, Brochard L. Sleep quality in mechanically ventilated patients: comparison of three ventilatory modes. Crit Care Med. 2008;36:1749–55.
25. Delisle S, Ouellet P, Bellemare P, Tetrault JP, Arsenault P. Sleep quality in mechanically ventilated patients: comparison between NAVA and PSV modes. Ann Intensive Care. 2011;1:42.
26. Alexopoulou C, Kondili E, Plataki M, Georgopoulos D. Patient-ventilator synchrony and sleep quality with proportional assist and pressure support ventilation. Intensive Care Med. 2013;39:1040–7.
27. Andrejak C, Monconduit J, Rose D, Toublanc B, Mayeux I, Rodenstein D, Jounieaux V. Does using pressure-controlled ventilation to rest respiratory muscles improve sleep in ICU patients? Respir Med. 2013;107:534–41.
28. Córdoba-Izquierdo A, Drouot X, Thille AW, Galia F, Roche-Campo F, Schortgen F, Prats-Soro E, Brochard L. Sleep in hypercapnic critical care patients under noninvasive ventilation: conventional versus dedicated ventilators. Crit Care Med. 2013;41:60–8.
29. Younes M, Ostrowski M, Thompson W, Leslie C, Shewchuk W. Chemical control stability in patients with obstructive sleep apnea. Am J Respir Crit Care Med. 2001;163:1181–90.
30. Hotchkiss JR Jr, Adams AB, Stone MK, Dries DJ, Marini JJ, Crooke PS. Oscillations and noise: inherent instability of pressure support ventilation? Am J Respir Crit Care Med. 2002;165:47–53.
31. Hotchkiss JR, Adams AB, Dries DJ, Marini JJ, Crooke PS. Dynamic behavior during noninvasive ventilation: chaotic support? Am J Respir Crit Care Med. 2001;163:374–8.
32. Poongkunran C, John SG, Kannan AS, Shetty S, Bime C, Parthasarathy S. A meta-analysis of sleep-promoting interventions during critical illness. Am J Med. 2015;128:1126–37.
33. Fan E, Del Sorbo L, Goligher EC, Hodgson CL, Munshi L, Walkey AJ, Adhikari NKJ, Amato MBP, Branson R, Brower RG, Ferguson ND, Gajic O, Gattinoni L, Hess D, Mancebo J, Meade MO, McAuley DF, Pesenti A, Ranieri VM, Rubenfeld GD, Rubin E, Seckel M, Slutsky AS, Talmor D, Thompson BT, Wunsch H, Uleryk E, Brozek J, Brochard LJ. An Official American Thoracic Society/European Society of Intensive Care Medicine/Society of Critical Care

Medicine Clinical Practice Guideline: mechanical ventilation in adult patients with acute respiratory distress syndrome. Am J Respir Crit Care Med. 2017;195:1253–63.
34. Brower RG, Matthay MA, Morris A, Schoenfeld D, Thompson BT, Wheeler A. Ventilation with lower tidal volumes as compared with traditional tidal volumes for acute lung injury and the acute respiratory distress syndrome. N Engl J Med. 2000;342:1301–8.
35. Parker JC, Hernandez LA, Peevy KJ. Mechanisms of ventilator-induced lung injury. Crit Care Med. 1993;21:131–43.
36. Tremblay LN, Slutsky AS. Pathogenesis of ventilator-induced lung injury: trials and tribulations. Am J Physiol Lung Cell Mol Physiol. 2005;288:L596–8.
37. Slutsky AS, Tremblay LN. Multiple system organ failure. Is mechanical ventilation a contributing factor? Am J Respir Crit Care Med. 1998;157:1721–5.
38. Parthasarathy S, Jubran A, Tobin MJ. Cycling of inspiratory and expiratory muscle groups with the ventilator in airflow limitation. Am J Respir Crit Care Med. 1998;158:1471–8.
39. Feihl F, Perret C, Permissive hypercapnia. How permissive should we be? Am J Respir Crit Care Med. 1994;150:1722–37.
40. Kallet RH, Campbell AR, Dicker RA, Katz JA, Mackersie RC. Effects of tidal volume on work of breathing during lung-protective ventilation in patients with acute lung injury and acute respiratory distress syndrome. Crit Care Med. 2006;34:8–14.
41. Gilstrap D, MacIntyre N. Patient-ventilator interactions. Implications for clinical management. Am J Respir Crit Care Med. 2013;188:1058–68.
42. Thille AW, Rodriguez P, Cabello B, Lellouche F, Brochard L. Patient-ventilator asynchrony during assisted mechanical ventilation. Intensive Care Med. 2006;32:1515–22.
43. Loring SH, Malhotra A. Driving pressure and respiratory mechanics in ARDS. N Engl J Med. 2015;372:776–7.
44. Beitler JR, Malhotra A, Thompson BT. Ventilator-induced Lung Injury. Clin Chest Med. 2016;37:633–46.
45. Gattinoni L. Counterpoint: Is low tidal volume mechanical ventilation preferred for all patients on ventilation? No. Chest. 2011;140:11–3.
46. Marini JJ, Capps JS, Culver BH. The inspiratory work of breathing during assisted mechanical ventilation. Chest. 1985;87:612–8.
47. Raschke RA, Stoffer B, Assar S, Fountain S, Olsen K, Heise CW, Gallo T, Padilla-Jones A, Gerkin R, Parthasarathy S, Curry SC. The relationship of tidal volume and driving pressure with mortality in hypoxic patients receiving mechanical ventilation. PLoS One. 2021;16:e0255812.
48. Tobin MJ. The dethroning of 6 ml/kg as the "Go-To" setting in acute respiratory distress syndrome. Am J Respir Crit Care Med. 2021;204:868–9.
49. Goligher EC, Costa ELV, Yarnell CJ, Brochard LJ, Stewart TE, Tomlinson G, Brower RG, Slutsky AS, Amato MPB. Effect of lowering Vt on mortality in acute respiratory distress syndrome varies with respiratory system elastance. Am J Respir Crit Care Med. 2021;203:1378–85.
50. Goligher EC, Costa ELV. Reply to Tobin. Am J Respir Crit Care Med. 2021;204:869–70.
51. Sanders RD, Maze M. Contribution of sedative-hypnotic agents to delirium via modulation of the sleep pathway. Can J Anaesth. 2011;58:149–56.
52. Pandharipande PP, Ely EW, Arora RC, Balas MC, Boustani MA, La Calle GH, Cunningham C, Devlin JW, Elefante J, Han JH, MacLullich AM, Maldonado JR, Morandi A, Needham DM, Page VJ, Rose L, Salluh JIF, Sharshar T, Shehabi Y, Skrobik Y, Slooter AJC, Smith HAB. The intensive care delirium research agenda: a multinational, interprofessional perspective. Intensive Care Med. 2017;43:1329–39.
53. Blissitt PA. Sleep and mechanical ventilation in critical care. Crit Care Nurs Clin North Am. 2016;28:195–203.
54. Spengler CM, Shea SA. Sleep deprivation per se does not decrease the hypercapnic ventilatory response in humans. Am J Respir Crit Care Med. 2000;161:1124–8.
55. Roche-Campo F, Thille AW, Drouot X, Galia F, Margarit L, Cordoba-Izquierdo A, Mancebo J, d'Ortho MP, Brochard L. Comparison of sleep quality with mechanical versus spontaneous ventilation during weaning of critically III tracheostomized patients. Crit Care Med. 2013;41:1637–44.

Sleep Disruption and its Relationship
to ICU Outcomes

Lauren Tobias, Margaret Pisani, and Carolyn D'Ambrosio

1   Introduction

For most ICU patients, critical illness and the ICU environment hinders sleep. Bright light at irregular times, loud noise, frequent clinical interventions and the state of critical illness contribute to insufficient sleep, sleep fragmentation, circadian rhythm disturbance, and a reduction in slow-wave as compared to lighter-stage sleep [1] (see chapter "Risk Factors for Disrupted Sleep in the ICU"). Critically ill patients also typically have multiple chronic comorbidities that predispose them to sleep disorders at baseline and the ICU experience may exacerbate this risk. Disrupted sleep may contribute to worsened neurocognitive, metabolic, cardiovascular, respiratory, and physical outcomes.

Sleep disruption in the ICU is a relatively new field of investigation. In 2018, the Society of Critical Care Medicine (SCCM) included sleep disruption in their practice guidelines for adult ICU patients [2]. Research in this domain must confront a challenge common in critically ill patients: demonstrating causality amid a sea of potential confounders mediating the relationship between risk factors and outcome. ICU patients frequently have complex comorbidities and present with wide-ranging disease states with varying prognoses, which makes it difficult to tease apart sleep's unique contribution to critical illness outcomes. Measuring sleep in the ICU is also

L. Tobias
Veterans Affairs Connecticut Healthcare System, West Haven, CT, USA

Section of Pulmonary, Critical Care and Sleep Medicine, Yale University School of Medicine, New Haven, CT, USA
e-mail: Lauren.Tobias@yale.edu

M. Pisani · C. D'Ambrosio (✉)
Section of Pulmonary, Critical Care and Sleep Medicine, Yale University School of Medicine, New Haven, CT, USA
e-mail: Margaret.Pisani@yale.edu; Carolyn.DAmbrosio@yale.edu

G. L. Weinhouse, J. W. Devlin (eds.), *Sleep in Critical Illness*,
https://doi.org/10.1007/978-3-031-06447-0_11

complicated, requiring equipment that is not standard in most ICUs, assessment of a multidimensional variable over a prolonged period, and yielding data that must be interpretated by specialially trained staff (eg. polysomnographers) (see chapter "Methods for Routine Sleep Assessment and Monitoring"). Interventions aimed at improving sleep during critical illness often require multidisciplinary collaboration; for example, implementation of a simple nap opportunity requires nurses and other staff to reschedule patient care activities such as medication administration, bathing, and transport for tests and imaging studies (see chapter "Best Practice for Improving Sleep in the ICU. Part I: Non-pharmacologic"). Finally, researchers must confront the lack of a gold standard for "normal" sleep quality in the ICU (see chapter "Normal Sleep Compared to Altered Consciousness During Sedation"). Our targets for optimal sleep—including duration, timing, and quality—are likely to be impacted by underlying disease processes that are pathophysiologically heterogeneous (see chapter "Biologic Effects of Disrupted Sleep").

Given the relatively few studies dedicated to examining sleep in critically ill patients, it is logical to generalize from what we have learned about the outcomes related to sleep disruption in the population of hospitalized patients at large. In most cases, the factors disrupting inpatients' sleep will only be intensified in the ICU setting, where vital sign monitoring occurs more frequently, blooddraws and imaging are obtained more often, and clinical instability necessitates more interruptions during times of potential rest. Perhaps the only aspect of sleep that may be superior in the ICU is the absence of a roomate, which patients often report to be the most important disruptor of sleep [3]. It also may be reasonable to extrapolate findings from healthy outpatients subject to acute stressors such as short-term sleep restriction or acute circadian disruption (See chapter "Characteristics of Sleep in Critically Ill Patients. Part II: Circadian Rhythm Disruption"). This chapter seeks to summarize what is known about the relationship between sleep and ICU health outcomes in critically ill patients. Chapter "Long-Term Outcomes: Sleep in Survivors of Critical Illness" reviews the long-term, post-ICU outcomes related to disrupted sleep.

2 Abnormal Sleep and Circadian Rhythms in Critical Illness

As highlighted in chapters "Characteristics of Sleep in Critically Ill Patients. Part I: Sleep Fragmentation and Sleep Stage Disruption", "Characteristics of Sleep in Critically Ill Patients. Part II: Circadian Rhythm Disruption", and "Biologic Effects of Disrupted Sleep", critically ill patients often have frequent arousals and awakenings during overnight sleep and brief naps during the daytime; a single consolidated period of sleep at night in the ICU rarely exists [4, 5]. As outlined in chapter "Atypical Sleep and Pathologic Wakefulness", when critically ill patients are able to sleep, they spend an inordinate time with "atypical" sleep, wherein the criteria for standard sleep stages including the presence of sleep spindles and K complexes are not met [1, 6]. For a regular circadian cycle, humans need exposure to certain external cues called zeitgebers (ie., light, meals, exercise, environmental temperature changes) (see chapter "Characteristics of Sleep in Critically Ill Patients. Part II: Circadian Rhythm Disruption"). Sleep disruption occurs when the circadian cycle of critically ill adults is altered by both derangements in these exogenous influences as well as endogenous disturbances. Exogenous factors contributing to sleep disruption in critically ill patients include excessive light, noise, nocturnal nursing interventions and medication, as described in chapters "Risk Factors for Disrupted Sleep in the ICU" and "Effects of Common ICU Medications on Sleep". Endogenous disturbances to the circadian cycle include pre-existing sleep disorders and the underlying critical illness, resulting in an abnormal melatonin secretion and often delayed circadian phase [7, 8]. Importantly, the loss of normal sleep architecture and circadian abnormalities are both markers of poor prognosis in critically ill adults. In one study, the degree of circadian disruption was directly related to severity of illness as measured by the APACHE-III score [9].

3   Association Between Pre-Existing Sleep Disorders and ICU Outcomes

Pre-existing sleep disorders likely contribute to poor sleep in critically ill patients. At least 10% of US adults are estimated to have some type of sleep disorder [10] and these rates are likely higher among hospitalized populations. Up to 40% of hospitalized patients are estimated to be at high risk for obstructive sleep apnea (OSA), one of the most common sleep disorders in adults [11]. The prevalence of OSA is increased in patients with certain comorbidities, such as COPD—a population frequently encountered in the ICU [12]. Patients with COPD also exhibit higher rates of insomnia and worse sleep quality during hospitalization [12]. Pre-existing sleep disorders may be overlooked at the time of ICU admission; lapses in treatment may result. For example, pre-existing OSA is often unrecognized on hospital admission and when recognized correct CPAP settings are infrequently prescribed [13]. A recent study examining the prevalence of various sleep disorders in patients hospitalized for COVID-19 found that OSA was present in 20%, insomnia in 11%, and restless leg syndrome (RLS) in 4% [14].

The presence of underlying sleep disorders may affect illness trajectory during critical illness. Several retrospective studies of ICU patients have found that OSA was independently associated with decreased ICU and hospital mortality, when adjusted for severity of illness [15, 16]. However, a recent study of over 5000 ICU patients found that pre-existing OSA did not impact ICU or hospital mortality or the risk of developing ventilator associated pneumonia, although patients with a body mass index (BMI) over 40 kg/m^2 had a significantly increased length of ICU stay [17]. Most recently, patients with comorbid OSA hospitalized with COVID-19 were found to have similar outcomes to non-OSA patients after adjustment for covariates [18]. The reason for these disparate findings is unclear but one potential explanation is the obesity paradox, which is the observation that elevated body mass index

(BMI) exerts protective effect on both ICU and hospital mortality. The presence of OSA does appear to confer elevated patient risk in certain populations (e.g., perioperative), where undiagnosed OSA is associated with higher postoperative rates of respiratory failure, ICU transfer, and cardiovascular complications [19, 20]. Patients with obesity hypoventilation syndrome are also at higher risk during hospitalization, with longer lengths of ICU admission and increased mortality.

Other sleep disorders commonly seen in hospitalized patients include insomnia, RLS, and hypersomnia disorders. These may be pre-existing or acquired. For example, RLS may be triggered during a hospitalization by immobility, sleep deprivation, and the use of antiemetics, antihistamines and antipsychotics [21].

4 Immune Function & Inflammation

A significant body of both experimental and clinical evidence supports a bidirectional relationship between immune function and sleep [22]. It is well-recognized that poor sleep has a detrimental effect on the immune system, affecting both adaptive and innate immunity [23–26]. Most research exploring this association has been conducted outside of the critical care setting. However, since critically ill patients' immune function is often compromised, we may reasonably speculate that they are particularly vulnerable to the impact of poor sleep on immune function. For example, a study of healthy volunteers found that antibody titers following influenza vaccination were more than twice as high in the group permitted a usual night of sleep as compared with those restricted to 4 h of sleep per night [27].

One of the mechanisms postulated to link sleep deprivation with adverse outcomes is increased levels of inflammation. Biochemically, acute and chronic sleep loss or sleep fragmentation results in a proinflammatory state with alterations in circulating pro- and anti-inflammatory cytokines, soluble receptors, and changes in inflammatory signaling pathways and innate immunity. This manifests as increased expression of interleukin (IL-1β) and tumor necrosis factor (TNF-α) and activation of NF-κB signaling in the brain and elevated circulating proinflammatory cytokine levels [28] (also see chapter "Biologic Effects of Disrupted Sleep").

The pro-inflammatory state associated with critical illness may also plausibly promote sleep. In humans, changes in sleep architecture may accompany systemic inflammation with increased NREM sleep, increased EEG delta-frequency and reduced REM. Research surrounding somnogenic substances in animal models led to the discovery that proinflammatory cytokines possess strong sleep-promoting activities [28]. Systemic infections, which are common at both the presentation of critical illness and also during it, may elicit production of endogenous pyrogens via endotoxin or other mechanisms. The effects of endogenous pyrogens on sleep have been investigated in several animal models, Table 1 lists the role these cytokines play in sleep. Most animal studies have demonstrated that sleep duration increases in response to infection. Pathways linking infection to sleep outcomes are likely to vary depending upon the specific infectious pathogens (e.g., viral, bacterial,

Table 1 Cytokines and neurohumoral regulators of sleep

	Effect on NREM Sleep
Interleukin-1	Increases
Interleukin-2	Increases
Interleukin-4	Decreases
Interleukin-6	Increases or decreases[a]
Interleukin-10	Decreases
Interleukin-18	Increases
Tumor necrosis factor-α (TNF-α)	Increases
Transforming growth factor-β (TGF-β)	Decreases
Insulin like growth Factor-1 (IGF-1)	Dose dependent Small dose decreases High dose increases
Growth hormone releasing hormone (GHRH)	Increases
Corticotropin releasing hormone (CRH)	Decreases
Nitric oxide (NO)	Increases
Ghrelin	Increases
Vasoactive Intestinal peptide (VIP)	Increases

[a]May play an important role in sleep regulation during pathologic states
References: [39, 80-83]

parasitic), its impact on immunological production of mediators (e.g., interleukins and cytokines), and responses of the neuroendocrine system to the secretion of substances (e.g., cortisol, epinephrine).

Other mechanisms linking sleep disturbance and adverse ICU outcomes include sympathetic activation and neuroendocrine effects. For example, patients whose sleep was curtailed to 4 h per night over a period of 6 nights demonstrated increased sympathetic activation and higher levels of evening cortisol, as compared with those provided a 12-h sleep opportunity [29]. In one healthy volunteer laboratory study, experimental sleep restriction resulted in dysregulation of the neuroendocrine control of appetite and satiety, a potential precursor to hyperglycemia and ultimately diabetes [30].

5 Disrupted Sleep and Organ System-Related Outcomes

There is growing evidence that sleep disruption in critically ill patients negatively affects both ICU and post-ICU outcomes [31–35] (see also chapter "Long-Term Outcomes: Sleep in Survivors of Critical Illness"). One of the first studies to highlight the importance of circadian alignment for recovery from critical illness was conducted in patients who sustained a myocardial infarction; those in sunny rooms had a shorter length of stay and lower mortality than those in darker rooms [36]. Since that time, subsequent work has demonstrated that chronic sleep deprivation is associated with several comorbidities including diabetes [37–39], hypertension

[40], heart disease/stroke [41, 42], obesity [43, 44], anxiety/depression, and increased mortality risk [38]. The loss of normal sleep architecture is a marker of poor prognosis in ICU patients; studies have demonstrated that the absence of sleep spindles and K-complexes in patients with respiratory failure, acute encephalopathy, posttraumatic coma and subarachnoid hemorrhage portend a worse prognosis [31]. A recent study found that greater circadian rhythm disorganization in critically ill patients corresponded to higher severity-of-illness as measured by the Sequential Organ Failure Assessment (SOFA) score [45]. Figure 1 proposes a conceptual framework linking ICU-related sleep disruption and adverse outcomes.

5.1 *Psychiatric and Neurocognitive Outcomes*

Delirium is the best studied clinical outcome that has been associated with sleep disruption in the ICU. Highly prevalent in intensive care units, delirium has become the target of much research that seeks to disentangle the shared characteristics between sleep disruption and delirium, to clarify bi-directional effects and mechanisms for this relationship, and to understand the impact of sleep disorders on outcomes of delirium in ICU patients. The relationship between sleep deprivation and delirium is likely bidirectional, where sleep deprivation can cause or worsen delirium and the presence of delirium can contribute to sleep disturbance resulting in a vicious cycle in critically ill patients. Studies of patients subjected to acute sleep deprivation note the presence of diminished psychomotor performance, short-term memory impairment and difficulties with executive function, all of which are symptoms associated with delirium [46]. A study of healthy subjects demonstrated that severe sleep deprivation led to perceptual disturbances, visual hallucinations, impaired attention, disordered thoughts and changes in mood that ranged from apathy to aggressive behavior; symptoms began as early as 24 h after the onset of sleep deprivation [47]. To date there have not been large, well-controlled studies examining the relationship between delirium and sleep disturbances. Many of the small studies have not controlled for important risk factors for sleep disruption or delirium such as ICU environmental factors (e.g., light and noise), in-room interruptions, and concomitant medications [48]. The relationship between sleep and delirium is discussed in chapters "Sleep Disruption and Its Relationship with Delirium: Electroencephalographic Perspectives" (physiologic perspective) and "Sleep Disruption and Its Relationship with Delirium: Clinical Perspectives" (clinical perspective).

Sleep disruption also impacts other neurocognitive outcomes beyond delirium. Multiple non-ICU studies have documented that acute total sleep deprivation results in significant cognitive deficits in terms of reduced cognitive processing speed, attention, verbal memory, difficulties with executive function, perceptual disturbances and emotional processing [46, 49]. Less extreme short-term sleep restriction also has dose-related effects neurocognitive function [50, 51]. Sleep-deprived patients may exhibit impaired recall of neutral and positive emotional stimuli; preserved recall negative stimuli predominates may precipitate the formation of false

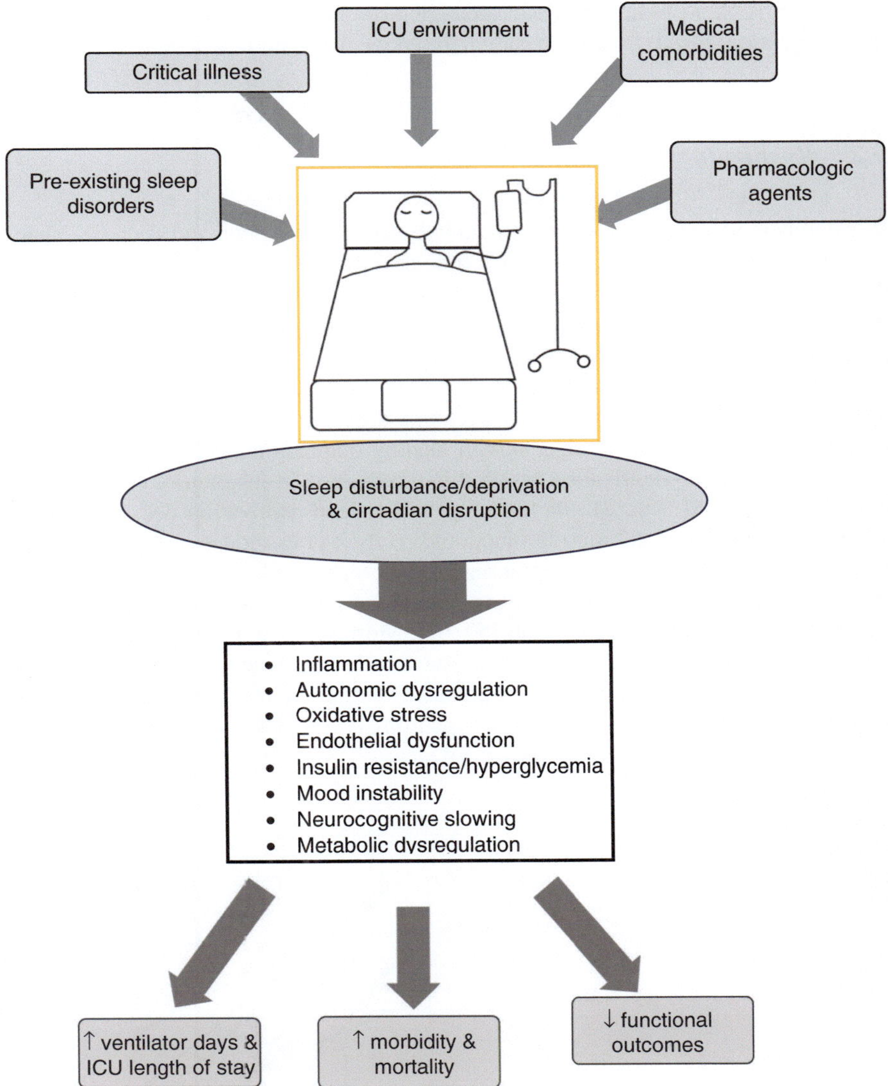

Fig. 1 Proposed mechanisms linking ICU sleep disruption adverse ICU outcomes

memories [52, 53]. These factors may compromise ICU experience processing and increase the risk for post-traumatic stress symptoms following critical illness [54].

Sleep and its related outcomes are one of the many reasons ICU pain management is important. Use of opioids and ketamine are linked to increased delirium. The failure to evaluated and treat pain will potentiate sleep disruption and worse ICU outcomes [55]. Recent papers demonstrate a protocolized approach to pain assessment and treatment in the ICU results in lower opioid use and better pain control [56]. Non-opioid analgesic strategies (including both non-pharmacologic and medication-based) have been shown to reduce ileus and ICU length of stay [57].

5.2 Respiratory Outcomes

While important interactions exist between ICU ventilatory support and sleep (see chapter "Mechanical Ventilation and Sleep"), little data exists regarding the impact of sleep deprivation on the respiratory system in critically ill adults. However, there are studies which have examined the impact of sleep deprivation or restriction on both healthy subjects and in patients with underlying lung disease.

Healthy participants have increased respiratory muscle fatigue and may have a decreased ventilatory response to hypercapnia after 24 h of sleep deprivation. For example, a recent study of subjects with healthy diaphragmatic function showed a single night of sleep deprivation resulted in a reduction in inspiratory endurance of more than half [58] (Fig. 2). Interestingly, while sleep deprivation does not appear impair respiratory skeletal muscle function directly it does reduce respiratory motor output from the cortex. These alterations to the control of breathing in critically ill adults may in turn impact the need for ventilatory support and the ability to wean patients from mechanical ventilation [59–61]. Mortality may be increased [62, 63]. Increased daytime sleep and reduced REM have been associated with late noninvasive ventilation failure [60]. Conversely, mechanical ventilation may impact sleep: several studies suggest that patient-ventilator dysynchrony is associated with sleep disruption

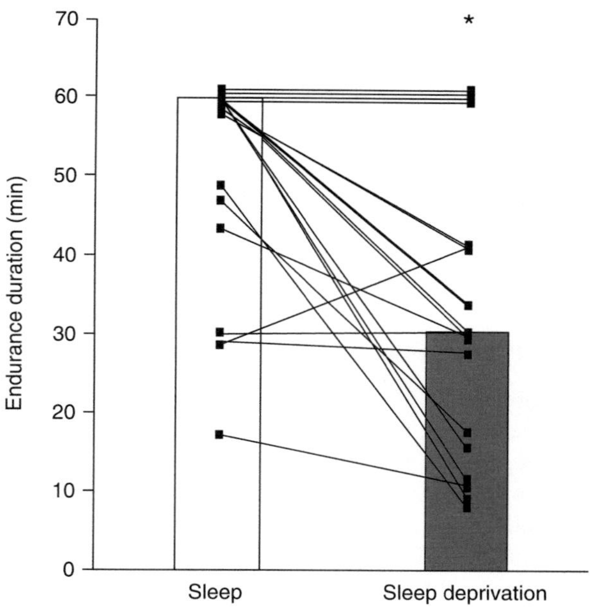

Fig. 2 Inspiratory endurance was twice as high after a normal sleep night than a sleepless night in healthy participants, suggesting that altered sleep could contribute to respiratory failure [58]

(see chapter "Mechanical Ventilation and Sleep"). Exacerbations of chronic pulmonary disease make up a significant proportion of ICU admissions; many of these patients also have comorbid sleep disorders that may influence prognosis. For instance, asthmatic patients with chronic insomnia tend to have poorer asthma control [64].

5.3 Cardiovascular Outcomes

The relationship between sleep disorders and cardiovascular morbidity has been extensively researched [65]. Sleep is typically associated with reduced sympathetic tone and subsequent reductions in heart rate, blood pressure and arrhythmias [66]. Investigators have observed stage-specific effects on heart rate variability, where parasympathetic modulation is greatest during NREM sleep and the sympathetic response is greatest during REM sleep [67].

Insufficient sleep has been linked to elevated cortisol levels, increased markers of sympathetic nervous system activity, increased metabolic rate and endothelial dysfunction [68]. Data from outpatient populations has shown that a chronic sleep deficit is associated with increased atrial fibrillation [69] which, in the ICU, is associated with a longer duration of ICU stay [70]. In community-based outpatient cohorts, rates of nocturnal ventricular arrythmias, sudden cardiac death and implanted defibrillator discharge are highest in the early morning hours, which suggests sleep-related fluctuations in autonomic activity are responsible [71, 72]. Circadian misalignment carries an increased risk for development of cardiovascular disease [73] and a small study showed that chronotherapeutic interventions may decrease cardiac arrhythmias [74].

Whether pre-existing sleep disorders such as OSA effect outcomes from an acute hospitalization is unclear. In outpatients, OSA is a well-documented independent risk factor for systemic hypertension, stroke, congestive heart failure and coronary artery disease [75, 76]. However, the use of positive airway pressure (PAP) therapy has not been shown to reduce cardiovascular outcomes or death [77]. In hospitalized patients overall, evidence is mixed regarding the impact of sleep apnea on short-term cardiovascular outcomes. For example, one study suggested that detection of OSA, and initiation of CPAP, among adults admitted for a heart failure exacerbation was associated with lower readmission rates at 6 months [78]. Another large prospective trial, however, found that patients admitted with acute coronary syndrome and OSA had similar 3-year outcomes to those without OSA, and in those with OSA, CPAP use did not reduce the risk of additional cardiovascular adverse events [79].

5.4 Metabolic Outcomes

Hyperglycemia in critically patients has been associated with poor clinical outcomes in epidemiological studies from a variety of patient populations [80]. Sleep restriction decreases insulin sensitivity and impairs glucose regulation and may thereby mediate the development of hyperglycemia in critically ill patients. In normal, healthy individuals, glucose tolerance varies across the day; plasma glucose responses to exogenous glucose is significantly higher in the evening than the morning and glucose tolerance is at its minimum in the middle of the night [81]. Glucose utilization is greatest during wake and lowest during NREM sleep with intermediate levels during REM sleep. Several studies have examined the impact of sleep restriction on glucose tolerance and insulin sensitivity [82]. One study in healthy humans subject to a 4-h sleep restriction over several nights demonstrated a 25% decrease in insulin sensitivity and a 30% decrease in acute insulin response to intravenous glucose [29]. Sleep fragmentation in patients with preserved total sleep time has also been associated with decreased insulin sensitivity [83–85]. Circadian misalignment, when subjects sleep out of normal circadian phase, has also been associated with an increase in glucose levels [86]. One study showed that intermittent gastric feeds resulted in lower insulin requirements among critically ill patients [87]. (Also see chapter "Biologic Effects of Disrupted Sleep").

5.5 Renal Function

Acute kidney injury (AKI) is a common consequence of critical illness and portends worse ICU outcomes. An emerging literature suggests OSA is a potential risk factor for the development and progression of chronic kidney disease, independent of other CKD risk factors [88, 89]. One proposed mechanism is that episodes of cyclic desaturation in OSA result in renal tissue hypoxia. While data in critically ill adults is limited, one retrospective cohort study found that OSA predisposes ICU patients to AKI; 57% of patients with pre-existing OSA developed AKI compared to only 46% when OSA was not present [90].

5.6 Physical Outcomes

The relationship between sleep and physical activity is bidirectional. On one hand, sleep deprivation can result in decreased energy and physical performance, a relationship documented in healthy outpatients [91, 92]. The existing physical performance of critically ill adults may impact their ability to participate in early mobilization programs (shown to improve outcome) and successful ventilator weaning trials [93]. On the other hand, participation in physical activity may have a salutary effect on sleep by strengthening the circadian differentiation between a physically active day and physically quiescent night. At this point, whether poor ICU sleep hinders early mobilization participation is largely speculative; one ICU study failed to find an association between sleep quality and willingness to participate in mobility efforts [94]. Future work examining the impact of sleep disruption in critical illness on early mobilization, physical therapy and functional outcomes is needed.

6   Outcomes after ICU Discharge

Chapter "Long-Term Outcomes: Sleep in Survivors of Critical Illness" reviews in detail how sleep disturbances in the ICU affect post-ICU outcomes. There is a growing body of data highlighting how Post-Intensive Care Unit Syndrome (PICS) [i.e., psychologic (e.g., anxiety, depression, post-traumatic stress disorder), cognitive (e.g., persistent delirium and long-term cognitive impairment) and physical function] can affect post-ICU outcomes [95]. Additionally, there exists an extensive non-ICU literature on the relationship between sleep duration and quality and depression, anxiety, fatigue and stress. Survivors of critical illness often report memories of poor sleep during their ICU stay [96]. In addition, delirium in the ICU appears to be associated with persistent post-ICU sleep disturbance [35, 97].

7   Areas for Future Research

Most studies to date have focused on how poor sleep impacts shorter-term outcomes in the ICU such as development of acute delirium, ICU or hospital length of stay, duration of mechanical ventilation, or organ-system-based outcomes such as glucose metabolism or the immune response. The consequences of poor sleep during critical illness may extend beyond the acute hospitalization. For example, survivors of acute respiratory failure demonstrated greater circadian disruption 3 months after discharge than community dwelling adults in one study [98]. Another study found that patients who developed insomnia disorder after treatment with extracorporeal membrane oxygenation (ECMO) had a 5 year mortality nearly double that of patients with pre-ECMO insomnia disorder [99].

Traditional ICU metrics such as ventilator-free days, length of stay, and delirium are important and easily measurable. These outcomes may not capture what is most important to patient; broader trajectories of recovery following critical illness including emotional and physical wellbeing [100]. Post-ICU clinics may be best positioned to evaluate these longer-term patient-centered outcomes in future studies.

8   Conclusion

The relationship between sleep and ICU outcomes in critically ill patients is impacted by both intrinsic and extrinsic factors. Intrinsic factors include pre-existing sleep disorders, psychiatric comorbidity, medical illness, pain/discomfort while extrinsic factors include environmental noise and lighting, repetitive clinical interventions such as vital sign checks, testing, examinations, and administration of medications. Mediated by inflammation, altered immune function, and neuro-endocrine effects, sleep disturbance in the ICU likely impacts a myriad of outcomes across different organ systems, and with important implications for patient recovery.

References

1. Cooper AB, Thornley KS, Young GB, Slutsky AS, Stewart TE, Hanly PJ. Sleep in critically ill patients requiring mechanical ventilation. Chest. 2000;117(3):809–18.
2. Yuksel D, Baker FC, Goldstone A, Claudatos SA, Forouzanfar M, Prouty DE, et al. Stress, sleep, and autonomic function in healthy adolescent girls and boys: findings from the NCANDA study. Sleep. Health. 2021;7(1):72–8.
3. Thomas KP, Salas RE, Gamaldo C, Chik Y, Huffman L, Rasquinha R, et al. Sleep rounds: a multidisciplinary approach to optimize sleep quality and satisfaction in hospitalized patients. J Hosp Med. 2012;7(6):508–12.
4. Friese RS, Diaz-Arrastia R, McBride D, Frankel H, Gentilello LM. Quantity and quality of sleep in the surgical intensive care unit: are our patients sleeping? J Trauma. 2007;63(6):1210–4.
5. Elliott R, Mckinley S, Cistulli P, Fien M. Characterisation of sleep in intensive care using 24-hour polysomnography: an observational study. Crit Care. 2013;17(2):R46.
6. Knauert MP, Yaggi HK, Redeker NS, Murphy TE, Araujo KL, Pisani MA. Feasibility study of unattended polysomnography in medical intensive care unit patients. Heart Lung. 2014;43(5):445–52.
7. Li C-X, Liang D-D, Xie G-H, Cheng B-L, Chen Q-X, Wu S-J, et al. Altered melatonin secretion and circadian gene expression with increased proinflammatory cytokine expression in early-stage sepsis patients. Mol Med Rep. 2013;7(4):1117–22.
8. Gehlbach BK, Chapotot F, Leproult R, Whitmore H, Poston J, Pohlman M, et al. Temporal disorganization of circadian rhythmicity and sleep-wake regulation in mechanically ventilated patients receiving continuous intravenous sedation. Sleep. 2012;35(8):1105–14.
9. Gazendam JAC, Van Dongen HPA, Grant DA, Freedman NS, Zwaveling JH, Schwab RJ. Altered circadian rhythmicity in patients in the ICU. Chest. 2013;144(2):483–9.
10. Ram S, Seirawan H, Kumar SKS, Clark GT. Prevalence and impact of sleep disorders and sleep habits in the United States. Sleep Breath. 2010;14(1):63–70.
11. Shear TC, Balachandran JS, Mokhlesi B, Spampinato LM, Knutson KL, Meltzer DO, et al. Risk of sleep apnea in hospitalized older patients. J Clin Sleep Med. 2014;10(10):1061–6.
12. Stewart NH, Walters RW, Mokhlesi B, Lauderdale DS, Arora VM. Sleep in hospitalized patients with chronic obstructive pulmonary disease: an observational study. J Clin Sleep Med. 2020;16(10):1693–9.
13. Saini P, Klada E, Patel V, Zaw M, Dubrovsky B, George L, et al. Continuous positive airway pressure usage in hospitalized patients with known obstructive sleep apnea: discrepancy between admission pressure settings and laboratory-determined settings. Sleep Breath. 2017;21(2):347–53.
14. Goldstein CA, Rizvydeen M, Conroy DA, O'Brien LM, Gupta G, Somers EC, et al. The prevalence and impact of pre-existing sleep disorder diagnoses and objective sleep parameters in patients hospitalized for COVID-19. J Clin Sleep Med. 2021;17(5):1039–50.
15. Bolona E, Hahn PY, Afessa B. Intensive care unit and hospital mortality in patients with obstructive sleep apnea. J Crit Care. 2015;30(1):178–80.
16. Wang H, Shao G, Rong L, Ji Y, Zhang K, Liu M, et al. Association between comorbid sleep apnoea–hypopnoea syndrome and prognosis of intensive care patients: a retrospective cohort study. BMJ Open. 2021;11(6):e048886.
17. Bailly S, Galerneau LM, Ruckly S, Seiller A, Terzi N, Schwebel C, et al. Impact of obstructive sleep apnea on the obesity paradox in critically ill patients. J Crit Care. 2020;56:120–4.
18. Mashaqi S, Lee-Iannotti J, Rangan P, Celaya MP, Gozal D, Quan SF, et al. Obstructive sleep apnea and COVID-19 clinical outcomes during hospitalization: a cohort study. J Clin Sleep Med. 2021;17(11):2197–204.
19. Memtsoudis SG, Stundner O, Rasul R, Chiu Y-L, Sun X, Ramachandran S-K, et al. The impact of sleep apnea on postoperative utilization of resources and adverse outcomes. Anesth Analg. 2014;118(2):407–18.

20. Chan MTV, Wang CY, Seet E, Tam S, Lai HY, Chew EFF, et al. Association of unrecognized obstructive sleep apnea with postoperative cardiovascular events in patients undergoing major noncardiac surgery. JAMA. 2019;321(18):1788–98.
21. Goldstein C. Management of Restless Legs Syndrome/Willis-Ekbom disease in hospitalized and perioperative patients. Sleep Med Clin. 2015;10(3):303–10, xiv.
22. Ibarra-Coronado EG, Pantaleón-Martínez AM, Velazquéz-Moctezuma J, Prospéro-García O, Méndez-Díaz M, Pérez-Tapia M, et al. The bidirectional relationship between sleep and immunity against infections. J Immunol Res. 2015;2015:1–14.
23. Irwin M, McClintick J, Costlow C, Fortner M, White J, Gillin JC. Partial night sleep deprivation reduces natural killer and cellular immune responses in humans. FASEB J. 1996;10(5):643–53.
24. Irwin M. Effects of sleep and sleep loss on immunity and cytokines. Brain Behav Immun. 2002;16(5):503–12.
25. Benca RM, Quintas J. Sleep and host defenses: a review. Sleep. 1997;20(11):1027–37.
26. Bryant PA, Trinder J, Curtis N. Sick and tired: does sleep have a vital role in the immune system? Nat Rev Immunol. 2004;4(6):457–67.
27. Spiegel K. Effect of sleep deprivation on response to Immunizaton. JAMA. 2002;288(12):1471.
28. Szentirmai E, Kapas L. Humoral and other sleep-promoting factors. In: Gozal D, editor. Pediatric sleep medicine. Cham: Springer; 2021. p. 123–32.
29. Spiegel K, Leproult R, Van Cauter E. Impact of sleep debt on metabolic and endocrine function. Lancet. 1999;354(9188):1435–9.
30. Van Cauter E, Holmbäck U, Knutson K, Leproult R, Miller A, Nedeltcheva A, et al. Impact of sleep and sleep loss on neuroendocrine and metabolic function. Horm Res Paediatr. 2007;67(1):2–9.
31. Knauert MP, Gilmore EJ, Murphy TE, Yaggi HK, Van Ness PH, Han L, et al. Association between death and loss of stage N2 sleep features among critically ill patients with delirium. J Crit Care. 2018;43:124–9.
32. Kamdar BB, King LM, Collop NA, Sakamuri S, Colantuoni E, Neufeld KJ, et al. The effect of a quality improvement intervention on perceived sleep quality and cognition in a medical ICU. Crit Care Med. 2013;41(3):800–9.
33. Sutter R, Barnes B, Leyva A, Kaplan PW, Geocadin RG. Electroencephalographic sleep elements and outcome in acute encephalopathic patients: a 4-year cohort study. Eur J Neurol. 2014;21(10):1268–75.
34. Altman MT, Knauert MP, Pisani MA. Sleep disturbance after hospitalization and critical illness: a systematic review. Ann Am Thorac Soc. 2017;14(9):1457–68.
35. Altman MT, Knauert MP, Murphy TE, Ahasic AM, Chauhan Z, Pisani MA. Association of intensive care unit delirium with sleep disturbance and functional disability after critical illness: an observational cohort study. Ann Intensive Care. 2018;8(1)
36. Beauchemin KM, Hays P. Dying in the dark: sunshine, gender and outcomes in myocardial infarction. J R Soc Med. 1998;91(7):352–4.
37. Holliday EG, Magee CA, Kritharides L, Banks E, Attia J. Short sleep duration is associated with risk of future diabetes but not cardiovascular disease: a prospective study and meta-analysis. PLoS One. 2013;8(11):e82305.
38. Cappuccio FP, D'Elia L, Strazzullo P, Miller MA. Quantity and quality of sleep and incidence of type 2 diabetes: a systematic review and meta-analysis. Diabetes Care. 2010;33(2):414–20.
39. Buxton OM, Cain SW, O'Connor SP, Porter JH, Duffy JF, Wang W, et al. Adverse metabolic consequences in humans of prolonged sleep restriction combined with circadian disruption. Sci Transl Med. 2012;4(129):129ra43.
40. Wang Q, Xi B, Liu M, Zhang Y, Fu M. Short sleep duration is associated with hypertension risk among adults: a systematic review and meta-analysis. Hypertens Res. 2012;35(10):1012–8.
41. Grandner MA, Chakravorty S, Perlis ML, Oliver L, Gurubhagavatula I. Habitual sleep duration associated with self-reported and objectively determined cardiometabolic risk factors. Sleep Med. 2014;15(1):42–50.

42. Shankar A, Koh WP, Yuan JM, Lee HP, Yu MC. Sleep duration and coronary heart disease mortality among Chinese adults in Singapore: a population-based cohort study. Am J Epidemiol. 2008;168(12):1367–73.

43. Patel SR, Blackwell T, Redline S, Ancoli-Israel S, Cauley JA, Hillier TA, et al. The association between sleep duration and obesity in older adults. Int J Obes. 2008;32(12):1825–34.

44. Patel SR, Hu FB. Short sleep duration and weight gain: a systematic review. Obesity (Silver Spring). 2008;16(3):643–53.

45. Maas MB, Lizza BD, Kim M, Abbott SM, Gendy M, Reid KJ, et al. Stress-induced behavioral quiescence and abnormal rest-activity rhythms during critical illness. Crit Care Med. 2020;48(6):862–71.

46. Pilcher JJ, Huffcutt AI. Effects of sleep deprivation on performance: a meta-analysis. Sleep. 1996;19(4):318–26.

47. Waters F, Chiu V, Atkinson A, Blom JD. Severe sleep deprivation causes hallucinations and a gradual progression toward psychosis with increasing time awake. Front Psych. 2018;9:303.

48. Flannery AH, Oyler DR, Weinhouse GL. The impact of interventions to improve sleep on delirium in the ICU: a systematic review and research framework. Crit Care Med. 2016;44(12):2231–40.

49. Goel N, Rao H, Durmer J, Dinges D. Neurocognitive consequences of sleep deprivation. Semin Neurol. 2009;29(04):320–39.

50. Van Dongen HP, Maislin G, Mullington JM, Dinges DF. The cumulative cost of additional wakefulness: dose-response effects on neurobehavioral functions and sleep physiology from chronic sleep restriction and total sleep deprivation. Sleep. 2003;26(2):117–26.

51. Belenky G, Wesensten NJ, Thorne DR, Thomas ML, Sing HC, Redmond DP, et al. Patterns of performance degradation and restoration during sleep restriction and subsequent recovery: a sleep dose-response study. J Sleep Res. 2003;12(1):1–12.

52. Frenda SJ, Patihis L, Loftus EF, Lewis HC, Fenn KM. Sleep deprivation and false memories. Psychol Sci. 2014;25(9):1674–81.

53. Sterpenich V, Albouy G, Boly M, Vandewalle G, Darsaud A, Balteau E, et al. Sleep-related Hippocampo-cortical interplay during emotional memory recollection. PLoS Biol. 2007;5(11):e282.

54. Elliott R, McKinley S, Fien M, Elliott D. Posttraumatic stress symptoms in intensive care patients: an exploration of associated factors. Rehabil Psychol. 2016;61(2):141–50.

55. Ouimet S, Kavanagh BP, Gottfried SB, Skrobik Y. Incidence, risk factors and consequences of ICU delirium. Intensive Care Med. 2007;33(1):66–73.

56. Skrobik Y, Ahern S, Leblanc M, Marquis F, Awissi DK, Kavanagh BP. Protocolized intensive care unit management of analgesia, sedation, and delirium improves analgesia and subsyndromal delirium rates. Anesth Analg. 2010;111(2):451–63.

57. Devlin JW, Skrobik Y, Gélinas C, Needham DM, Slooter AJC, Pandharipande PP, et al. Clinical practice guidelines for the prevention and Management of Pain, agitation/sedation, delirium, immobility, and sleep disruption in adult patients in the ICU. Crit Care Med. 2018;46(9):e825–e73.

58. Rault C, Sangaré A, Diaz V, Ragot S, Frat J-P, Raux M, et al. Impact of sleep deprivation on respiratory motor output and endurance. A physiological study. Am J Respir Crit Care Med. 2020;201(8):976–83.

59. Roche-Campo F, Thille AW, Drouot X, Galia F, Margarit L, Córdoba-Izquierdo A, et al. Comparison of sleep quality with mechanical versus spontaneous ventilation during weaning of critically III tracheostomized patients. Crit Care Med. 2013;41(7):1637–44.

60. Roche Campo F, Drouot X, Thille AW, Galia F, Cabello B, d'Ortho MP, et al. Poor sleep quality is associated with late noninvasive ventilation failure in patients with acute hypercapnic respiratory failure. Crit Care Med. 2010;38(2):477–85.

61. Chen HI, Tang YR. Sleep loss impairs inspiratory muscle endurance. Am Rev Respir Dis. 1989;140(4):907–9.

62. Boyko Y, Toft P, Ørding H, Lauridsen JT, Nikolic M, Jennum P. Atypical sleep in critically ill patients on mechanical ventilation is associated with increased mortality. Sleep Breath. 2019;23(1):379–88.

63. Thille AW, Reynaud F, Marie D, Barrau S, Rousseau L, Rault C, et al. Impact of sleep alterations on weaning duration in mechanically ventilated patients: a prospective study. Eur Respir J. 2018;51(4)

64. Alanazi TM, Alghamdi HS, Alberreet MS, Alkewaibeen AM, Alkhalefah AM, Omair A, et al. The prevalence of sleep disturbance among asthmatic patients in a tertiary care center. Sci Rep. 2021;11(1)

65. Grandner MA, Alfonso-Miller P, Fernandez-Mendoza J, Shetty S, Shenoy S, Combs D. Sleep. Curr Opin Cardiol. 2016;31(5):551–65.

66. Gula LJ, Krahn AD, Skanes AC, Yee R, Klein GJ. Clinical relevance of arrhythmias during sleep: guidance for clinicians. Heart. 2004;90(3):347–52.

67. Boudreau P, Yeh WH, Dumont GA, Boivin DB. Circadian variation of heart rate variability across sleep stages. Sleep. 2013;36(12):1919–28.

68. Khan MS, Aouad R. The effects of insomnia and sleep loss on cardiovascular disease. Sleep Med Clin. 2017;12(2):167–77.

69. Morovatdar N, Ebrahimi N, Rezaee R, Poorzand H, Bayat Tork MA, Sahebkar A. Sleep duration and risk of atrial fibrillation: a systematic review. J Atr Fibrillation. 2019;11(6):2132.

70. Valderrábano RJ, Blanco A, Santiago-Rodriguez EJ, Miranda C, Rivera-Del Rio Del Rio J, Ruiz J, et al. Risk factors and clinical outcomes of arrhythmias in the medical intensive care unit. J Intensive Care 2016;4(1).

71. Lavery CE, Mittleman MA, Cohen MC, Muller JE, Verrier RL. Nonuniform nighttime distribution of acute cardiac events: a possible effect of sleep states. Circulation. 1997;96(10):3321–7.

72. Cowie MR. Sleep apnea: state of the art. Trends Cardiovasc Med. 2017;27(4):280–9.

73. Fishbein AB, Knutson KL, Zee PC. Circadian disruption and human health. J Clin Investig. 2021;131(19)

74. Ono H, Taguchi T, Kido Y, Fujino Y, Doki Y. The usefulness of bright light therapy for patients after oesophagectomy. Intensive Crit Care Nurs. 2011;27(3):158–66.

75. Sheikh M, Kuperberg S. An organ systems-based review of outcomes associated with sleep apnea in hospitalized patients. Medicine (Baltimore). 2021;100(34):e26857.

76. Somers VK, White DP, Amin R, Abraham WT, Costa F, Culebras A, et al. Sleep apnea and cardiovascular disease: an American Heart Association/American College of Cardiology Foundation scientific statement from the American Heart Association Council for high blood pressure research professional education committee, council on clinical cardiology, stroke council, and council on cardiovascular nursing. J Am Coll Cardiol. 2008;52(8):686–717.

77. Yu J, Zhou Z, Mcevoy RD, Anderson CS, Rodgers A, Perkovic V, et al. Association of Positive Airway Pressure with Cardiovascular Events and Death in adults with sleep apnea. JAMA. 2017;318(2):156.

78. Kauta SR, Keenan BT, Goldberg L, Schwab RJ. Diagnosis and treatment of sleep disordered breathing in hospitalized cardiac patients: a reduction in 30-day hospital readmission rates. J Clin Sleep Med. 2014;10(10):1051–9.

79. Sánchez-de-la-Torre M, Sánchez-de-la-Torre A, Bertran S, Abad J, Duran-Cantolla J, Cabriada V, et al. Effect of obstructive sleep apnoea and its treatment with continuous positive airway pressure on the prevalence of cardiovascular events in patients with acute coronary syndrome (ISAACC study): a randomised controlled trial. Lancet Respir Med. 2020;8(4):359–67.

80. Yamada T, Shojima N, Noma H, Yamauchi T, Kadowaki T. Glycemic control, mortality, and hypoglycemia in critically ill patients: a systematic review and network meta-analysis of randomized controlled trials. Intensive Care Med. 2017;43(1):1–15.

81. Knutson KL, Spiegel K, Penev P, Van Cauter E. The metabolic consequences of sleep deprivation. Sleep Med Rev. 2007;11(3):163–78.

82. Buxton OM, Pavlova M, Reid EW, Wang W, Simonson DC, Adler GK. Sleep restriction for 1 week reduces insulin sensitivity in healthy men. Diabetes. 2010;59(9):2126–33.
83. Tasali E, Leproult R, Ehrmann DA, Van Cauter E. Slow-wave sleep and the risk of type 2 diabetes in humans. Proc Natl Acad Sci U S A. 2008;105(3):1044–9.
84. Tasali E, Leproult R, Spiegel K. Reduced sleep duration or quality: relationships with insulin resistance and type 2 diabetes. Prog Cardiovasc Dis. 2009;51(5):381–91.
85. Stamatakis KA, Punjabi NM. Effects of sleep fragmentation on glucose metabolism in normal subjects. Chest. 2010;137(1):95–101.
86. Scheer FAJL, Hilton MF, Mantzoros CS, Shea SA. Adverse metabolic and cardiovascular consequences of circadian misalignment. Proc Natl Acad Sci. 2009;106(11):4453–8.
87. Sjulin TJ, Strilka RJ, Huprikar NA, Cameron LA, Woody PW, Armen SB. Intermittent gastric feeds lower insulin requirements without worsening dysglycemia: a pilot randomized crossover trial. Int J Crit Illn Inj Sci. 2020;10(4):200–5.
88. Voulgaris A, Marrone O, Bonsignore MR, Steiropoulos P. Chronic kidney disease in patients with obstructive sleep apnea. A narrative review. Sleep Med Rev. 2019;47:74–89.
89. Beaudin AE, Raneri JK, Ahmed SB, Hirsch Allen AJM, Nocon A, Gomes T, et al. Risk of chronic kidney disease in patients with obstructive sleep apnea. Sleep. 2022;45(2):zsab267.
90. Dou L, Lan H, Reynolds DJ, Gunderson TM, Kashyap R, Gajic O, et al. Association between obstructive sleep apnea and acute kidney injury in critically ill patients: a propensity-matched study. Nephron. 2017;135(2):137–46.
91. Dam TT, Ewing S, Ancoli-Israel S, Ensrud K, Redline S, Stone K. Association between sleep and physical function in older men: the osteoporotic fractures in men sleep study. J Am Geriatr Soc. 2008;56(9):1665–73.
92. Goldman SE, Stone KL, Ancoli-Israel S, Blackwell T, Ewing SK, Boudreau R, et al. Poor sleep is associated with poorer physical performance and greater functional limitations in older women. Sleep. 2007;30(10):1317–24.
93. Schweickert WD, Pohlman MC, Pohlman AS, Nigos C, Pawlik AJ, Esbrook CL, et al. Early physical and occupational therapy in mechanically ventilated, critically ill patients: a randomised controlled trial. Lancet. 2009;373(9678):1874–82.
94. Kamdar BB, Combs MP, Colantuoni E, King LM, Niessen T, Neufeld KJ, et al. The association of sleep quality, delirium, and sedation status with daily participation in physical therapy in the ICU. Crit Care. 2016;20(1)
95. Wang S, Meeker JW, Perkins AJ, Gao S, Khan SH, Sigua NL, et al. Psychiatric symptoms and their association with sleep disturbances in intensive care unit survivors. Int J Gen Med. 2019;12:125–30.
96. Rotondi AJ, Chelluri L, Sirio C, Mendelsohn A, Schulz R, Belle S, et al. Patients' recollections of stressful experiences while receiving prolonged mechanical ventilation in an intensive care unit. Crit Care Med. 2002;30(4):746–52.
97. Novaes MAFP, Knobel E, Bork AM, Pavão OF, Nogueira-Martins LA, Bosi FM. Stressors in ICU: perception of the patient, relatives and health care team. Intensive Care Med. 1999;25(12):1421–6.
98. Oldham MA, Lee HB, Desan PH. Circadian rhythm disruption in the critically ill: an opportunity for improving outcomes. Crit Care Med. 2016;44(1):207–17.
99. Yang PL, Ward TM, Burr RL, Kapur VK, McCurry SM, Vitiello MV, et al. Sleep and circadian rhythms in survivors of acute respiratory failure. Front Neurol. 2020;11:94.
100. Park HY, Song IA, Cho HW, Oh TK. Insomnia disorder and long-term mortality in adult patients treated with extracorporeal membrane oxygenation in South Korea. J Sleep Res. 2022;31(2):e13454.

Long-Term Outcomes: Sleep in Survivors of Critical Illness

Sharon McKinley, Rosalind Elliott, Wade Stedman, and Julia Pilowsky

1 Introduction

Intensive care units and models for the care of the critically ill evolved from the polio epidemic of the mid-twentieth century. Since then, survival rates have increased steadily, and the focus on the outcome of mortality has changed to include a holistic consideration of the quality of recovery from critical illness. ICU survivorship is of critical importance to most ICU survivors given how much it affects important patient determinants of health (including quality of life, happiness and economic stability). Therefore, how patients recover from critical illness, and the key mechanisms/symptoms that affect this recovery, is a growing area of interest and practice for critical care clinicians and researchers. The objectives of this chapter are to outline the key challenges for ICU survivors, the incidence of sleep disturbance and the potential causes and recommendations to improve sleep in this population.

S. McKinley
University of Technology Sydney, Sydney, Australia

R. Elliott (✉) · J. Pilowsky
Malcolm Fisher Intensive Care Unit, Royal North Shore Hospital, Northern Sydney Local Health District and Faculty of Health, University of Technology Sydney, Sydney, Australia
e-mail: Rosalind.Elliott@health.nsw.gov.au; Julia.Pilowsky@health.nsw.gov.au

W. Stedman
Faculty of Medicine, University of Sydney, Sydney, Australia
e-mail: Wade.Stedman@health.nsw.gov.au

G. L. Weinhouse, J. W. Devlin (eds.), *Sleep in Critical Illness*,
https://doi.org/10.1007/978-3-031-06447-0_12

191

2 Recovery from Critical Illness

Recovery from critical illness may present important physical, psychological, cognitive and social challenges to both patients and their families. A frequently used term for new or worsening impairments in physical, cognitive, or mental health status arising after critical illness and persisting beyond acute care hospitalization experienced by ICU survivors is post intensive care syndrome (PICS) [1]. New sleep disturbances, or an exacerbation of pre-ICU sleep disorder, are common during recovery [2]. A conceptual framework of ICU survivorship incorporating features of PICS plus sleep assessment and interventions is presented in Table 1.

2.1 ICU Recovery Frameworks

Various frameworks for intensive care recovery have been published, usually across a sequential timeline or pathway of pre-intensive care illness (premorbidity), the episode of critical illness (intensive care outcomes), the ward or general hospital unit period (hospital outcomes) and the post-hospital discharge period of 3–6 months. Frameworks include all aspects of physical health and functioning, psychological health and functioning and quality of life. Recommendations are included for assessments and individualized care and treatment at each stage and referral to specialist services when indicated. Some recovery pathways focus on physical disability and recovery [3, 4], while others are more focused on cognitive health and psychological morbidity (e.g., anxiety and depression) with an emphasis in the interrelated benefits for outcomes of critically ill patients [5]. The symptom of fatigue is often assessed, as well as post-traumatic stress symptoms (PTSS) [4] and delusional memories and hallucinations [5].

These matters were recommended in the 2020 Society of Critical Care Medicine's International Consensus Conference on Prediction and Identification of Long-Term Impairments After Critical Illness, but somewhat surprisingly sleep and its assessment was not included [6]. As sleep is important in its own right and known to be associated with other impairments seen after critical illness it has been included in the present recovery framework. Sleep assessment and its relationship to recovery usually is not explicitly proposed for formalised assessment and follow up. In this chapter it is proposed that sleep screening, referral for assessment and treatment of sleep disorders should be integrated into formalized frameworks to promote recovery from critical illness such as part of specific ICU follow up services (Table 1).

3 Assessment of Sleep during the ICU Recovery Period

Sleep is a complex behavioural and physiological state classically characterised by perceptual disengagement, unresponsiveness, postural recumbence, inactivity, eye closure, reversibility and specific brain waveforms and ocular

Table 1 Framework encompassing considerations for the assessment and treatment of sleep during the critical illness recovery trajectory

Domain	Phase			
	Pre-critical illness (Before ICU admission)	Critical illness (During ICU admission)	Hospital ward/floor (After ICU discharge)	Post-hospital discharge (Home, rehabilitation, convalescence, nursing home setting)
Physical health and functioning	Assess: Comorbidities Usual functioning/quality of life Prehospital sleep (e.g., ISI)	Treat: Organ failures Concurrent physical problems Complications Assess: Sleep self-report (e.g., RCSQ) Objective actigraphy Maintain: Physical function Nutrition	Maintain: Supportive treatments Nutrition Assess: Physical disability Fatigue Weight loss Sleep (e.g., RCSQ) Commence: Graded physical therapy Sleep hygiene practices Refer: Specialist support	Maintain: Graded physical therapy Sleep hygiene practices Assess: Medical treatment needs Physical functioning mobility, pain Sleep (e.g., PSQI) Refer: Medical specialists Physiotherapy/occupational therapy Sleep specialists /sleep investigation clinic
Psychological health	Assess: History Self-report Or psychiatric/psychology report	Maintain: Frequent communication ICU diaries (if appropriate) Refer: Specialist assessment	Maintain: Frequent communication Refer: Specialist assessment	Assess: Post-traumatic stress symptoms Anxiety Depression Refer: Specialist psychological support or sleep psychologist for CBT-I

(continued)

Table 1 (continued)

Domain	Phase			
	Pre-critical illness (Before ICU admission)	Critical illness (During ICU admission)	Hospital ward/floor (After ICU discharge)	Post-hospital discharge (Home, rehabilitation, convalescence, nursing home setting)
Cognitive functioning	Assess History Self-report or by proxy See previous formal screening if available	Assess: Delirium (CAM/CAM-ICU) (& treat cause)	Assess: Delirium (CAM) (& treat cause)	Assess: Cognitive function (CAM) Refer: Specialist support
Social functioning	Informally assess	Provide support/involve family	Provide support/involve family	Assess: HRQoL

Notes: Domains are the accepted dimensions of health contributing to wellbeing, *CAM* confusion assessment method, *CAM-ICU* confusion assessment method for the ICU, *CBT-I* cognitive behavioural therapy for insomnia, *HRQoL* health related quality of life, *ISI* Insomnia Severity Index, *RCSQ* Richards-Campbell Sleep Questionnaire, *PSQI* Pittsburgh Sleep Quality Index movements [7]. The restorative outcomes and quality of sleep are highly subjective. Consequently, the measurement of sleep quality and quantity is complicated even for healthy individuals. In the general population polysomnography (PSG) is the gold standard for objective sleep assessment but self-assessment of sleep quality is always obtained because sleep is so subjective. The characteristics of sleep measured by PSG in critically ill adults are thoroughly explored in chapters "Characteristics of Sleep in Critically Ill Patients. Part I: Sleep Fragmentation and Sleep Stage Disruption", "Atypical Sleep and Pathologic Wakefulness" and "Best Practice for Improving Sleep in the ICU. Part I: Non-pharmacologic". An alternative objective measure which provides less detailed information is actigraphy. Subjective measures include self-administered questionnaires and sleep logs.

The selection of an objective sleep assessment measure in the post-ICU period is dependent on whether a suspected sleep disorder is present. Actigraphy is unable to provide estimates of sleep architecture or respiratory function but may be sufficient for long term monitoring for circadian and insomnia disorders. As for any individual, consultation with a sleep medicine specialist is advised if sleep disruption is on-going. In this section we review methods for sleep assessment commonly used in the post-ICU period. The Chapter "Methods for Routine Sleep Assessment and Monitoring" describes methods of sleep measurement during the ICU admission.

3.1 Objective Methods

3.1.1 Polysomnography

Many challenges exist with using PSG during critical illness in the ICU including its application and maintenance of the electrode montage and how atypical brain wave activity (see chapter "Atypical Sleep and Pathologic Wakefulness") is interpreted. During the post-ICU recovery period, the ICU-specific limitations of using PSG are far less of a concern but the ability to accurately capture an abbreviated PSG montage in the natural setting in ambulatory patients has its own limitations. PSG assessment in a sleep laboratory may be impractical and costly and not representative of sleep quality and quantity in the patient's natural setting. In addition, there are problems with interference and loss of data for unattended PSG recordings. However, an abbreviated unattended PSG recording under the direction of a sleep medicine specialist may be the most appropriate sleep assessment method when sleep disordered breathing (SDB) is suspected and may be useful for diagnosing other sleep disorders. Adequate reliability and validity and safety of an abbreviated unattended montage has been established for diagnosis of SDB in the absence of significant cardiopulmonary disease or respiratory dysfunction [8].

3.1.2 Actigraphy

Actigraphy devices incorporate either a piezoelectric or a microelectromechanical accelerometer and may be worn on the wrist, ankle, or waist and therefore actigraphy is a simple, cost-effective method of estimating sleep quality and quantity. While actigraphy may be used to monitor rest and activity it does not measure time spent in sleep stages and other potentially important metrics. Estimates of some sleep parameters, such as total sleep time (TST) and sleep efficiency index (SEI) may be obtained, with graphical representations of wakefulness and sleep patterns. Circadian rhythm may be estimated using rest/activity algorithms [9], in particular inter-daily stability and intra-daily variability [10]. Although actigraphy provides limited information and differentiation between sleep and inactivity (a common condition during both the ICU and post-ICU recovery periods) it may be useful for identifying insomnia and circadian rhythm sleep-wake disorders, insufficient sleep syndrome and even SDB if integrated with home sleep apnoea testing (i.e., an integrated portable monitor recording oxygen saturations, expired gas flow and rise and fall of the chest wall) [9]. Commercially available fitness trackers such as Fitbit may play a role for monitoring trends in sleep quality as well as measuring restoration of normal activity for individuals recovering from critical illness [11], but they cannot be used to assess specific sleep parameters or to diagnose sleep disorders.

3.2 Subjective Measures

Given sleep quality is inherently subjective, self-assessment (with or without objective measurement) is considered by sleep medicine experts to be a key component of sleep assessment in any population [8]. Subjective assessment and history taking are the mainstays for sleep assessment in patients with chronic insomnia [12]. Subjective sleep assessment may include both sleep logs and self-administered questionnaires.

3.2.1 Sleep Logs

Sleep logs or diaries such as the Consensus Sleep Diary [13] allow individuals to record qualitative aspects of their sleep such as 'bedtime', sleep quality, night-time awakenings and daytime fatigue. They provide useful insights about the primary complaint, sleep behaviours, sleep-wake schedule, nocturnal symptoms (particularly if bed partner reports are considered), daytime activities and function and total sleep time [14].

3.2.2 Self-Administered Questionnaires

Sleep quality is a multifaceted construct so it is essential that validated assessment instruments are used. There are many self-administered instruments with demonstrated validity and reliability for assessing sleep including Richards Campbell Sleep Questionnaire [RCSQ] [15], numerical rating scale (NRS) [16], Pittsburgh Sleep Quality Index [PSQI] [17] and Insomnia Severity Index [ISI] [18]. There are no instruments specifically validated for assessing sleep for patients recovering from critical illness. The RCSQ is sometimes reported as being used in the intensive care patient population but often the authors are referring to interactive and cooperative patients who are extubated and sedation-free.

The selection of self-administered questionnaire depends on the purpose of the assessment, the suspected disorder, the cognitive function of the patient and the duration of assessment that is required (or possible). For example, instruments such as the RCSQ [15] and PSQI [18] are designed to assess the quality and quantity of sleep; the RCSQ provides an assessment of sleep domains for the night before while the PSQI provides an assessment of sleep domains over the previous month. In addition, the PSQI incorporates input from a sleeping partner if available. This is particularly useful if SDB is suspected. However multi-domain instruments like the PSQI are too challenging for patients with poor cognitive function; the simpler RCSQ [15] or even a one-dimensional scale like the NRS [16] would be advised in this situation. Some sleep instruments provide the ability to assess just a few sleep domains such as the ISI [18], whereas instruments such as the Functional Outcomes of Sleep [19] and the Epworth Sleepiness Scale [ESS] [20] provide information about the qualitative effect of sleep quality and quantity on daytime function.

4 Sleep Quality and Quantity during ICU Recovery

While sleep quality and quantity is generally poor throughout recovery, it does tend to improve in later recovery stages, with sleep quality and quantity 6 months after ICU discharge returning to pre-critical illness levels. The prevalence of post-ICU sleep disturbance varies between 20 and 67% and depends predominately on gender (female), age, chronic disease (especially respiratory), and pre-illness sleep quality [2]. Additionally, sleep quality often fluctuates over the post-ICU recovery period if acute exacerbations of chronic diseases occur, and particularly if rehospitalization is required. Interestingly a small proportion (10–12%) of patients report poor sleep at each time point in the critical illness and recovery assessment period [21]. Tables 2 and 3 provide summaries of the subjective and objective characteristics of sleep during ICU recovery and their potential variation from expected population norms. Sleep disturbance may be the result of a breathing disorder, circadian rhythm disruption or conditioned insomnia and is associated with varying degrees of fragmentation and functional impacts [2, 22].

Table 2 Summary of subjective sleep characteristics during recovery: potential variation from expected population norm

	Early (during hospitalisation)	Within 1 month in the community	At 6 months in the community
Sleep duration	Reduced	Reduced	Sufficient / reduced
Perceived quality	Very poor	Poor	Poor / good
Fragmentation / awakenings	Very frequent	Frequent	Infrequent / frequent
Daytime dysfunction e.g., sleepiness	Extensive	Moderate	Low

Table 3 Summary of objective sleep characteristics (PSG and actigraphy) during recovery: potential variation from expected population norm

	Early (during hospitalisation)	Within 1 month in the community	At 6 months in the community
TST/SEI	Reduced/normal/ prolonged	Reduced/normal	Normal
NREM sleep stage 1 & 2	Prolonged	Prolonged	Near normal
NREM stage 3	Significantly reduced	Reduced	Near normal
REM	Reduced	Reduced	Near normal
Fragmentation/ awakenings	Severe	Moderate	Low
Daytime sleep, %	Up to 50%	Unknown	Unknown

Notes: *NREM* non-rapid eye movement, *REM* rapid eye movement, *SEI* sleep efficiency index

4.1   Potential Sleep Disturbances during the ICU Recovery Period

A number of different sleep disturbances may occur during the ICU recovery period. These disturbances may differ depending on whether the patient remains institutionalized (e.g., acute or chronic care) or has transitioned to home.

4.1.1   Sleep Disordered Breathing (SDB)

Many patients treated for respiratory failure have concomitant comorbidities including SDB [23]. However, new onset SDB has been detected in survivors both early and later in recovery and was not found to be related to lung function [24].

4.1.2   Circadian Rhythm

As described in chapter "Characteristics of Sleep in Critically Ill Patients. Part II: Circadian Rhythm Disruption", the sleep-wake cycle is partially under the control of the circadian rhythm. Environmental cues (zeitgebers) and an internal clock (the suprachiasmatic nucleus in the anterior hypothalamus) are key determinants of circadian entrainment in humans i.e., nocturnal sleep and daytime wakefulness. However, during critical illness sleep may be distributed equally across night and day [25]. During early critical illness recovery circadian disruption does not appear to be overtly evident on actigraphy [26] and has not been subjectively assessed.

4.1.3   Insomnia

Insomnia is the subjective report of difficulty going to sleep, staying asleep or experiencing non-restorative sleep with functional daytime impacts [27]. This appears to be the most frequently reported type of sleep disturbance during recovery from critical illness and is also the most common sleep disorder in the general public. Conditioned insomnia (also referred to as psychophysiologic insomnia) may be the predominate sub-type in this population. In other words, the condition began after treatment in ICU where the patient experienced sleeplessness resulting in a state of conditioned arousal [28].

4.2   Sleep while Still Hospitalized but after the ICU

The quality and quantity of sleep early during recovery from critical illness (while in the hospital) may show signs of improvement but most often remains unchanged from that during the ICU stay with reduced TST and SEI and evidence of significant sleep disruption [29]. Likewise, as patients transition to a rehabilitation setting and home, TST may be prolonged, normal or reduced, with prolonged stage 1 and 2 sleep and concomitant reduced slow wave and REM sleep and fragmentation observed [24, 26, 30]. Patients self-report slightly improved sleep compared to their ICU experiences; however, most still report disrupted, poor quality and low quantity sleep [21, 29] and daytime sleepiness [30].

4.3   Sleep after Hospital/Institutional Discharge

The quality and quantity of sleep improves later during ICU recovery as patients return home but may not return to the pre-illness quality and quantity for some patients. Specifically, PSG and actigraphy data indicates that both TST and SEI, and slow wave sleep, are near population norms at 6 months after ICU treatment [22, 24]. However subjective reports of sleep quality remain below population norms.

5   Factors Associated with Disturbed Sleep during Recovery

Sleep during recovery from critical illness in the post-discharge period, either at home or in convalescence care, may be affected by physical, psychological, cognitive and social factors. Many of these are features of the patterns of signs and symptoms seen alone or in combination in the constellation known as the post-intensive care syndrome (PICS). The associated factors may include pre-existing problems, the effects of critical illness and the ICU admission, and post-discharge experiences. The evidence about factors associated with post-discharge sleep is limited by few small sample sized studies and the inconsistency of methods of sleep assessment, which prevent meta-analyses in the systematic reviews that have been performed.

5.1   Prehospital

As described in chapter "Risk Factors for Disrupted Sleep in the ICU", multiple prehospital and ICU factors affect sleep quality in the ICU. Patients who are older and female are at greater risk of poor posthospital sleep. Other risk factors for disrupted sleep after discharge are prehospital concurrent disease such as asthma and heart failure [31] and the presence of ≥3 chronic diseases such as diabetes, hypertension and heart disease [32]. Prehospital sleeping problems, including clinical insomnia at home (ISI), have been retrospectively reported by nearly 20% of ICU survivors and found to be independently associated with worse sleep quality six months after discharge [21].

5.2   During Critical Illness and Hospitalization

Severity of illness (APACHE II) on admission [22, 32] and sleep quality (RCSQ) during the periods of ICU admission and post-ICU hospitalization [21] have been shown to be independently associated with sleep disturbances after hospital discharge. In one series of seven patients with acute respiratory distress syndrome (ARDS), overnight PSG in a sleep laboratory was used to diagnose new self-reported sleeping problems between 22 and 168 months (median 50) after ICU discharge [28]. Most (5) had conditioned insomnia, a heightened arousal response that the insomniac has become conditioned to associate with poor sleep and triggered by environmental stimuli that become associated with poor sleep during the ICU stay. Another patient had parasomnia, typically initiated by stress, and one was reported to have mild obstructive sleep apnoea which was diagnosed after discharge from hospital [28].

5.3   After Discharge from Hospital

Several factors affecting sleep present after hospital discharge have commonalities with the features of PICS, although sleep does not feature in constellation of symptoms described in PICS. Some factors related to the critical illness that necessitated intensive care, may potentially affect sleep quality during recovery. Prominent amongst these are health-related quality of life and bodily pain. Because of the bidirectional nature of the associations, with health-related quality of life (HRQoL) and/or pain simultaneously impairing sleep, and sleep disturbances following on from pain and reduced quality of life, the evidence related to these is briefly discussed here but is described more fully below in the impact on outcomes.

Following discharge from hospital after critical illness, HRQoL has been found in several studies when evaluated using either the SF-36 or EuroQol-5D to be associated with sleep disturbances [21, 22, 31, 33, 34]. Multivariate analyses controlling for potential confounders known to affect sleep, including anxiety and depression, found HRQoL to be significantly associated with sleep quality both 3 months [22] and 6 months [21] after ICU discharge.

Some investigators have reported a relationship between pain (and its related symptoms) and sleep in survivors of critical illness after hospital discharge. A significant bivariate relationship between pain and sleep disturbance was found 2 months after discharge in a small sample of medical ICU patients who had required long durations of ventilation [35]. Langerud and colleagues [36] also found chronic, post-ICU pain was associated with a greater risk for sleep disturbance three and 12 months after discharge. Bodily pain on the SF-36 has also been reported to be independently associated with post discharge sleep in several other studies [21, 22, 33, 34].

6   Impact of Disturbed Sleep after Critical Illness on Recovery Outcomes

Posthospital sleep disturbances are known to affect the outcomes associated with recovery from critical illness. As noted above, there are many features in the patterns of signs and symptoms seen alone or in combination in the constellation known as the post-intensive care syndrome (PICS). These factors are often interrelated and likely bidirectional. As noted in the prior section, reduced quality of life and chronic pain are important risk factors for poor post-ICU sleep. Poor post-ICU sleep may also worsen quality of life and increase pain. Disrupted sleep in the post-ICU recovery period will also worsen HRQoL and psychological symptoms such as those of posttraumatic stress, and may impair cognitive function. A cause-and-effect relationship is sometimes claimed, e.g., that observed sleep disturbances *affected* mental health and bodily pain domains [31]. However, the evidence equally could support a bidirectional relationship.

6.1 Health-Related Quality of Life

Assessment of HRQoL after critical illness and intensive care has mostly been studied with the SF-36 [37] and the EuroQol-5D (EQ-5D) [38] in combination with a range of self-report sleep instruments. Various sleep parameters have been found to be independently associated with both global measures and specific domains of HRQoL. Solverson and colleagues [22] reported associations between sleep quality assessed with the PSQI 3 months after discharge and anxiety (HADS), perceived health status, mobility and self-care (EQ-5D), and with the Physical (PCS) and Mental composite scores (MCS) of the SF-36). (The composite scores, both PCS and MCS, are made up of each of the eight SF-36 subscale scores with the subscale scores weighted differently in calculating the total score according to its contribution to the two major physical and mental domains). Investigators who used the Basic Nordic Sleep Questionnaire (3 items) in former ICU patients at 6 months found correlations with the SF-36 scales for mental health, bodily pain, general health, vitality and role limitations due to physical problems. Relationships have also been found between sleep assessed at 12 months [34] and 6 months (PSQI) after general ICU and the PCS and MCS of the SF-36 [21, 39], and in postoperative coronary artery bypass graft patients who had a median stay of 2 days in the ICU [40].

6.2 Psychological Symptoms

Psychological symptoms are commonly observed in critical illness survivors with symptoms of anxiety, depression and posttraumatic stress symptoms (PTSS) often detected. (Posttraumatic stress symptoms is used to indicate reporting of posttraumatic symptoms as distinct from diagnosis of posttraumatic stress disorder—PTSD). The relationship between mental health symptoms and disordered sleep is complex. Up to 40% of the general population who report insomnia have also been diagnosed with a psychiatric condition [41], while up to 90% of people with depression report some type of sleep disturbance [42]. There is substantial overlap between disordered sleep and mental health disorders. Critical illness survivors are a unique population, but this relationship between mental health symptoms and disordered sleep appears to be present.

The association of PTSS and post-discharge sleep in ICU patients has been studied using the Impact of Events Scale -Revised (IES-R) which assesses the post-trauma symptoms of intrusion, avoidance and hyperarousal [43]. It was found in multivariate analyses that PTS symptoms were related to worse sleep 6 months [33] and 12 months [34] after ICU.

In two studies [22, 44] data were collected on anxiety, depression and trauma-related symptoms, and on sleep (PSQI or self-report on sleep disturbances) at 3 months after ICU. Anxiety or trauma-related symptoms were found to correlate most strongly with poorer quality sleep, but symptoms of depression were not associated with sleep disturbances. In a secondary analysis of patients enrolled in a rehabilitation study out to 6 months after ICU discharge [33], sleep disturbances were associated with anxiety, stress, and depression (DASS-21).

The prevalence of mental health symptomatology and sleep disturbances in patients with specific physical conditions or comorbidities has also been studied. One study [45] performing follow-up of participants with sepsis aftercare reported an increase in PTSS in some participants 24 months after ICU discharge. There was no commensurate increase in reported sleep disturbances.

7 Strategies for Sleep Promotion during Recovery

As outlined above, the factors related to sleep disturbance post-ICU are multifactorial, change over time, and can persist for 6–12 months after ICU discharge. The environment for recovery is varied and can include an existing or new home, a rehabilitation facility or a long-term acute care hospital.

Sleep disorders are common in the general population, with more than half (59.4%) of adult Australians affected by at least one chronic sleep symptom [46] and 14.8% of people have symptoms of chronic insomnia, as classified by the International Classification of Sleep Disorders. Almost half (48.8%) report that all or most of the time their daily routine does not provide adequate opportunity to sleep.

The high prevalence of disordered sleep, heterogeneity of patients and lack of data makes a single specific strategy for sleep promotion during ICU recovery difficult to recommend. However, clinicians should start with some understanding of whether the disturbance is pre-existing and/or related to the recent episode of critical illness.

For sleep disturbance that appears related to the recent critical illness, a multidisciplinary ICU follow-up clinic provides an opportunity and the time required to identify new sleep issues. Prior to, or during the clinic visit, a subjective sleep screening tool such as the PSQI or ESS (for cognitively impaired patients a unidimensional instrument such as the RCSQ or NRS can be used to assess global sleep quality). Other assessment methods, particularly mental health screening tools, can help identify factors associated with sleep disturbance. This allows for patients with significant symptoms of anxiety, depression and/or PTSS to be identified and referred for specialized mental health services in parallel to general sleep recommendations. As sleep affects and is affected by all domains of health a holistic approach is advised; see Table 1 for guidance.

7.1   Assessment and Referral

Pre-existing disordered sleep or chronic insomnia may be best directed to the patient's treating general practitioner or, if known to one, their sleep physician. In referring to their treating clinician, referral communication should acknowledge the role critical illness can have in precipitating an acute deterioration, as this may not be appreciated by all non-ICU clinicians. Patients should also be assessed for sleep-altering effects from common medications prescribed in ICU (see chapter "Effects of Common ICU Medications on Sleep"). SDB should be treated by a sleep expert, but insomnia treatment may be provided by other health professionals such as the ICU follow up team or the primary provider. A brief summary of examples of insomnia treatments follows.

7.2   Treatment for Chronic Insomnia

Generally, chronic insomnia can be difficult to treat and is often relapsing. However reasonable sleep improvements can be expected when non-pharmacological, single component treatments such as relaxation therapy and sleep hygiene techniques (SHTs) are implemented. More lasting improvements may be achieved with multi-component treatments such as cognitive behavioral therapy for insomnia (CBT-I). The potential harms associated with pharmacological interventions, i.e. sedatives and hypnotics, such as dependency, worsening cognitive function and falls particularly in the elderly preclude their use for insomnia. Current recommendation from sleep experts is that sedatives and hypnotics should be avoided and prescribed only in the short term by sleep experts [47]. Generalized recommendations about pharmacological treatments are usually not provided by sleep experts, with selection of the type and dose of medication based on the individual patient's needs and health status [27].

7.2.1   Single Component Treatments

Relaxation Therapy
Relaxation therapy includes structured exercises to reduce body tension, using techniques such as abdominal breathing, autogenic (desensitization-relaxation) training, systematic and progressive muscle relaxation, and mental stimulation e.g., meditation, guided imagery. Specific sleep experts are not required to deliver this safe and cost-effective single component treatment. Relaxation therapy is a vital first step in assisting ICU survivors experiencing poor quality sleep and may be all that is required to enable restorative sleep [47].

Stimulus Control

This single component treatment has some supporting low level research evidence [47] and requires some expertise to deliver (i.e., motivational techniques) but could be learned by the ICU clinician. The objective is to reduce conditioned insomnia by providing instructions to ameliorate the association between the bed/bedroom and wakefulness and re-establish the association of bed/bedroom with sleep and ensure a consistent wake-time. Therefore, stimulus control instructions are:

1. Wake and get up at the same time each morning
2. Go to bed only when sleepy
3. When unable to sleep get out of bed
4. Use the bed/bedroom for sleep and sex only (all reading, TV and social media activity should be conducted in other rooms)
5. Do not nap during the daytime

Sleep Restriction

This technique is designed to enhance the urge to sleep and consolidate sleep by constraining time in bed to the patient's average sleep time [47]. The sleep time is often derived from self-administered sleep logs. Initially time in bed is restricted to average sleep time and subsequently increased or decreased based on sleep efficiency, until adequate sleep time is achieved. This is typically based on overall sleep satisfaction and daytime function. Sleep restriction is best administered by a sleep expert.

Sleep Hygiene Techniques (SHTs)

SHTs are a single component treatment focused on educating the patient on creating the most conducive ambiance, physical condition, and psychological status for sleep. Empirically supported SHTs include instruction on a range of strategies which the patient can implement at home. Strategies such as a regular bedtime, avoiding screens (e.g., phone and computer screens), avoiding coffee and alcohol and minimizing sleep medications are effective and safe to recommend [48]. It is recommended that SHTs are not used in isolation but in combination with CBT-I [47].

7.2.2 Multicomponent Treatments

Cognitive Behavior Therapy for Insomnia (CBT-I)

CBT-I is a multicomponent evidence-based [49], cost effective [50] approach to treat insomnia. The effect can match hypnotic drugs and persist after completion of therapy [49]. It is the mainstay for insomnia treatment [47]. For patients living remote from a large referral hospital, CBT-I can be as effective when delivered online or via telephone [51] and may also be delivered effectively by the primary care provider [52].

CBT-I is generally delivered over 4–10 sessions and includes sleep hygiene education, stimulus control, sleep-restriction therapy, relaxation techniques and cognitive therapy. Four or more sessions appears to be more effective than a single consultation [53] but even a single session can be powerful and reassuring for patients and families in acknowledging any sleep disturbance and normalizing the process. This allows the start of a patient-centered approach to sleep education that will be critical in recovery. Patients can leave the consult empowered with increased knowledge as well as educational material and reliable resources to manage their condition.

Brief Therapies for Insomnia (BTIs)

BTIs are an abbreviated version of CBT-I [47]. They usually comprise up to 4 sessions in which the behavioral components of sleep promotion are emphasized. Components of BTIs include education about sleep and circadian rhythm, factors that influence sleep quality, and behaviors that adversely affect or promote sleep, combined with an individualized behavioral prescription based on self-administered sleep diaries/logs, comprising stimulus control and sleep restriction therapy. Cognitive and relaxation therapies are other key components. Although not as effective as CBT-I, BTIs may be an achievable component of an ICU follow-up service and could be provided as a bridge to CBT-I if access to this is constrained by cost or availability.

8   Concluding Remarks and Future Directions

This chapter has presented a summary of the research to date on sleep in survivors of critical illness that is broad in its scope though necessarily brief in description. The means of assessing sleep, the nature of sleep during recovery and factors associated with this and strategies for improving sleep in ICU survivors have benefitted from the science and scholarship published to date. Nevertheless, there remains a paucity of published sleep research to guide practitioners in the assessment and treatment of sleep in ICU survivors. Therefore, in the absence of strong evidence, the use of assessment methods (i.e., history taking, screening and sleep assessment for the most likely sleep disorder with an abbreviated PSG montage if required) and interventions (e.g. CBT-I) used by sleep medicine experts is advised. Pharmacological interventions are not generally recommended. It is imperative that this vital aspect of health is considered during the holistic follow up of ICU survivors and that appropriate care, support and treatment is offered.

Further research to investigate the most appropriate time in the recovery trajectory to screen and assess sleep, assessment methods, the impact of sleep disturbance on outcomes and interventions for improvement would be beneficial. For example, software on commercially available fitness trackers may be a low cost and burdenless method of continuously assessing trends in sleep quality and providing an indication of a potential sleep disorder. More scientific information on the sources and mechanisms of sleep disturbance during recovery from critical illness, and trialling of novel interventions to improve outcomes will be beneficial for patients and their treating practitioners.

References

1. Elliott D, et al. Exploring the scope of post-intensive care syndrome therapy and care: engagement of non-critical care providers and survivors in a second stakeholders meeting. Crit Care Med. 2014;42(12):2518–26.
2. Altman MT, Knauert MP, Pisani MA. Sleep disturbance after hospitalization and critical illness: a systematic review. Ann Am Thorac Soc. 2017;14(9):1457–68.
3. Denehy L, Hough CL. Critical illness, disability, and the road home. Intensive Care Med. 2017;43(12):1881–3.
4. Ramsay P, et al. A rehabilitation intervention to promote physical recovery following intensive care: a detailed description of construct development, rationale and content together with proposed taxonomy to capture processes in a randomised controlled trial. Trials. 2014;15:38.
5. Hopkins RO, Wade D, Jackson JC. What's new in cognitive function in ICU survivors. Intensive Care Med. 2017;43(2):223–5.
6. Mikkelsen ME, et al. Society of Critical Care Medicine's International Consensus Conference on Prediction and Identification of Long-Term Impairments After Critical Illness. Crit Care Med. 2020;48(11):1670–9.
7. Carskadon MA, Dement WC. Chapter 2. Normal Human Sleep: An overview. In: Kryger MH, Roth T, Dement WC, editors. Principles and practice of sleep medicine. Philadelphia, PA: Elsevier; 2017.
8. Kapur VK, et al. Clinical practice guideline for diagnostic testing for adult obstructive sleep apnea: an American Academy of sleep medicine clinical practice guideline. J Clin Sleep Med. 2017;13(3):479–504.
9. Smith MT, et al. Use of Actigraphy for the evaluation of sleep disorders and circadian rhythm sleep-wake disorders: an American Academy of sleep medicine clinical practice guideline. J Clin Sleep Med. 2018;14(7):1231–7.
10. Goncalves BS, et al. Nonparametric methods in actigraphy: an update. Sleep Sci. 2014;7(3):158–64.
11. Louzon PR, et al. Characterisation of ICU sleep by a commercially available activity tracker and its agreement with patient-perceived sleep quality. BMJ Open Respir Res. 2020;7(1)
12. Riemann D, et al. European guideline for the diagnosis and treatment of insomnia. J Sleep Res. 2017;26(6):675–700.
13. Carney CE, et al. The consensus sleep diary: standardizing prospective sleep self-monitoring. Sleep. 2012;35(2):287–302.
14. Dietch JR, Taylor DJ. Evaluation of the consensus sleep diary in a community sample: comparison with single-channel EEG, actigraphy, and retrospective questionnaire. J Clin Sleep Med. 2021;17(7):1389–99.
15. Richards K. Techniques for measurement of sleep in critical care. Focus Crit Care. 1987;14(4):34–40.
16. Rood P, et al. Development and daily use of a numeric rating score to assess sleep quality in ICU patients. J Crit Care. 2019;52:68–74.
17. Buysse DJ, et al. The Pittsburgh sleep quality index: a new instrument for psychiatric practice and research. Psychiatry Res. 1989;28(2):193–213.

18. Morin CM, et al. The insomnia severity index: psychometric indicators to detect insomnia cases and evaluate treatment response. Sleep. 2011;34(5):601–8.
19. Weaver TE, et al. An instrument to measure functional status outcomes for disorders of excessive sleepiness. Sleep. 1997;20(10):835–43.
20. Johns M, Hocking B. Daytime sleepiness and sleep habits of Australian workers. Sleep. 1997;20(10):844–9.
21. McKinley S, et al. Sleep and psychological health during early recovery from critical illness: an observational study. J Psychosom Res. 2013;75(6):539–45.
22. Solverson KJ, Easton PA, Doig CJ. Assessment of sleep quality post-hospital discharge in survivors of critical illness. Respir Med. 2016;114:97–102.
23. Adler D, et al. Comorbidities and subgroups of patients surviving severe acute Hypercapnic respiratory failure in the intensive care unit. Am J Respir Crit Care Med. 2017;196(2):200–7.
24. Alexopoulou C, et al. Sleep quality in survivors of critical illness. Sleep Breath. 2019;23(2):463–71.
25. Gao CA, Knauert MP. Circadian biology and its importance to intensive care unit care and outcomes. Semin Respir Crit Care Med. 2019;40(5):629–37.
26. Wilcox ME, et al. Sleep fragmentation and cognitive trajectories after critical illness. Chest. 2021;159(1):366–81.
27. Sateia MJ, et al. Clinical practice guideline for the pharmacologic treatment of chronic insomnia in adults: an American Academy of sleep medicine clinical practice guideline. J Clin Sleep Med. 2017;13(2):307–49.
28. Lee CM, et al. Chronic sleep disorders in survivors of the acute respiratory distress syndrome. Intensive Care Med. 2009;35(2):314–20.
29. Elias MN, Munro CL, Liang Z. Sleep quality associated with motor function among older adult survivors of critical illness. Nurs Res. 2020;69(4):322–8.
30. Dhooria S, et al. Sleep after critical illness: study of survivors of acute respiratory distress syndrome and systematic review of literature. Ind J Crit Care Med. 2016;20(6):323–31.
31. Orwelius L, et al. Prevalence of sleep disturbances and long-term reduced health-related quality of life after critical care: a prospective multicenter cohort study. Crit Care. 2008;12(4):R97.
32. Chen CJ, et al. Predictors of sleep quality and successful weaning from mechanical ventilation among patients in respiratory care centers. J Nurs Res. 2015;23(1):65–74.
33. McKinley S, et al. Sleep and other factors associated with mental health and psychological distress after intensive care for critical illness. Intensive Care Med. 2012;38(4):627–33.
34. Parsons EC, et al. Post-discharge insomnia symptoms are associated with quality of life impairment among survivors of acute lung injury. Sleep Med. 2012;13(8):1106–9.
35. Choi J, et al. Self-reported physical symptoms in intensive care unit (ICU) survivors: pilot exploration over four months post-ICU discharge. J Pain Symptom Manag. 2014;47(2):257–70.
36. Langerud AK, et al. Intensive care survivor-reported symptoms: a longitudinal study of survivors' symptoms. Nurs Crit Care. 2018;23(1):48–54.
37. Ware JE Jr. SF-36 health survey update. Spine (Phila Pa 1976). 2000;25(24):3130–9.
38. Rabin R, de Charro F. EQ-5D: a measure of health status from the EuroQol group. Ann Med. 2001;33(5):337–43.
39. McKinley S, et al. Health-related quality of life and associated factors in intensive care unit survivors 6 months after discharge. Am J Crit Care. 2016;25(1):52–8.
40. Caruana N, et al. Sleep quality during and after cardiothoracic intensive care and psychological health during recovery. J Cardiovasc Nurs. 2018;33(4):E40–e49.
41. Anderson KN, Bradley AJ. Sleep disturbance in mental health problems and neurodegenerative disease. Nat Sci Sleep. 2013;5:61–75.
42. Fang H, et al. Depression in sleep disturbance: a review on a bidirectional relationship, mechanisms and treatment. J Cell Mol Med. 2019;23(4):2324–32.
43. Weiss D, Marmar C. The impact of event scale-revised. In: Wilson JP, Keane TM, editors. Assessing psychological trauma and PTSD: a Practitioner's handbook New York. Guilford Press; 1997.

44. Wang S, et al. Psychiatric symptoms and their association with sleep disturbances in intensive care unit survivors. Int J General Med. 2019;12:125–30.
45. Schmidt KF, et al. Long-term courses of sepsis survivors: effects of a primary care management intervention. Am J Med. 2020;133(3):381–385. e5.
46. Reynolds A, et al. Chronic insomnia disorder in Australia: a report to the sleep Health Foundation. North Strathfield, NSW: Sleep Health Foundation; 2019.
47. Edinger JD, et al. Behavioral and psychological treatments for chronic insomnia disorder in adults: an American Academy of sleep medicine clinical practice guideline. J Clin Sleep Med. 2021;17(2):255–62.
48. Irish LA, et al. The role of sleep hygiene in promoting public health: a review of empirical evidence. Sleep Med Rev. 2015;22:23–36.
49. Edinger JD, et al. Behavioral and psychological treatments for chronic insomnia disorder in adults: an American Academy of sleep medicine systematic review, meta-analysis, and GRADE assessment. J Clin Sleep Med. 2021;17(2):263–98.
50. Natsky AN, et al. Economic evaluation of cognitive behavioural therapy for insomnia (CBT-I) for improving health outcomes in adult populations: a systematic review. Sleep Med Rev. 2020;54:101351.
51. Espie CA, et al. A randomized, placebo-controlled trial of online cognitive behavioral therapy for chronic insomnia disorder delivered via an automated media-rich web application. Sleep. 2012;35(6):769–81.
52. Davidson JR, Dickson C, Han H. Cognitive behavioural treatment for insomnia in primary care: a systematic review of sleep outcomes. Br J Gen Pract. 2019;69(686):e657–64.
53. van Straten A, et al. Cognitive and behavioral therapies in the treatment of insomnia: a meta-analysis. Sleep Med Rev. 2018;38:3–16.

Methods for Routine Sleep Assessment and Monitoring

Alexander O. Pile, Erica B. Feldman, Jennifer L. Martin, and Biren B. Kamdar

1   Introduction

The role of sleep and sleep disruption in critical illness is an emerging topic of interest. While it is widely accepted that sleep is important for recovery from critical illness, this field is challenged by a lack of effective methods to measure sleep in the context of factors such as patient illness, sleep-altering medications, other monitoring devices, and staff availability. This chapter reviews methods to evaluate sleep in critically ill patients, including polysomnography, bispectral index (BIS), actigraphy, questionnaires and novel methods such as commercially available smartwatches.

A. O. Pile
Department of Biological Sciences, University of California San Diego, La Jolla, CA, USA
e-mail: apile@ucsd.edu

E. B. Feldman · B. B. Kamdar (✉)
Division of Pulmonary, Critical Care, Sleep Medicine and Physiology,
UC San Diego School of Medicine, La Jolla, CA, USA
e-mail: e2feldman@health.ucsd.edu; bkamdar@health.ucsd.edu

J. L. Martin
VA Greater Los Angeles Healthcare System, Geriatric Research, Education and Clinical Center and David Geffen School of Medicine at the University of California,
Los Angeles, CA, USA
e-mail: Jennifer.martin@va.gov

2 Objective Methods to Measure Sleep

2.1 Polysomnography

Polysomnography (PSG), widely considered the "gold standard" for sleep measurement, involves the objective measurement of physiological and electrical changes based on simultaneous electroencephalogram (EEG), electro-oculogram (EOG), electrocardiogram (ECG) and electromyogram (EMG) recordings [1]. PSG provides data on total sleep duration, sleep architecture (sleep stages), and frequency and duration of awakenings [1]. Typically, PSG is conducted in a controlled sleep laboratory where patients are monitored overnight. In comparison, use of PSG in critically ill adults is challenging for a number of reasons including cumbersome equipment, high cost, need for close monitoring, patient intolerance, frequent ICU-related disruptions, and difficulties with interpretation. As highlighted in chapters "Risk Factors for Disrupted Sleep in the ICU", "Effects of Common ICU Medications on Sleep" and "Mechanical Ventilation and Sleep", critically ill patients often receive mechanical ventilation, sedative infusions, steroids, analgesics, and vasoactive medications, all of which can alter signals obtained during PSG recordings [2–6].

2.1.1 Data from ICU Application

As noted in chapter "Characteristics of Sleep in Critically Ill Patients. Part I: Sleep Fragmentation and Sleep Stage Disruption", PSG has been used widely in the ICU setting, in particular in seminal studies describing sleep in critically ill patients (Fig. 1) [7]. In one observational study involving mechanically ventilated patients, PSG was used to demonstrate that patients experience markedly disrupted sleep architecture, with skipped stages, reduced rapid eye movement (REM) sleep, and frequent daytime and nighttime arousals and awakenings [8]. Additionally, 24-h portable PSG recordings revealed sleep architecture disruptions in non-ventilated ICU patients similar to those observed in mechanically ventilated patients [1].

Numerous PSG studies have observed that critically ill patients often exhibit EEG patterns that are uninterpretable using traditional scoring criteria, due to reduced REM, a lack of K complexes and sleep spindles, and a preponderance of monomorphic delta and theta waves [8–11]. Using modified EEG cutoffs and automated spectral analysis, several studies proposed modified ICU-specific sleep scoring strategies [11–14]. One such study noted that critically ill patients who appeared awake had PSG patterns suggesting sleep, and vice versa, and proposed a new scoring system that included traditional stages along with pathologic wakefulness and six "atypical" designations of non-normal sleep (Fig. 2) [15]. (Chapter "Atypical Sleep and Pathologic Wakefulness" provides additional background on atypical sleep and pathologic wakefulness). This adapted scoring system has been used in various studies, including one investigating the effect of a "quiet routine" intervention that did not yield improvements in patient sleep [16].

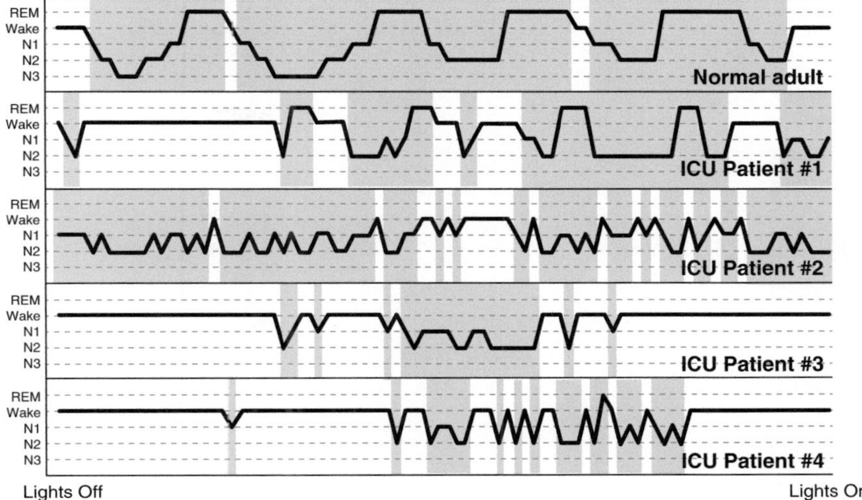

Fig. 1 Polysomnography in one healthy and four critically ill patients. Gray areas represent sleep while white areas represent wake. Notable in critically ill patients is the fragmentation and near-lack of REM and N3 sleep [7]. From "Sleep and Sleep Disordered Breathing in Hospitalized Patients", by M. P. Knauert, 2014, *Semin Respir Crit Care Med, 35*(5), 582–92. Copyright 2014 by Georg Thieme Verlag KG Stuttgart. Reprinted with permission

In addition to describing sleep rhythms, PSG has also been used to evaluate the influence of environmental factors on sleep in the ICU, including unnatural and inconsistent levels of light, loud sounds, and patient care interactions [17]. (Chapter "Risk Factors for Disrupted Sleep in the ICU" reviews risk factors for disrupted sleep). For example, a prospective cohort analysis of 22 ICU patients undergoing PSG demonstrated that all patients experienced sleep-wake cycle abnormalities, with noise being the primary contributor to about 17% of awakenings [9]. Another study comparing PSG in mechanically ventilated and healthy adults exposed to an ICU environment demonstrated that 21% of arousals and awakenings were attributed to sounds exceeding guideline-recommended levels, while 7% were attributed to interruptions such as visitations and treatment [18].

2.1.2 Limitations in the ICU

Various ICU-related factors can alter PSG patterns and thus complicate sleep measurement. Commonly used sedatives such as benzodiazepines and propofol are associated with changes in EEG amplitude and frequency, and analgesics and antipsychotics have been associated with EEG slowing and altered sleep architecture [19–21] as described in greater detail in chapter "Effects of Common ICU Medications on Sleep". Illness itself can also alter and complicate PSG interpretation, specifically common ICU conditions such as encephalopathy, sepsis, and electrolyte derangements [22, 23].

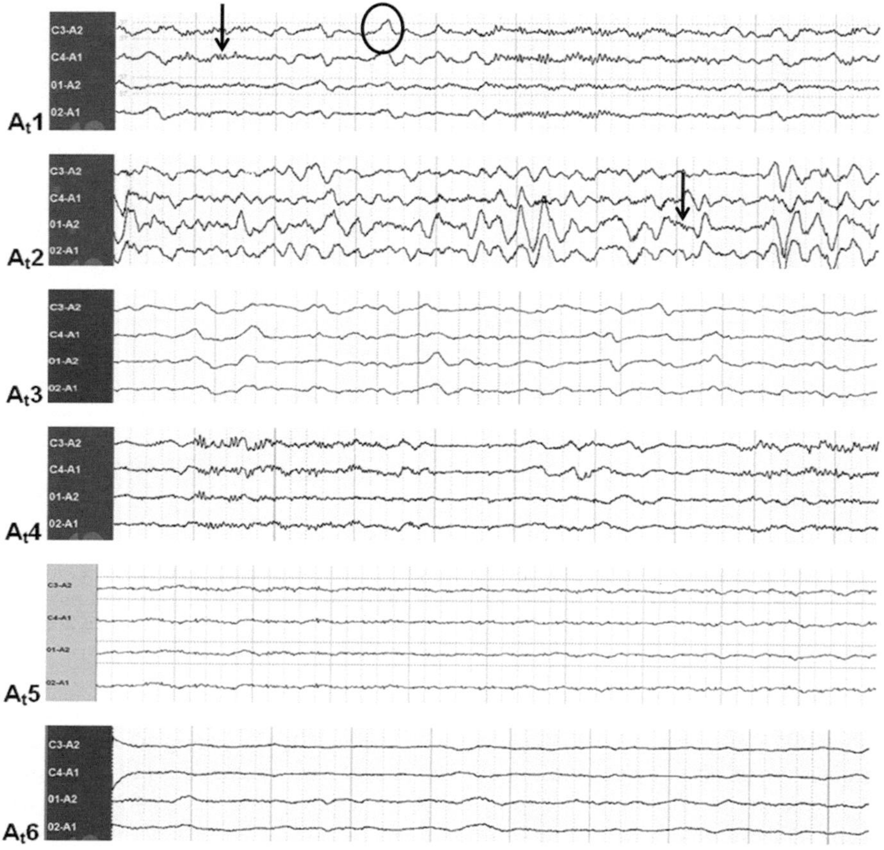

Fig. 2 Atypical PSG recording from a critically ill patient, scored using modified criteria (A_t1–6) as follows: atypical stage 1 (A_t1): ≥10% alpha and/or theta activity (arrow) and some delta activity (circle), frontal intermittent rhythmic delta activity (FIRDA), and/or triphasic activity; A_t2: intermittent alpha, beta, or theta complexes (arrow) without polymorphic delta activity; A_t3: polymorphic delta activity without alpha, beta or theta complexes; A_t4: EEG amplitude <5 μV mixed with burst suppression (isoelectric activity); A_t5: burst suppression patterns similar to A_t4 with EEG amplitude <20 μV; A_t6: no EEG activity (isoelectric). Last, a sleep stage was proposed to capture atypical but pathologic wakefulness, characterized by wakefulness devoid of alpha and beta activity [15]. From "Atypical Sleep in Ventilated Patients: Empirical Electroencephalography Findings and the Path Toward Revised ICU Sleep Scoring Criteria," by P. L. Watson, 2013, *Critical Care Medicine, 41*(8), 1958–67. Copyright 2013 by the Society of Critical Care Medicine and Lippincott Williams. Reprinted with permission

From a usability standpoint, large-scale application of PSG is not feasible due to its high cost, cumbersome equipment, and the need for trained personnel for setup and interpretation. Consequently, few ICU-based studies have obtained PSG beyond 24 h [24]. An evaluation of 24-h unattended portable PSG yielded usable data from 27 of 29 enrolled patients, however nine prematurely discontinued participation while 5 experienced inadvertent removal and dislodged electrodes [25]. Notably, a low enrollment rate was observed in the study, with family and staff declining to participate, presumably due to perceived invasiveness of PSG and the presence of extra monitoring equipment required. In other studies, common reasons for PSG discontinuation include electrical or respiratory artifact [8] and device malfunction [12]. Given these challenges, the 2018 Clinical Practice Guidelines for the Prevention and Management of Pain, Agitation/Sedation, Delirium, Immobility, and Sleep Disruption in the ICU (PADIS) do not recommend the routine use of PSG in the ICU [25, 26].

2.2 Bispectral Index

Bispectral Index (BIS) poses another option for objective sleep measurement. Typically used in the operating room to guide titration of general anesthesia, BIS integrates data from EEG electrodes contained within a single forehead sensor to generate a value of 0 to 100, with 100 representing maximum wakefulness [27, 28].

2.2.1 Data from ICU Application

BIS has been evaluated in several ICU studies. Using a previously-established BIS sleep scoring system (>85 = awake, 60–85 = light sleep, <60 = slow wave sleep, and REM scored by combining EMG recordings with BIS) [29], a 2001 study of 27 minimally sedated ICU patients used BIS to confirm poor sleep in the patients who averaged 98 min of sleep across the 10-h recording period [30]. Subsequently, a randomized trial of melatonin versus placebo in 24 mechanically ventilated patients used BIS to evaluate nighttime sleep quality [31]. Using a BIS cutoff of 80 to represent sleep, the study found that patients receiving melatonin had a higher sleep efficiency, however simultaneous actigraphy, nurse assessment, and Richards Campbell Sleep Questionnaire (RCSQ) recordings did not corroborated this result [31]. Finally, a cross-sectional study aiming to evaluate BIS for ICU sleep measurement found that 29 critically ill adults experienced an average total nighttime sleep duration of 234 min, with 1.7 min of deep sleep [32]. Notably, in these mostly awake patients, BIS was limited in its ability to identify lighter stages of sleep, suggesting that BIS was infeasible as a method to estimate ICU sleep [32].

2.2.2 Limitations in the ICU

While BIS is less cumbersome than PSG, it requires an electrode which can easily fall off or be removed [27]. Further, patients in the ICU are often sedated, ventilated, hemodynamically unstable or cognitively impaired, all of which can affect the EEG data necessary for BIS. As such, several studies involving BIS excluded delirious patients [31–33]. While BIS may be more affordable and feasible to use than PSG, it shares many of its limitations and unlike PSG is substantially limited in its ability to differentiate between sleep stages and light sleep and wakefulness [27, 28]. Robust, large-scale studies are required to evaluate BIS as a measure of sleep in the ICU.

2.3 Actigraphy

Actigraphy involves use of an accelerometer to measure physical activity, usually by applying a wristwatch-type device on the wrist or ankle [34–36]. Low cost and easy to apply, actigraphy rest-activity data have been used for decades to estimate sleep [37–43], including in the ICU where it has been shown to be feasible and well tolerated for continuous use [31, 34, 36, 44–49].

While actigraphy has been validated against PSG as a measure of sleep in healthy outpatients [42, 43], a study of 12 mechanically ventilated hospitalized patients revealed that actigraphy overestimated total sleep time and efficiency as compared to PSG, with <65% agreement [50].

2.3.1 Data from ICU Application

Despite its potential for sleep misestimation, actigraphy has been used to estimate differences in sleep in several ICU-based intervention studies, including those involving melatonin [31, 44, 45], valerian acupressure [49], and bright light therapy [51, 52]. Actigraphy-based measurements have also been used to describe circadian rest-activity rhythms in diverse critically ill populations, including sedated and non-sedated patients and those in medical, surgical and neurological ICUs [51, 53, 54]. Like studies involving PSG, most of these studies were small but given its feasibility and low cost, large-scale efforts should consider actigraphy as an outcome measure, particularly those involving an intervention to improve sleep-wake or rest-activity rhythms. Future studies are warranted to develop ICU-specific algorithms to score sleep using actigraphy data.

2.3.2 Limitations in the ICU

As critically ill patients are often inactive, actigraphy interpretation, when scored using traditional algorithms, is prone to misclassification of motionless wakefulness as sleep [34]. For example, a study of actigraphy feasibility in 35 critically ill patients demonstrated that 64% and 83% of 30-second wrist and ankle measurements, respectively, equaled zero, with 72% and 93% scored as "sleep" by a traditional scoring algorithm (Fig. 3) [34]. Unsurprisingly, patients with higher organ failure scores, restraints, or those receiving mechanical ventilation or continuous sedation registered more zero-activity epochs and lower non-zero activity levels, rest-activity patterns that could be misclassified as sleep by traditional scoring algorithms [55]. Nevertheless, if not for sleep estimation, wrist actigraphy in the ICU can be used to collect large-scale activity measurements.

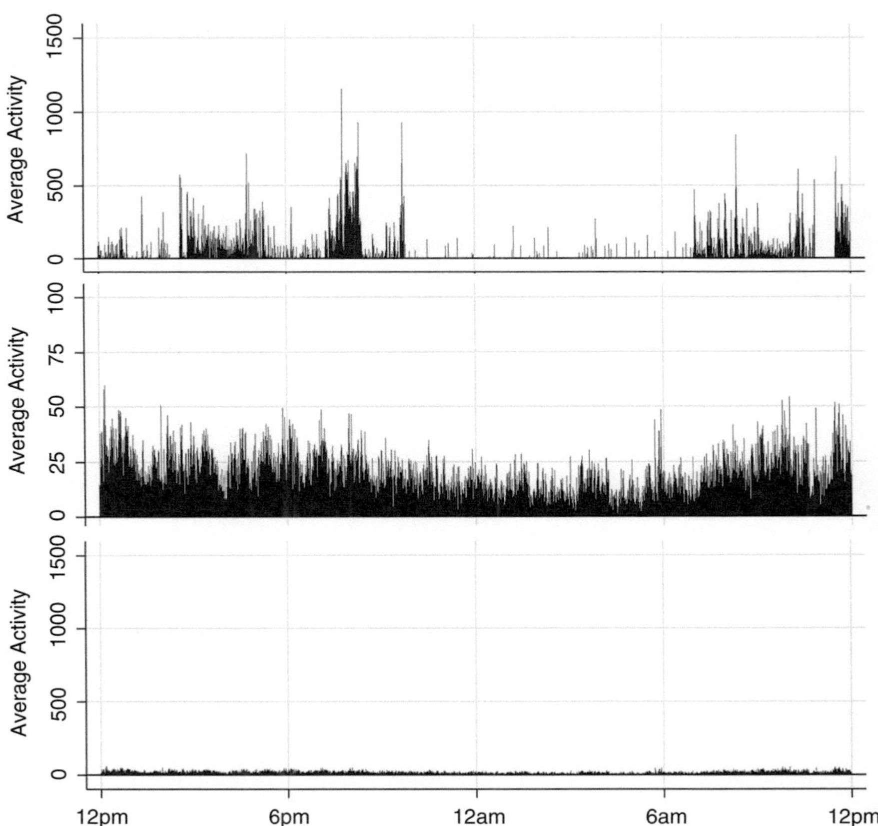

Fig. 3 Twenty-four-hour wrist actigraphy in a healthy adult (top panel) as compared to critically ill patients in a medical ICU (middle and bottom panels). Notably, the healthy adult exhibits rest-activity fluctuations corresponding to circadian sleep-wake cycles, with activity peaks exceeding 1000 movements per 30-second epoch. Alternatively, aggregate activity data from 35 critically ill patients demonstrate near absent rest-activity rhythmicity and activity peaks rarely exceeding 50 movements per epoch. Displaying critically ill patient activity on a 0 to 1500 scale highlights the profound immobility affecting this population [34]. From "Feasibility of Continuous Actigraphy in Patients in a Medical Intensive Care Unit," by B. B. Kamdar, 2017, *American Journal of Critical Care, 26*(4), 329–35. Copyright 2017 by the American Association of Critical-Care Nurses. Reprinted with permission

3 Subjective Methods to Measure Sleep (Table 1)

3.1 Clinician Observation

One 1993 study compared PSG recordings with Sleep Observation Tool (SOT) assessments (a clinician-based evaluation of sleep and wake states) in critically ill adults [56]. From 1 am to 5 am, every 15 min, fifteen nurses logged whether 21 patients (all but one mechanically ventilated) who were undergoing PSG were "Asleep," "Awake," or "Could Not Tell". Over 272 sleep-wake observations, nurses recorded "sleep" accurately 88% of the time (145 of 165 observations) and "awake" 70% of the time (55 of 79 observations) when compared with PSG [56].

As an alternative to the SOT, other studies have evaluated customized sleep evaluation tools. A study involving 12 mechanically ventilated patients compared nurse observation, actigraphy and PSG and concluded that nurse assessments were both inaccurate and unreliable; however, this study lacked a specific observation protocol, with nurses estimating hours slept and number of awakenings at the end of the recording period [50]. Another study evaluating PSG versus nurse assessment in 9 surgical ICU patients, with observations made every 5 min, suggested that nurses tend to overestimate sleep time compared to PSG [57]. Hence, while bedside staff are capable of logging sleep-wake observations in busy ICU settings, current methods may be too labor intensive and/or unreliable for widespread use.

3.2 Patient-Perception: Richards-Campbell Sleep Questionnaire

The Richards-Campbell Sleep Questionnaire (RCSQ) is the most commonly used subjective method of sleep measurement in the ICU setting, and the only one validated against PSG [58, 59]. The RCSQ is comprised of five items, each on a 0 mm to 100 mm visual-analogue scale (VAS), inquiring about sleep depth, onset latency (the time spent in bed for sleep before actually falling asleep), number of awakenings, time spent awake, and overall sleep quality, with an average of the five items equaling a total sleep score (0 = bad sleep and 100 = good sleep). Several studies that used the RCSQ also added a sixth 0 to 100 mm VAS inquiring about perceived nighttime ICU noise levels [60–62].

3.2.1 Data from ICU Application

Low cost, feasible to perform by a patient or proxy, and available in multiple languages [63–67], the RCSQ has been used to measure sleep in many ICU-based studies [60, 63, 67–72]. Notably, in a 2008 study involving 104 surgical patients, the RCSQ was used to confirm that patients experience suboptimal sleep quality and

Table 1 Subjective Methods to Evaluate Sleep in Critically Ill Patients

Instrument (Year Developed)	Rater	Assessment Frequency	Items	Question Topics	Scoring Method	ICU Validation Studies	Key Intervention Studies
Sleep observation tool (SOT) (1993) [56]	ICU provider	Every 15 min	1	Sleep versus wake	3 options: "Asleep", "awake" or "could not tell"	88% and 70% agreement recording "sleep" versus "wake" as compared to PSG	None
Richards-Campbell sleep questionnaire (RCSQ) (2000) [59]	Patient[a]	Daily	5 (or 6)	Nighttime sleep quality[b] (with optional perceived noise rating)	100 mm visual-analog scales	Good content and criterion validity against PSG	Multiple quality improvement efforts, n = 300 [62], n = 421 [71], n = 646 [73]
Leeds sleep evaluation questionnaire (LSEQ) (1978) [83, 84]	Patient	Daily	10	Nighttime sleep quality[b]	100 mm visual-analog scales	None	Phase II RCT comparing nocturnal dexmedetomidine to placebo [75]
St. Mary's hospital sleep questionnaire (SMHSQ) (1981) [77, 85]	Patient	Daily	14	Nighttime sleep quality[b]	Likert scale and free response questions	None	Valerian oil acupressure [76]
Verran/ Snyder-Halpern (VSH) Sleep Scale (1987) [87]	Patient	Every 3 nights	9 to 15	Nighttime sleep quality[b]	100 mm visual-analog scales	None	Earplugs [88], eye masks [79], back massages [89], aromatherapy [80], music therapy [90]
Sleep in the ICU questionnaire (SICUQ) (1998) [82]	Patient	Periodically during or after ICU stay	27	Sleep quality during entire ICU stay[b,c]	1 (poor) to 10 (excellent) Likert scale	None	Multiple quality improvement efforts to improve ICU sleep [61, 62, 91]
Numeric rating scale for sleep (NRS-sleep) (2019) [98]	Patient	Daily	1	Nighttime sleep quality[b]	0 to 10 Likert scale	Strong correlation with RCSQ in defining sleep as "good"	None

Abbreviations: *ICU* Intensive Care Unit; *PSG* Polysomnography; *RCT* Randomized Controlled Trial
[a]Can also be performed by proxy (e.g., nurse) rater, however nurse raters have been shown to overestimate patient sleep quality [69, 74]
[b]Addresses various domains of sleep and wake including sleep depth, sleep onset latency, number of awakenings, time spent awake, overall sleep quality, behavior following wakefulness, morning alertness
[c]Also addresses specific causes of sleep disruption (i.e., noise, light)

frequent awakenings in the ICU [69]. On a larger scale, RCSQ scores have been used to evaluate the effect of sleep-improvement interventions, including a multi-stage intervention involving 300 medical ICU patients [62], a nighttime noise reduction intervention involving 421 patients in a mixed medical-surgical ICU [71], and a comprehensive sleep-wake promotion intervention involving 646 patients in two surgical ICUs [73]. While these interventions did not yield significant pre-post RCSQ improvements, the studies confirmed the feasibility of collecting many RCSQs on a large scale.

3.2.2   Limitations in the ICU

An overarching limitation of the RCSQ is its feasibility in sedated patients or those experiencing cognitive impairments such as delirium or coma. A 2003 study evaluating patient and nurse perceptions of sleep in the ICU found no significant patient-nurse differences in RCSQ ratings, suggesting that nurses could act as proxies for patients unable to complete the RCSQ [60]. However, more recent studies demonstrated that nurse-patient interrater reliability on the RCSQ was poor, with nurses tending to overestimate patient sleep quality (Fig. 4) [69, 74]. Methodological differences may explain these discrepant results, as the former study evaluated 13

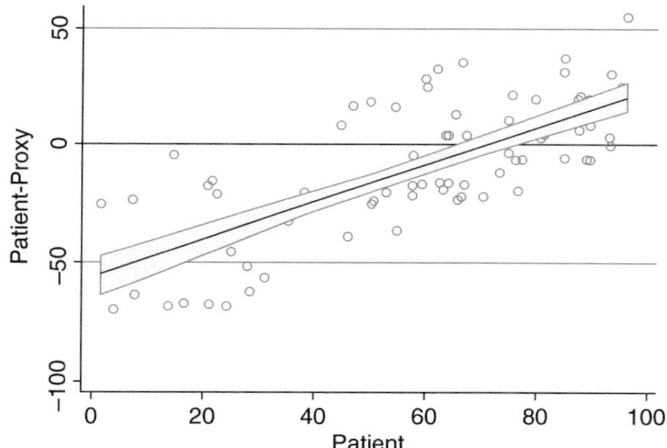

Fig. 4 Bland-Altman plot depicting Richards-Campbell Sleep Questionnaire (RCSQ) ratings from 33 medical ICU (MICU) patients whose nurse proxies completed the questionnaire simultaneously as part of an interrater reliability evaluation. The RCSQ is a five-question instrument evaluating sleep depth, sleep latency, number of nighttime awakenings, sleep efficiency and sleep quality via 100 mm visual-analogue scales, with higher scores representing better sleep quality and an average of the 5 items representing overall sleep quality. The linear regression plot and 95% confidence interval depicts the difference between nurse and patient scores, demonstrating that nurses tended to overestimate patient sleep quality when completed the RCSQ [74]. From "Patient-nurse interrater reliability and agreement of the Richards-Campbell sleep questionnaire," by B. B. Kamdar, 2012, *American Journal of Critical Care, 21*(4), 261–269. Copyright 2012 by American Association of Critical-Care Nurses. Reprinted with permission

nurse-patient RCSQ pairs in 13 patients and the latter 92 pairs in 33 patients, repeated assessments which may have been vulnerable to rater fatigue. Further, the latter occurred during an ICU-wide sleep improvement project that may have positively biased nurses' perception of their patients' sleep quality. Hence, while the RCSQ is validated, inexpensive and easy to perform, its use is primarily confined to awake and alert patients, a shortcoming limiting its ability to evaluate sleep on large, diverse populations of critically ill patients.

3.3 Patient-Perception: Other Methods

A variety of other subjective methods of sleep measurement have been used in the ICU setting, including the Leeds Sleep Evaluation Questionnaire (LSEQ) [75], St. Mary's Hospital Sleep Questionnaire (SMHSQ) [76, 77], Verran/Snyder-Halpern (VSH) Sleep Scale [78–81], and Sleep in the Intensive Care Unit Questionnaire [82]. Like the RCSQ, each method affords the ability to measure sleep at a low cost and on a large scale while lacking the physiologic, objective data provided by PSG, BIS and actigraphy.

3.3.1 Leeds Sleep Evaluation Questionnaire

The Leeds Sleep Evaluation Questionnaire (LSEQ) is a 10-item tool involving 100 mm visual analogue scales like the RCSQ [83, 84]. Capturing the domains of "ease of initiating asleep", "quality of sleep", "ease of awaking" and "behavior following wakefulness", the LSEQ was developed to evaluate patient changes in sleep following the receipt of psychoactive drugs. Notably, the LSEQ was used to evaluate nighttime sleep in a recent phase II randomized trial comparing nocturnal dexmedetomidine to placebo in 100 adults without delirium, demonstrating no difference in perceived sleep quality despite a lower incidence of delirium in the experimental group [75].

3.3.2 St. Mary's Hospital Sleep Questionnaire

The St. Mary's Hospital Sleep Questionnaire (SMHSQ) was developed in London in 1981 as a more feasible option than PSG in hospitalized patients [77, 85]. Consisting of 14 Likert scale and fill-in-the-blank questions, the SMHSQ addresses sleep latency, restlessness, nighttime awakenings, and morning alertness. In the ICU setting, the SMHSQ was used to demonstrate improved perceived sleep quality in patients receiving acupressure with valerian oil as compared to controls [76]. While the SMHSQ can effectively evaluate sleep duration and quality, some questions, specifically those inquiring about specific sleep/wake times and sleep duration may not be feasible for critically ill patients.

3.3.3 Verran/Snyder-Halpern Sleep Scale

The Verran/Snyder-Halpern (VSH) Sleep Scale was developed in 1987 to evaluate sleep disturbances and effectiveness (such as rest upon awakening and perception of sleep quality) in healthy and hospitalized patients [86]. The VSH uses a 100 mm visual analogue scale, like the 5-item RCSQ, but includes 9 to 15 items (depending on the version) and evaluates sleep three nights, with a 0 to 1500 total score [87]. The VSH has been used to evaluate sleep quality improvements in various studies [81], including interventions suggesting improved sleep quality when patients wore earplugs [88] and/or eye masks [79], received back massages [89] or were exposed to aromatherapy [80] or music therapy [90]. Like the RCSQ, the VSH is simple to administer, but has yet to be validated in the ICU setting and may be vulnerable to recall bias when focusing on the past three nights.

3.3.4 Sleep in the ICU Questionnaire

A 1998 cross-sectional study introduced the Sleep in the Intensive Care Unit Questionnaire (SICUQ), a 27-component one-time evaluation of sleep quality, daytime sleepiness, and causes of wake and arousal over a patient's entire ICU stay [82]. Completion of the SICUQ by 203 patients at discharge from four ICUs confirmed that patients experienced poorer sleep than home while in the ICU, with more interruptions in the medical ICU than surgical and cardiac ICU settings. The SICUQ has been used in quality improvement efforts to assess intervention-related differences in sleep quality ratings [61, 62, 91]. While the number of SICUQ components render it infeasible for daily use, it provides a valuable source of patient feedback when planning efforts to improve sleep disruption in the ICU.

4 Evolving and Future Assessment Methods

Various tools and technologies may gain popularity for sleep measurement in the ICU setting. For example, single-use EEG sensors pose a more feasible cost-effective option than traditional electrodes, with the advantage of being disposable and faster and easier to apply [92]. Other wearable EEG sensors include the Flex-printed forehead EEG (fEEGrid), which can yield several hours of recordings [93]. While promising, these devices are in the testing phase and have not been validated for use in critically ill patients.

In the area of motion-based technologies, the greatest attention has been paid to commercial devices manufactured by Apple, FitBit, Samsung, Huawei, and Oura. Affordable, equipped with Bluetooth capabilities and physiologic measures such as heart rate, and undergoing rapid development and validation by advanced technology companies [94], these devices carry tremendous potential as alternatives to traditional wired actigraphy devices. However, these devices have limited battery life, minimal to no access to raw data and/or ICU-specific sleep scoring algorithms and have yet to be rigorously evaluated in the ICU setting. Notably, one study involving Fitbit recordings in non-mechanically ventilated and non-delirious critically ill adults observed this device was often unable to detect sleep interruptions and sleep phases and had poor agreement with the RCSQ [95]. Finally, because the Oura ring is made of titanium, it could get stuck on edematous digits, putting patients at risk for injury.

As alternatives to wrist- and finger-based measurement, the Nemuri SCAN (NSCAN) is an under-mattress pressure sensor that can measure awakenings, sleep, body motion, heart rate and respiratory rate [96]. When evaluated against PSG and the RCSQ for 24 h in eleven critically ill patients, NSCAN demonstrated 68% agreement with PSG, with 90% sensitivity and 39% specificity, with low specificity likely due to inability to detect motionless wakefulness [96]. Alternatively, non-invasive sensors have been evaluated in the ICU setting, specifically the Microsoft Kinect, a wall sensor and camera-based technology which demonstrated strong agreement in measuring patient mobility levels as compared to manual recordings [97]. Though not yet used to measure sleep in critically ill patients, these technologies carry potential for non-invasive measurement in ICU patients, particularly when paired with machine-learning based scoring algorithms.

Finally, from a subjective standpoint, to address rater fatigue imposed by repeated daily RCSQ measurements, a research group developed a simple 0 to 10 Numeric Rating Scale for Sleep (NRS-Sleep), observing a strong RCSQ-NRS correlation ($r = 0.88$) in 194 ICU patients rating the previous night's sleep [98]. Moreover, using an NRS cutoff >5 to define "good sleep" yielded an area under the ROC curve of 0.81, with a sensitivity and specificity of 83% and 79%, respectively. Given its convenience and comparability to routine daily assessments (e.g., pain) the NRS could be considered for incorporation into daily bedside practice.

5 Conclusion

Measuring sleep in the ICU is a challenge for both clinical and research purposes. While PSG has been performed for decades in the ICU setting, it has lost popularity due to cost, infeasibility, and challenges with interpretation, and for this reason is not recommended for routine use in critically ill patients. As a more promising objective measurement option, wrist actigraphy is affordable, feasible for large-scale use and can inform intervention efforts, but currently has limited utility in mostly inactive patients, especially in the absence of ICU-specific actigraphy sleep-wake scoring algorithms. Subjective options such as nurse observation and questionnaires can inform sleep intervention efforts but lack the ability to detect physiologic sleep in critically ill patients. Emerging tools and technologies for sleep assessment in the ICU setting may gain popularity but require validation and large-scale evaluation.

To conclude, based on the advantages, disadvantages, time and labor costs of each measurement tool, we recommend that small- to medium-sized ICU investigations and interventions utilize actigraphy but analyze granular (unprocessed) rest-activity data until ICU-specific software packages become available. If actigraphy is unavailable or infeasible, or large-scale ICU measurement is desired, the RCSQ represents a practical and affordable option but carries significant limitations given its subjectivity. Nevertheless, to better understand or optimize sleep in critically ill patients, providers and investigators are encouraged to select one or multiple measurement tools and should engage interdisciplinary stakeholder teams in the selection process.

Acknowledgements None.

Funding Information B.B.K. is currently supported by a Paul B. Beeson Career Development Award through the National Institutes of Health/National Institute on Aging [grant number K76AG059936].

References

1. Elliott R, McKinley S, Cistulli P, Fien M. Characterisation of sleep in intensive care using 24-hour polysomnography: an observational study. Crit Care. 2013;17(2):R46. https://doi.org/10.1186/cc12565.
2. Delisle S, Ouellet P, Bellemare P, Tetrault JP, Arsenault P. Sleep quality in mechanically ventilated patients: comparison between NAVA and PSV modes. Ann Intensive Care. 2011;1(1):42. https://doi.org/10.1186/2110-5820-1-42.
3. Oto J, Yamamoto K, Koike S, Imanaka H, Nishimura M. Effect of daily sedative interruption on sleep stages of mechanically ventilated patients receiving midazolam by infusion. Anaesth Intensive Care. 2011;39(3):392–400.
4. Trompeo AC, Vidi Y, Locane MD, Braghiroli A, Mascia L, Bosma K, et al. Sleep disturbances in the critically ill patients: role of delirium and sedative agents. Minerva Anestesiol. 2011;77(6):604–12.
5. Kondili E, Alexopoulou C, Xirouchaki N, Georgopoulos D. Effects of propofol on sleep quality in mechanically ventilated critically ill patients: a physiological study. Intensive Care Med. 2012;38(10):1640–6. https://doi.org/10.1007/s00134-012-2623-z.
6. Watson PL, Pandharipande P, Gehlbach BK, Thompson JL, Shintani AK, Dittus BS, et al. Atypical sleep in ventilated patients. Crit Care Med. 2013;41(8):1958–67. https://doi.org/10.1097/ccm.0b013e31828a3f75.
7. Knauert MP, Malik V, Kamdar BB. Sleep and sleep disordered breathing in hospitalized patients. Semin Respir Crit Care Med. 2014;35(5):582–92. https://doi.org/10.1055/s-0034-1390080.
8. Cooper AB, Thornley KS, Young GB, Slutsky AS, Stewart TE, Hanly PJ. Sleep in critically ill patients requiring mechanical ventilation. Chest. 2000;117(3):809–18.
9. Freedman NS, Gazendam J, Levan L, Pack AI, Schwab RJ. Abnormal sleep/wake cycles and the effect of environmental noise on sleep disruption in the intensive care unit. Am J Respir Crit Care Med. 2001;163(2):451–7. https://doi.org/10.1164/ajrccm.163.2.9912128.
10. Cordoba-Izquierdo A, Drouot X, Thille AW, Galia F, Roche-Campo F, Schortgen F, et al. Sleep in hypercapnic critical care patients under noninvasive ventilation: conventional versus dedicated ventilators. Crit Care Med. 2013;41(1):60–8. https://doi.org/10.1097/CCM.0b013e31826764e3.

11. Ambrogio C, Koebnick J, Quan SF, Ranieri M, Parthasarathy S. Assessment of sleep in ventilator-supported critically Ill patients. Sleep. 2008;31(11):1559–68.
12. Hardin KA, Seyal M, Stewart T, Bonekat HW. Sleep in critically ill chemically paralyzed patients requiring mechanical ventilation. Chest. 2006;129(6):1468–77. https://doi.org/10.1378/chest.129.6.1468.
13. Drouot X, Roche-Campo F, Thille AW, Cabello B, Galia F, Margarit L, et al. A new classification for sleep analysis in critically ill patients. Sleep Med. 2012;13(1):7–14. https://doi.org/10.1016/j.sleep.2011.07.012.
14. Gehlbach BK, Chapotot F, Leproult R, Whitmore H, Poston J, Pohlman M, et al. Temporal disorganization of circadian rhythmicity and sleep-wake regulation in mechanically ventilated patients receiving continuous intravenous sedation. Sleep. 2012;35(8):1105–14. https://doi.org/10.5665/sleep.1998.
15. Watson PL, Pandharipande P, Gehlbach BK, Thompson JL, Shintani AK, Dittus BS, et al. Atypical sleep in ventilated patients: empirical electroencephalography findings and the path toward revised ICU sleep scoring criteria. Crit Care Med. 2013;41(8):1958. https://doi.org/10.1097/CCM.0b013e31828a3f75.
16. Boyko Y, Jennum P, Nikolic M, Holst R, Oerding H, Toft P. Sleep in intensive care unit: the role of environment. J Crit Care. 2017;37:99–105. https://doi.org/10.1016/j.jcrc.2016.09.005.
17. Elliott R, McKinley S, Cistulli P. The quality and duration of sleep in the intensive care setting: an integrative review. Int J Nurs Stud. 2011;48(3):384–400. https://doi.org/10.1016/j.ijnurstu.2010.11.006.
18. Gabor JY, Cooper AB, Crombach SA, Lee B, Kadikar N, Bettger HE, et al. Contribution of the intensive care unit environment to sleep disruption in mechanically ventilated patients and healthy subjects. Am J Respir Crit Care Med. 2003;167(5):708–15. https://doi.org/10.1164/rccm.2201090.
19. Banoczi W. How some drugs affect the electroencephalogram (EEG). Am J Electroneurodiagnostic Technol. 2005;45(2):118–29.
20. Herkes GK, Wszolek ZK, Westmoreland BF, Klass DW. Effects of midazolam on electroencephalograms of seriously ill patients. Mayo Clin Proc. 1992;67(4):334–8. https://doi.org/10.1016/s0025-6196(12)61548-1.
21. Rabelo FA, Kupper DS, Sander HH, Fernandes RM, Valera FC. Polysomnographic evaluation of propofol-induced sleep in patients with respiratory sleep disorders and controls. Laryngoscope. 2013;123(9):2300–5. https://doi.org/10.1002/lary.23664.
22. Nielsen RM, Urdanibia-Centelles O, Vedel-Larsen E, Thomsen KJ, Møller K, Olsen KS, et al. Continuous EEG monitoring in a consecutive patient cohort with sepsis and delirium. Neurocrit Care. 2020;32(1):121–30. https://doi.org/10.1007/s12028-019-00703-w.
23. Semmler A, Widmann CN, Okulla T, Urbach H, Kaiser M, Widman G, et al. Persistent cognitive impairment, hippocampal atrophy and EEG changes in sepsis survivors. J Neurol Neurosurg Psychiatry. 2013;84(1):62–9. https://doi.org/10.1136/jnnp-2012-302883.
24. Richards KC, Wang Y-Y, Jun J, Ye L. A systematic review of sleep measurement in critically ill patients. Front Neurol. 2020;11 https://doi.org/10.3389/fneur.2020.542529.
25. Knauert MP, Yaggi HK, Redeker NS, Murphy TE, Araujo KL, Pisani MA. Feasibility study of unattended polysomnography in medical intensive care unit patients. Heart Lung. 2014;43(5):445–52. https://doi.org/10.1016/j.hrtlng.2014.06.049.
26. Devlin JW, Skrobik Y, Gelinas C, Needham DM, Slooter AJC, Pandharipande PP, et al. Clinical practice guidelines for the prevention and Management of Pain, agitation/sedation, delirium, immobility, and sleep disruption in adult patients in the ICU. Crit Care Med. 2018;46(9):e825–e73. https://doi.org/10.1097/CCM.0000000000003299.
27. Benissa MR, Khirani S, Hartley S, Adala A, Ramirez A, Fernandez-Bolanos M, et al. Utility of the bispectral index for assessing natural physiological sleep stages in children and young adults. J Clin Monit Comput. 2016;30(6):957–63. https://doi.org/10.1007/s10877-015-9800-x.
28. Giménez S, Romero S, Alonso JF, Mañanas MÁ, Pujol A, Baxarias P, et al. Monitoring sleep depth: analysis of bispectral index (BIS) based on polysomnographic recordings

and sleep deprivation. J Clin Monit Comput. 2017;31(1):103–10. https://doi.org/10.1007/s10877-015-9805-5.

29. Sleigh JW, Andrzejowski J, Steyn-Ross A, Steyn-Ross M. The bispectral index: a measure of depth of sleep? Anesth Analg. 1999;88(0003–2999; 0003–2999; 3):659.

30. Nicholson T, Patel J, Sleigh JW. Sleep patterns in intensive care unit patients: a study using the bispectral index. Crit Care Resusc. 2001;3(1441–2772; 1441–2772; 2):86.

31. Bourne RS, Mills GH, Minelli C. Melatonin therapy to improve nocturnal sleep in critically ill patients: encouraging results from a small randomised controlled trial. Crit Care. 2008;12(2):R52. https://doi.org/10.1186/cc6871.

32. Pedrao RAA, Riella RJ, Richards K, Valderramas SR. Viability and validity of the bispectral index to measure sleep in patients in the intensive care unit. Rev Bras Ter Intensiva. 2020;32(4):535–41. https://doi.org/10.5935/0103-507X.20200083.

33. Lu W, Fu Q, Luo X, Fu S, Hu K. Effects of dexmedetomidine on sleep quality of patients after surgery without mechanical ventilation in ICU. Medicine (Baltimore). 2017;96(23):e7081. https://doi.org/10.1097/MD.0000000000007081.

34. Kamdar BB, Kadden DJ, Vangala S, Elashoff DA, Ong MK, Martin JL, et al. Feasibility of continuous Actigraphy in patients in a medical intensive care unit. Am J Crit Care. 2017;26(4):329–35. https://doi.org/10.4037/ajcc2017660.

35. Grap MJ, Borchers CT, Munro CL, Elswick RK Jr, Sessler CN. Actigraphy in the critically ill: correlation with activity, agitation, and sedation. Am J Crit Care. 2005;14(1):52–60.

36. Verceles AC, Hager ER. Use of Accelerometry to monitor physical activity in critically ill subjects: a systematic review. Respir Care. 2015;60(9):1330–6. https://doi.org/10.4187/respcare.03677.

37. Kripke DF, Mullaney DJ, Messin S, Wyborney VG. Wrist actigraphic measures of sleep and rhythms. Electroencephalogr Clin Neurophysiol. 1978;44(5):674–6. https://doi.org/10.1016/0013-4694(78)90133-5.

38. Mullaney DJ, Kripke DF, Messin S. Wrist-Actigraphic estimation of sleep time. Sleep. 1980;3(1):83–92. https://doi.org/10.1093/sleep/3.1.83.

39. Webster JB, Kripke DF, Messin S, Mullaney DJ, Wyborney G. An activity-based sleep monitor system for ambulatory use. Sleep. 1982;5(4):389–99. https://doi.org/10.1093/sleep/5.4.389.

40. Hauri PJ, Wisbey J. Wrist Actigraphy in insomnia. Sleep. 1992;15(4):293–301. https://doi.org/10.1093/sleep/15.4.293.

41. Sadeh A, Hauri PJ, Kripke DF, Lavie P. The role of Actigraphy in the evaluation of sleep disorders. Sleep. 1995;18(4):288–302. https://doi.org/10.1093/sleep/18.4.288.

42. Cole RJ, Kripke DF, Gruen W, Mullaney DJ, Gillin JC. Automatic sleep/wake identification from wrist activity. Sleep. 1992;15(5):461–9. https://doi.org/10.1093/sleep/15.5.461.

43. Sadeh A, Sharkey M, Carskadon MA. Activity-based sleep-wake identification: an empirical test of methodological issues. Sleep. 1994;17(3):201–7. https://doi.org/10.1093/sleep/17.3.201.

44. Shilo L, Dagan Y, Smorjik Y, Weinberg U, Dolev S, Komptel B, et al. Effect of melatonin on sleep quality of COPD intensive care patients: a pilot study. Chronobiol Int. 2000;17(1):71–6.

45. Shilo L, Dagan Y, Smorjik Y, Weinberg U, Dolev S, Komptel B, et al. Patients in the intensive care unit suffer from severe lack of sleep associated with loss of Normal melatonin secretion pattern. Am J Med Sci. 1999;317(5):278–81. https://doi.org/10.1016/s0002-9629(15)40528-2.

46. Taguchi T, Yano M, Kido Y. Influence of bright light therapy on postoperative patients: a pilot study. Intensive Crit Care Nurs. 2007;23(5):289–97. https://doi.org/10.1016/j.iccn.2007.04.004.

47. Kroon K, West S. 'Appears to have slept well': assessing sleep in an acute care setting. Contemp Nurse. 2000;9(3–4):284–94.

48. Mistraletti G, Taverna M, Sabbatini G, Carloni E, Bolgiaghi L, Pirrone M, et al. Actigraphic monitoring in critically ill patients: preliminary results toward an "observation-guided sedation". J Crit Care. 2009;24(4):563–7. https://doi.org/10.1016/j.jcrc.2009.05.006.

49. Chen JH, Chao YH, Lu SF, Shiung TF, Chao YF. The effectiveness of valerian acupressure on the sleep of ICU patients: a randomized clinical trial. Int J Nurs Stud. 2012;49(8):913–20. https://doi.org/10.1016/j.ijnurstu.2012.02.012.

50. Beecroft JM, Ward M, Younes M, Crombach S, Smith O, Hanly PJ. Sleep monitoring in the intensive care unit: comparison of nurse assessment, actigraphy and polysomnography. Intensive Care Med. 2008;34(11):2076–83. https://doi.org/10.1007/s00134-008-1180-y.

51. Schwab KE, Ronish B, Needham DM, To AQ, Martin JL, Kamdar BB. Actigraphy to evaluate sleep in the intensive care unit. A systematic review. Ann Am Thorac Soc. 2018;15(9):1075–82. https://doi.org/10.1513/AnnalsATS.201801-004OC.

52. Ono H, Taguchi T, Kido Y, Fujino Y, Doki Y. The usefulness of bright light therapy for patients after oesophagectomy. Intensive Crit Care Nurs. 2011;27(3):158–66. https://doi.org/10.1016/j. iccn.2011.03.003.

53. Osse RJ, Tulen JH, Bogers AJ, Hengeveld MW. Disturbed circadian motor activity patterns in postcardiotomy delirium. Psychiatry Clin Neurosci. 2009;63(1):56–64. https://doi. org/10.1111/j.1440-1819.2008.01888.x.

54. Duclos C, Dumont M, Blais H, Paquet J, Laflamme E, de Beaumont L, et al. Rest-activity cycle disturbances in the acute phase of moderate to severe traumatic brain injury. Neurorehabil Neural Repair. 2014;28(5):472–82. https://doi.org/10.1177/1545968313517756.

55. Gupta P, Martin JL, Needham DM, Vangala S, Colantuoni E, Kamdar BB. Use of actigraphy to characterize inactivity and activity in patients in a medical ICU. Heart Lung. 2020;49(4):398–406 https://doi.org/10.1016/j.hrtlng.2020.02.002.

56. Edwards GB, Schuring LM. Pilot study: validating staff nurses' observations of sleep and wake states among critically ill patients, using polysomnography. Am J Crit Care. 1993;2(2):125–31.

57. Aurell J, Elmqvist D. Sleep in the surgical intensive care unit: continuous polygraphic recording of sleep in nine patients receiving postoperative care. Br Med J. 1985;290(6474):1029–32.

58. Shahid A, Wilkinson K, Marcu S, Shapiro C. Richards–Campbell Sleep Questionnaire (RCSQ). In: Shahid A, Wilkinson K, Marcu S, Shapiro CM, editors. STOP, THAT and one hundred other sleep scales. Springer: New York; 2012. p. 299–302.

59. Richards KC, O'Sullivan PS, Phillips RL. Measurement of sleep in critically ill patients. J Nurs Meas. 2000;8(2):131–44.

60. Frisk U, Nordstrom G. Patients' sleep in an intensive care unit--patients' and nurses' perception. Intensive Crit Care Nurs. 2003;19(6):342.

61. Li S-Y, Wang T-J, Vivienne Wu SF, Liang S-Y, Tung H-H. Efficacy of controlling night-time noise and activities to improve patients' sleep quality in a surgical intensive care unit. J Clin Nurs. 2011;20(3–4):396–407. https://doi.org/10.1111/j.1365-2702.2010.03507.x.

62. Kamdar BB, King LM, Collop NA, Sakamuri S, Colantuoni E, Neufeld KJ, et al. The effect of a quality improvement intervention on perceived sleep quality and cognition in a medical ICU. Crit Care Med. 2013;41(3):800–9. https://doi.org/10.1097/CCM.0b013e3182746442.

63. Chen LX, Ji DH, Zhang F, Li JH, Cui L, Bai CJ, et al. Richards-Campbell sleep questionnaire: psychometric properties of Chinese critically ill patients. Nurs Crit Care. 2019;24(6):362–8. https://doi.org/10.1111/nicc.12357.

64. Al-Sulami GS, Rice AM, Kidd L, O'Neill A, Richards KC, McPeake J. An Arabic translation, reliability, validity, and feasibility of the Richards-Campbell sleep questionnaire for sleep quality assessment in ICU: prospective-repeated assessments. J Nurs Meas. 2019;27(3):E153–E69. https://doi.org/10.1891/1061-3749.27.3.E153.

65. Krotsetis S, Richards KC, Behncke A, Kopke S. The reliability of the German version of the Richards Campbell sleep questionnaire. Nurs Crit Care. 2017;22(4):247–52. https://doi. org/10.1111/nicc.12275.

66. Murata H, Oono Y, Sanui M, Saito K, Yamaguchi Y, Takinami M, et al. The Japanese version of the Richards-Campbell sleep questionnaire: reliability and validity assessment. Nurs Open. 2019;6(3):808–14. https://doi.org/10.1002/nop2.252.

67. Biazim SK, Souza DA, Carraro Junior H, Richards K, Valderramas S. The Richards-Campbell sleep questionnaire and sleep in the intensive care unit questionnaire: translation to Portuguese

and cross-cultural adaptation for use in Brazil. J Bras Pneumol. 2020;46(4):e20180237. https://doi.org/10.36416/1806-3756/e20180237.

68. Williamson JW. The effects of ocean sounds on sleep after coronary artery bypass graft surgery. Am J Crit Care. 1992;1(1):91.

69. Nicolas A, Aizpitarte E, Iruarrizaga A, Vazquez M, Margall A, Asiain C. Perception of nighttime sleep by surgical patients in an intensive care unit. Nurs Crit Care. 2008;13(1):25–33. https://doi.org/10.1111/j.1478-5153.2007.00255.x.

70. Kamdar BB, Combs MP, Colantuoni E, King LM, Niessen T, Neufeld KJ, et al. The association of sleep quality, delirium, and sedation status with daily participation in physical therapy in the ICU. Crit Care. 2016;19:261. https://doi.org/10.1186/s13054-016-1433-z.

71. van de Pol I, van Iterson M, Maaskant J. Effect of nocturnal sound reduction on the incidence of delirium in intensive care unit patients: an interrupted time series analysis. Intensive Crit Care Nurs. 2017;41:18–25. https://doi.org/10.1016/j.iccn.2017.01.008.

72. Simons KS, Verweij E, Lemmens PMC, Jelfs S, Park M, Spronk PE, et al. Noise in the intensive care unit and its influence on sleep quality: a multicenter observational study in Dutch intensive care units. Crit Care. 2018;22(1) https://doi.org/10.1186/s13054-018-2182-y.

73. Tonna JE, Dalton A, Presson AP, Zhang C, Colantuoni E, Lander K, et al. The effect of a quality improvement intervention on sleep and delirium in critically ill patients in a surgical intensive care unit. Chest. 2021; https://doi.org/10.1016/j.chest.2021.03.030.

74. Kamdar BB, Shah PA, King LM, Kho ME, Zhou X, Colantuoni E, et al. Patient-nurse interrater reliability and agreement of the Richards-Campbell sleep questionnaire. Am J Crit Care. 2012;21(4):261–9. https://doi.org/10.4037/ajcc2012111.

75. Skrobik Y, Duprey MS, Hill NS, Devlin JW. Low-dose nocturnal Dexmedetomidine prevents ICU delirium. A randomized, placebo-controlled trial. Am J Respir Crit Care Med. 2018;197(9):1147–56. https://doi.org/10.1164/rccm.201710-1995OC.

76. Bagheri-Nesami M, Gorji MA, Rezaie S, Pouresmail Z, Cherati JY. Effect of acupressure with valerian oil 2.5% on the quality and quantity of sleep in patients with acute coronary syndrome in a cardiac intensive care unit. J Tradit Complement Med. 2015;5(4):241–7. https://doi.org/10.1016/j.jtcme.2014.11.005.

77. Ellis BW, Johns MW, Lancaster R, Raptopoulos P, Angelopoulos N, Priest RG. The St. Mary's hospital sleep questionnaire: a study of reliability. Sleep. 1981;4(1):93–7. https://doi.org/10.1093/sleep/4.1.93.

78. Snyder-Halpern R, Verran JA. Instrumentation to describe subjective sleep characteristics in healthy subjects. Res Nurs Health. 1987;10(3):155–63.

79. Yazdannik AR, Zareie A, Hasanpour M, Kashefi P. The effect of earplugs and eye mask on patients' perceived sleep quality in intensive care unit. Iran J Nurs Midwifery Res. 2014;19(6):673–8.

80. Cho MY, Min ES, Hur MH, Lee MS. Effects of aromatherapy on the anxiety, vital signs, and sleep quality of percutaneous coronary intervention patients in intensive care units. Evid Based Complement Alternat Med. 2013;2013:381381. https://doi.org/10.1155/2013/381381.

81. Frighetto L, Marra C, Bandali S, Wilbur K, Naumann T, Jewesson P. An assessment of quality of sleep and the use of drugs with sedating properties in hospitalized adult patients. Health Qual Life Outcomes. 2004;2:17. https://doi.org/10.1186/1477-7525-2-17.

82. Freedman NS, Kotzer N, Schwab RJ. Patient perception of sleep quality and etiology of sleep disruption in the intensive care unit. Am J Respir Crit Care Med. 1999;159(4 Pt 1):1155–62. https://doi.org/10.1164/ajrccm.159.4.9806141.

83. Parrott AC, Hindmarch I. The Leeds sleep evaluation questionnaire in psychopharmacological investigations–a review. Psychopharmacology. 1980;71(2):173–9. https://doi.org/10.1007/BF00434408.

84. Shahid A, Wilkinson K, Marcu S, Shapiro CM. Leeds Sleep Evaluation Questionnaire (LSEQ). In: Shahid A, Wilkinson K, Marcu S, Shapiro CM, editors. STOP, THAT and one hundred other sleep scales. New York, NY: Springer New York; 2011. p. 211–3.

85. Shahid A, Wilkinson K, Marcu S, Shapiro CM. St. Mary's hospital sleep questionnaire. In: Shahid A, Wilkinson K, Marcu S, Shapiro CM, editors. STOP, THAT and one hundred other sleep scales. New York, NY: Springer New York; 2011. p. 363–5.
86. Shahid A, Wilkinson K, Marcu S, Shapiro C. Verran and Snyder-Halpern Sleep Scale (VSH). In: Shahid A, Wilkinson K, Marcu S, Shapiro CM, editors. STOP, THAT and one hundred other sleep scales. Springer: New York; 2012. p. 397–8.
87. Shahid A, Wilkinson K, Marcu S, Shapiro CM. Verran and Snyder-Halpern sleep scale (VSH). New York: Springer; 2011. p. 397–8.
88. Scotto CJ, McClusky C, Spillan S, Kimmel J. Earplugs improve patients' subjective experience of sleep in critical care. Nurs Crit Care. 2009;14(4):180–4. https://doi.org/10.1111/j.1478-5153.2009.00344.x.
89. Hsu WC, Guo SE, Chang CH. Back massage intervention for improving health and sleep quality among intensive care unit patients. Nurs Crit Care. 2019;24(5):313–9. https://doi.org/10.1111/nicc.12428.
90. Su CP, Lai HL, Chang ET, Yiin LM, Perng SJ, Chen PW. A randomized controlled trial of the effects of listening to non-commercial music on quality of nocturnal sleep and relaxation indices in patients in medical intensive care unit. J Adv Nurs. 2013;69(6):1377–89. https://doi.org/10.1111/j.1365-2648.2012.06130.x.
91. Patel J, Baldwin J, Bunting P, Laha S. The effect of a multicomponent multidisciplinary bundle of interventions on sleep and delirium in medical and surgical intensive care patients. Anaesthesia. 2014;69(6):540–9. https://doi.org/10.1111/anae.12638.
92. Sohrt A, Maerkedahl A, Padula WV. Cost-effectiveness analysis of single-use EEG cup electrodes compared with reusable EEG cup electrodes. Pharmacoecon Open. 2019;3(2):265–72. https://doi.org/10.1007/s41669-018-0090-3.
93. Blum S, Emkes R, Minow F, Anlauff J, Finke A, Debener S. Flex-printed forehead EEG sensors (fEEGrid) for long-term EEG acquisition. J Neural Eng. 2020;17(3):034003. https://doi.org/10.1088/1741-2552/ab914c.
94. Roberts DM, Schade MM, Mathew GM, Gartenberg D, Buxton OM. Detecting sleep using heart rate and motion data from multisensor consumer-grade wearables, relative to wrist actigraphy and polysomnography. Sleep. 2020;43(7) https://doi.org/10.1093/sleep/zsaa045.
95. Louzon PR, Andrews JL, Torres X, Pyles EC, Ali MH, Du Y, et al. Characterisation of ICU sleep by a commercially available activity tracker and its agreement with patient-perceived sleep quality. BMJ open. Respir Res. 2020;7(1) https://doi.org/10.1136/bmjresp-2020-000572.
96. Nagatomo K, Masuyama T, Iizuka Y, Makino J, Shiotsuka J, Sanui M. Validity of an under-mattress sensor for objective sleep measurement in critically ill patients: a prospective observational study. J Intensive Care. 2020;8(1) https://doi.org/10.1186/s40560-020-0433-x.
97. Ma AJ, Rawat N, Reiter A, Shrock C, Zhan A, Stone A, et al. Measuring patient mobility in the ICU using a novel noninvasive sensor. Crit Care Med. 2017;45(4):630–6. https://doi.org/10.1097/CCM.0000000000002265.
98. Rood P, Frenzel T, Verhage R, Bonn M, van der Hoeven H, Pickkers P, et al. Development and daily use of a numeric rating score to assess sleep quality in ICU patients. J Crit Care. 2019;52:68–74. https://doi.org/10.1016/j.jcrc.2019.04.009.

Best Practice for Improving Sleep in the ICU. Part I: Non-pharmacologic

Amy S. Korwin and Melissa P. Knauert

1 Introduction

Recent advances have expanded our understanding of the importance of restorative sleep and maintenance of circadian rhythms in promoting recovery from acute illness. However, the hospital setting and especially the intensive care unit (ICU) remain poorly conducive to achieving adequate sleep for patients. As noted in chapter "Characteristics of Sleep in Critically Ill Patients. Part I: Sleep Fragmentation and Sleep Stage Disruption", ICU patients have a reduced sleep duration as well as significantly impaired sleep quality [1–5]. Furthermore, sleep architecture is severely distorted with a reduction or absence of restorative N3 and REM stages, or even atypical sleep that is unclassifiable by standard criteria [2, 3, 6] (see chapter "Atypical Sleep and Pathologic Wakefulness").

In addition to disrupted sleep duration and quality, ICU patients are also at risk for misaligned or abolished circadian rhythms (chapter "Characteristics of Sleep in Critically Ill Patients. Part II: Circadian Rhythm Disruption"). Sleep is best and of the highest quality when it occurs at an optimized circadian time [7]; thus, sleep promotion must, de facto, include promotion of circadian alignment (Fig. 1). Alignment of the circadian system is accomplished via networked signaling between external circadian cues (i.e., zeitgebers), the central clock in the suprachiasmatic nucleus, and peripheral clocks in nearly all cells of the body. Studies have demonstrated that ICU patients often have misaligned (usually delayed type) or even absent circadian rhythms. This has been described in multiple ICU patient cohorts

A. S. Korwin · M. P. Knauert (✉)
Department of Internal Medicine, Section of Pulmonary, Critical Care and Sleep Medicine, Yale School of Medicine, New Haven, CT, USA
e-mail: Amy.Korwin@yale.edu; Melissa.Knauert@yale.edu

G. L. Weinhouse, J. W. Devlin (eds.), *Sleep in Critical Illness*,
https://doi.org/10.1007/978-3-031-06447-0_14

231

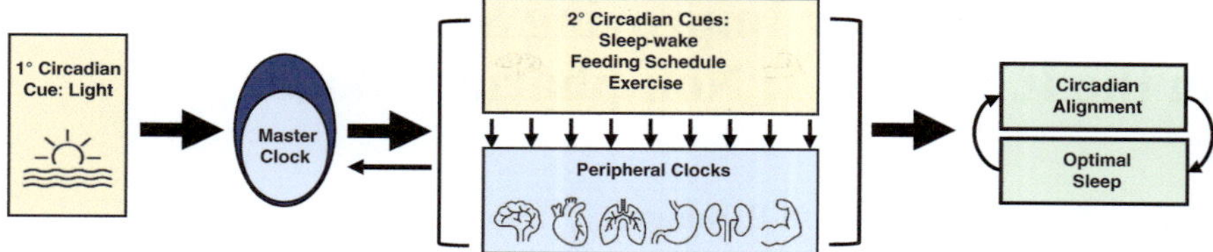

Fig. 1 Conceptual model depicting primary (1°) and secondary (2°) circadian cues that contribute to circadian alignment and sleep optimization

including patients with sepsis, intracerebral hemorrhage, and those requiring mechanical ventilation with intravenous sedation [8–13].

As emphasized in chapters "Mechanical Ventilation and Sleep", "Sleep Disruption and Its Relationship with ICU Outcomes", and "Long-Term Outcomes–Sleep in Survivors of Critical Illness", it is important to acknowledge and address sleep and circadian disruption in ICU patients as they are associated with significant clinical consequences. Among other outcomes, abnormal sleep architecture has been associated with late failure of noninvasive ventilation and prolonged mechanical ventilator weaning [6, 14]. Aside from respiratory effects, sleep deficiency in non-critically ill patient populations has been associated with poor glycemic control [15], and impaired immunologic function [16, 17]. As highlighted in chapters "Sleep Disruption and Its Relationship with Delirium: Electroencephalographic Perspectives" and "Sleep Disruption and Its Relationship with Delirium: Clinical Perspectives", sleep disruption has also been proposed as a risk factor for delirium [18], and, in delirious medical ICU patients, the loss of sleep features (i.e., loss of K-complexes) is associated with increased in-hospital mortality [19].

As highlighted in chapter "Risk Factors for Disrupted Sleep in the ICU", sleep and circadian disruption in the hospital result from multifactorial etiologies and include patient characteristics (e.g., psychological distress, discomfort or pain, sleep comorbidities, and sleep preferences), environmental factors (e.g., noise, light, and interruptions for provision of care), and acute illness and treatment-related factors (e.g., severity of illness, medications, mechanical ventilation, immobility and continuous feeding) [20, 21]. Each of these impediments to healthy sleep and normal circadian rhythms represents a potential therapeutic target, and an opportunity to improve overall and sleep-specific patient outcomes.

Currently, multicomponent non-pharmacologic therapies are guideline-recommended as the first-line approach to addressing sleep disruption in the ICU [22]. As noted in chapter "Best Practices for Improving Sleep in the ICU. Part II: Pharmacologic", there is a lack of evidence to support significant clinical benefit from sleep-promoting medications, and there are potential harms related to their use [22]. Therefore, it is important to be aware of non-pharmacologic interventions that may improve patients' sleep duration and quality, as well as promote circadian alignment. These non-pharmacologic interventions aim to improve sleep opportunity by addressing patient characteristics, environmental exposures, and effects related to acute illness and medical treatments. Non-pharmacologic interventions also promote maintenance of circadian alignment through the use of circadian cues. This chapter will review best practice in non-pharmacologic therapies to improve sleep and circadian disruption in ICU patients and highlight emerging strategies that hold promise as future interventions.

2   Patient Factors that Disrupt Sleep

Patient characteristics that contribute to poor sleep in the ICU include psychological distress, pain or discomfort, sleep comorbidities, and sleep preferences chapter "Risk Factors for Disrupted Sleep in the ICU". Psychological distress is common and most frequently refers to anxiety, stress or fear experienced by ICU patients; however, patients also report being in an unfamiliar place, loneliness, and lack of privacy as sleep disruptors [20]. In one qualitative survey study, more than half of patients endorsed psychological issues such as worry about health and uncertainty about prognosis as more important than the ICU environment as a sleep disruptor [23].

2.1   Psychologic Distress

Various non-pharmacologic interventions have aimed to improve psychologic distress. Music therapy, mind-body practices, and other psychological interventions have all been attempted with critically ill patients. When studies evaluating these interventions have been systematically reviewed, they have been found to be potentially beneficial. However, heterogeneity precluded meta-analysis, many studies had high risk of bias, and studies were underpowered to detect clinical effects [24]. Among these interventions, music therapy has been reproducibly implemented with success. A systematic review of eleven ICU studies demonstrated a consistent association between music therapy and reduced anxiety and stress [25]. In one randomized, controlled trial of mechanically ventilated adults, patient-directed music therapy was associated with reduced anxiety and sedation intensity compared to usual care [26]. Among investigations exploring sleep outcomes directly, one small study using polysomnographic data found that music therapy was associated with longer stage N3 in the first two hours of nocturnal sleep, though no differences were seen in total sleep time or sleep efficiency [27]. Another study reported a greater reduction in bispectral index in patients receiving music therapy versus usual care [28]; however, the exact relationship between bispectral index and sleep remains unclear [29]. Other relaxation techniques have also been studied, including relaxing imagery prior to bedtime [30], foot massage or bath [31], and valerian acupressure [32]. These interventions have been associated with improved subjective sleep quality and, in some studies, an increase in total sleep time. Overall quality of evidence to support these complementary medicine techniques remains very low.

2.2 Pain and Discomfort

Physical pain has a bidirectional relationship with sleep in which pain disrupts sleep and sleep disruption increases perceived pain [33–35]. Non-pharmacologic approaches to reduce pain in hospitalized patients include repositioning the patient, adjusting bedding or medical equipment, applying ice or heat packs, and using complementary techniques including massage therapy, hypnosis, acupuncture, and natural sounds. A recent review of 12 studies evaluating non-pharmacologic pain interventions in the ICU found reduction in pain intensity was conferred by hypnosis, acupuncture, and natural sounds [36]. It should be acknowledged the evidence supporting the use of non-pharmacologic pain reduction strategies in the ICU remains limited, and most studies of these interventions did not evaluate sleep-specific outcomes. If pharmacologic analgesia is required, providers should consider optimization non-opioid analgesics first. If opioids are required, they should be used at the minimum necessary dose and for the shortest duration necessary given opioids negatively impact sleep architecture (see chapter "Effects of Common ICU Medications on Sleep") and increase delirium [22, 37]. Other sources of discomfort such as hunger, thirst, a need to void or defecate, and nausea have also been named by patients as sleep disruptors [20] and can be addressed if the care team remain vigilant for these needs.

2.3 Sleep History

A lack of attention to patient sleep history and sleep preferences can also contribute to sleep deficiency in the ICU. These factors are often overlooked by critical care providers and may be easily treated or accommodated to improve patient sleep. For example, obstructive sleep apnea (OSA) is common in critically ill elderly patients and associated with poor outcomes, yet is under-diagnosed and often goes untreated during hospital admissions [38–41]. One hospital study found that positive airway pressure therapy was provided to only 5% of patients with a history of OSA [42]. Notably, acute sleep deprivation in the ICU can worsen OSA-associated obstruction, thus forming a vicious cycle of obstruction and sleep disruption [43]. Restless legs syndrome, a sensorimotor disorder that affects sleep initiation and maintenance, is often exacerbated or unmasked by factors associated with critical illness including blood loss, immobility, sleep deprivation, cessation of therapeutic medications, or initiation of provoking drugs [44]. Medications that increase the risk of restless legs symptoms include antidopaminergic antipsychotics, many classes of antidepressants, anti-emetics (i.e., prochlorperazine, metoclopramide), and diphenhydramine [45]. Attention to underlying sleep-associated disorders, and providing patients with their pre-existing outpatient treatments, should improve sleep duration and quality during ICU admission.

Attending to patients' sleep preferences in the ICU, including their habitual home sleep time, body position, arrangement of bedding, room lighting, and temperature, may improve sleep although rigorous evidence to support these practices is lacking. A recent project at the Hospital of the University of Pennsylvania piloted the use of asking patients how they wanted their room arranged (e.g., lights on or off, blinds up or down) and offering items from a "comfy cart" which included a variety of items that patients could use at bedtime (e.g., blankets, tea, snacks). This pilot was low cost and associated with patient reported sleep improvement [46].

3 Environmental Factors that Disrupt Sleep

Environmental features of the ICU conflict with sleep opportunity and provide poor circadian signaling to ICU patients. Addressing these issues is a promising target for non-pharmacologic interventions. Salient disturbances include high sound levels, abnormal light exposure, and frequent patient care interactions during the overnight period.

3.1 *Noise*

Noise, defined as disturbing sound, is often cited by patients as the most frequent cause of disturbed sleep in the ICU sleep [20]. Sound levels in the ICU significantly exceed nocturnal limits recommended by the World Health Organization [47]. Staff conversations, medical equipment noises, equipment alarms, television sound, telephones, and care processes are the most common sources of noise in this setting. ICU polysomnographic studies suggest up to 20% of arousals are attributable to ambient noise [48].

3.2 *Light*

Abnormal light exposure in the ICU is also believed to impact sleep. Studies of the relationship between ICU light and sleep are more limited than those evaluating sounds and have focused on overnight illumination as a potential source of sleep disruption. One environmental survey of 990 ICU patient-nights found that 21% of rooms had bright light illumination on and 48% had the television on at a midnight timepoint [49]. Despite these findings, overnight studies of ICU light reveal low average illuminance (e.g., less than 20 lux) with high variability including several light peaks per hour [2, 50–52]. Importantly, these studies have also demonstrated remarkably dim daytime light levels (e.g., less than 100 lux). Bright daytime light is a key determinant of circadian entrainment and therefore an important sleep promotion strategy in the ICU [53].

3.3 Bedside Care Interactions

As noted in chapter "Risk Factors for Disrupted Sleep in the ICU", ICU patient care tasks can be disruptive to sleep. One study of 147 patient-nights found that patients had an average of 43 care interactions per overnight period (19:00–7:00) [54]. This finding is consistent with other studies showing a high frequency of care interactions, often for non-urgent care [55, 56].

3.4 Multicomponent Sleep Improvement

Methods of controlling the environment, clustering care delivery, or combining elements of both strategies have been studied to improve sleep in ICU patients [57]. In fact, as noted above, multicomponent, sleep promotion bundles are guideline-recommended for ICU patients [22].

Mitigation of overnight sound via "quiet time" protocols typically aims to reduce staff/visitor talking, minimize or eliminate overhead announcements, adjust patient equipment to decrease nuisance alarms, and close the doors to patient rooms [58, 59]. Clustering care means to move non-urgent care outside of designated protected sleep times, as well as to consolidate tasks that are not time-sensitive into fewer interruptions. Targets of rescheduling include a broad array of tasks such as routine ventilator checks, suctioning, medication administration, diagnostic testing, bathing, linen changes, skin and wound care, routine equipment care such as intravenous medication tubing changes, stocking of room supplies, and room cleaning [60].

Quiet time interventions may be effective at reducing environmental disturbances. For example, one comprehensive staff educational intervention was found to be feasible and effective at reducing the loudest sound peaks (over 80 dBA) [61], and a multifaceted sound intervention reported a 10% decrease in noise levels over 70 dBA [59]. Similarly, a neurocritical care unit "quiet time" protocol from 02:00–04:00 and 14:00–16:00 effectively decreased sound and light levels during these periods and increased the likelihood of patient sleep (based on nurse observation) [62]. One pilot randomized controlled trial of an ICU sleep promotion protocol focused on restricting nonurgent patient care between 00:00–4:00 reduced in-room activity by 9 min per hour, increased rest time between care interactions from 26 to 46 minutes, and reduced average A-weighted sound levels by 2.5 decibels (approaching a difference of one sound doubling) [56]. In contrast to the above studies, Boyko et al. report that a structured ICU "quiet time" protocol from 22:00 to 6:00 did not alter the unit's soundscape [63].

Improvements in sleep-related outcomes due to non-pharmacologic sleep promotion interventions have been more difficult to demonstrate. A multi-component protocol that emphasized environmental control but also included earplugs (see below) did demonstrate increased delirium/coma-free days despite not showing sleep changes [64]. Similarly, a more recent non-pharmacologic multi-component sleep promotion intervention conducted in surgical ICUs was associated with a significant reduction in the proportion of days patients experienced delirium, but also did not show a change in patient-reported perceived sleep quality [65].

3.5 Earplugs and Eye Masks

Earplugs and eye masks have been used alone or as an adjunct to the bundled approaches described above. Earplug use has been shown to be feasible and well-tolerated by both sedated and non-sedated intensive care unit patients, with an estimated mean sound abatement of 10 decibels [66]. One randomized controlled trial investigating the use of both earplugs and eye masks in the ICU found patients whose earplugs remained appropriately positioned all night experienced an increased duration of N3 sleep and had fewer prolonged awakenings; however, 30% of the patients declined to use earplugs [66]. One other ICU study reported earplug and/or eye mask use to be associated with an increased duration of REM, N2, and N3 sleep [67]. Meta-analyses suggest earplug and eye mask use in the ICU is associated with increased total sleep time and reduced delirium [68, 69]. While noise-cancelling headphones are associated with only a mild reduction in noise exposure, their use has also been reported to improve patient-reported sleep [70].

3.6 Light Interventions

As highlighted in chapter "Characteristics of Sleep in Critically Ill Patients. Part II: Circadian Rhythm Disruption", entrainment and maintenance of circadian alignment depends upon diurnal variation of light, and, as noted in the introduction, sleep is of the longest duration and best quality when it is aligned properly with circadian phase [7]. Accordingly, increased daytime lighting has been studied as a strategy to promote normal circadian alignment and thus improve ICU sleep. Factors influencing the robustness of circadian entrainment include light intensity, duration, spectra, and history [71]. Specifically, daytime light must be of sufficient intensity and duration and contain high proportions of circadian active wavelengths (e.g., 250 lux for several hours with a light source that is similar in spectral composition to natural sunlight) [71, 72]. Theses light metrics are not currently being met in most ICUs (Fig. 2) [50, 52].

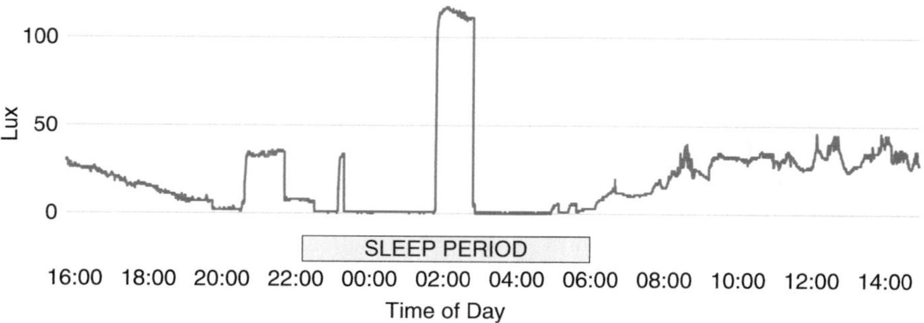

Fig. 2 24-hour light profile for a single intensive care unit patient. Monitoring period starts in the afternoon at 16:00 and continues for 24 hours. Notably, the highest light exposure occurs during the 02:00 to 04:00 hours. Maximum daytime light does not exceed an intensity of 50 lux. A normal sleep period is indicated below the plot by the labeled rectangle

Cycled lighting and bright daytime light interventions seek to provide patients with circadian- appropriate diurnal variation in light exposures and have been shown in small ICU studies to improve patient satisfaction with their sleep [73], foster earlier postoperative mobility [74], and reduce postoperative delirium [74–76]. A pilot randomized controlled trial in critically ill adults with a delayed circadian phase found that a timed light intervention was associated with a 3.6-h correction towards normal circadian phase at study day 3 (versus study day 1). In contrast, usual care patients had an additional 2.4-h circadian delay by study day 3 [77]. However, other bright light daytime studies have failed to show benefit. The use of high lighting levels in the control group [78] and inappropriate timing, duration, and spectra of the light intervention [79] may have accounted for the lack of sleep improvement. In sum, control of the disruptive ICU environment is necessary but not sufficient for critical illness sleep promotion. The addition of circadian guided light therapies is a promising intervention currently under investigation.

4 Acute Illness and Treatment Factors that Disrupt Sleep

As reviewed in chapters "Risk Factors for Disrupted Sleep in the ICU" and "Effects of Common ICU Medications on Sleep", there are many factors related to critical illness or admission to the ICU that impact sleep and circadian rhythms. Physiologic abnormalities related to critical illness can directly alter sleep architecture and circadian function [5]. Furthermore, ICU patients are often immobile and may require various forms of sleep disruptive life-sustaining therapy. These can include invasive monitoring, medical support devices, mechanical ventilation, enteral nutrition, and a high burden of medications that disrupt sleep architecture. Vis a vis sleep promotion, monitoring and support devices should be optimally positioned for patient comfort as noted above under pain and discomfort. For a thorough discussion on the relationship between mechanical ventilation and sleep please refer to chapter "Mechanical Ventilation and Sleep". In this chapter we focus on mitigating sleep disruption caused by ICU sedative use, continuous enteral nutrition, and immobility.

4.1 Sedation

An ICU patient who is sedated may not necessarily have good sleep. As reviewed in chapters "Normal Sleep Compared to Altered Consciousness During Sedation" and "Effects of Common ICU Medications on Sleep", many sedating medications commonly used in the critical care setting can change sleep architecture. Narcotics and benzodiazepines suppress Stage REM and NREM 3 sleep [80]. Similarly, propofol decreases Stage REM. In contrast, dexmedetomidine has been associated with improved sleep parameters including higher sleep efficiency and reduced sleep fragmentation when measured via polysomnography [81]. Pharmacologic strategies to promote sleep are discussed in chapter "Best Practices for Improving Sleep in the ICU. Part II: Pharmacologic". Benzodiazepines and opioids each increase the risk for delirium occurrence [37, 82]. Most mechanically ventilated, critically ill adults do not require continuous sedation; comfort and safety can often be maintained with intermittent analgesia/sedative therapy [83]. To maintain patients at a light level of sedation, reduce coma and delirium, facilitate mechanical ventilation liberation, and also improve sleep, practice guidelines recommend the use of a spontaneous awakening trial or sedation protocolization [22].

4.2 Enteral Nutrition Schedule

Continuous enteral feeding, commonly administered to ICU patients, may worsen circadian misalignment. The timing of nutrition provision is an influential zeitgeber, particularly for peripheral clocks in the gut, liver, and pancreas. Misalignment of the peripheral clocks with the central clock and/or day-night is termed "internal circadian dyssynchrony." Internal circadian dyssynchrony is associated with circadian disruption, poor sleep, and poor glucose tolerance [21, 84, 85]. Thus, optimal feeding would occur during the day in a time-restricted manner. A recent pilot study of 70 critically ill adults found that implementation of a 12-hour overnight enteral nutrition interruption resulted in a nocturnal fasting response that improved metabolic parameters including a reduction in the insulin requirements [86]. One small ICU pilot study demonstrated that use of a time-restricted intermittent enteral nutrition schedule is feasible in mechanically ventilated, medically ill, adults [87]. Qualitative analysis of the study found total nutritional delivery to be unchanged [88]. Time-restricted (daytime) enteral feeding has strong biologic plausibility for benefit in ICU patients and is feasible. An ICU randomized controlled trial investigating circadian phase alignment and additional clinical outcomes is ongoing (NCT04437264).

4.3 Mobilization

Despite the consequences of immobility and ICU-acquired weakness, critically ill adults often remain bed-bound due to the severity of their clinical condition and the physical barriers imposed by medical support devices. In healthy individuals, bed rest, particularly in the setting of hypoxemia, results in breathing instability during sleep and greater time with N1 sleep [89]. Daytime exercise is known to be important for the maintenance of circadian alignment and has been shown to increase nighttime sleep [90, 91]. Early ICU mobilization is guideline recommended as it will increase muscle strength, reduce delirium, and shorten the ICU stay [22]. Although a key part of the ABCDEF bundle, many barriers to ICU early mobilization exist [92]. In the setting of a bundled sleep promotion intervention, patient engagement in physical therapy sessions was associated with reduced incidence of delirium and continuous sedation infusions but was not associated with any change in patient perception of sleep quality [93]. Further study of early mobility in this population and related effects on sleep and circadian outcomes may provide evidence for novel, mobility-related methods to promote sleep in the ICU.

4.4 Naps

Napping (i.e., sleep during daytime hours) is common in critically ill patients. Propensity to nap may be affected by several variables, including sedating medications, residual sleepiness due to poor overnight sleep quality and short nocturnal sleep duration, and lack of stimulating daytime activity. Napping reduces homeostatic sleep drive, and thus may contribute to difficulty achieving nocturnal sleep and alterations in sleep architecture. Sleeping during daytime hours may also negatively impact circadian alignment. Naps have been associated with both beneficial and detrimental clinical outcomes in healthy adult populations [94]. The impact of napping on overall clinical outcomes and on sleep and circadian health in ICU patients has not been well-studied. For patients suffering from insomnia, it may be reasonable to minimize long duration naps particularly in the later afternoon as this may contribute to insufficient sleep drive in the evening. Strategies for achieving this could include engaging patients with cognitive stimulation and/or physical activity.

5 Summary of Strategies to Improve ICU Sleep

Non-pharmacologic interventions offer many opportunities for clinicians to make practice changes to improve patients' sleep and circadian health (Table 1, Intervention Checklist). Key areas include meeting patient needs, controlling environmental disturbances, and modifying treatment- and acute illness-related factors. Current practice guidelines recommend a sleep-promotion protocol or bundle that encompasses many of these domains. Engagement of multidisciplinary care team members may increase successful implementation, with recent research suggesting an integral role for pharmacists [95]. The clinical team should optimize patient-related sleep impediments, including psychosocial distress and pain.

Table 1 Checklist for improving sleep and circadian health in the ICU

Patient Factors	
Reduce psychological distress, pain, and discomfort.	Address pain via repositioning, ice or heat packs, or alternative techniques where available. Address stress and anxiety via communication about medical condition, reassurance, or alternative techniques where available. Minimize pharmacologic pain and anxiety therapies as possible. Address toileting needs.
Treat underlying sleep disorders.	History of OSA: Continue PAP therapy History of RLS: Continue outpatient therapy, avoid provoking medications
Accommodate habitual sleep preferences.	Allow patient's preferred sleep time, body position, bedding, room lighting and temperature as possible.
Environmental factors	
Reduce noise stimulus and perception.	Decrease volume on medical equipment Reduce staff/visitor conversation Close patient room doors Offer ear plugs, sound-masking headphones
Improve day-night light pattern.	Daytime: Bright light with goal >250 lux for several hours, high proportion of blue light (i.e., mimic sunlight, 460–480 nm) Nighttime: Minimize overnight light exposure and variability Offer eye masks
Reduce overnight care interactions.	Cluster urgent care during designated sleep period Complete non-urgent care outside of designated sleep period
Treatment-related factors	
Mitigate medication effects	Protocolize sedation interruption Avoid pharmacologic sleep aids and, if prescribed, discontinue prior to ICU discharge.
Optimize mobility	Promote early mobilization including rehabilitation and physical therapy

Non-pharmacologic strategies to address these issues include various complementary medicine interventions and relaxation techniques. Pharmacologic analgesia and anxiolysis may be necessary and is discussed elsewhere. Patients' habitual sleep preferences should be elicited and accommodated to the extent possible. A sleep disorder history should be taken to inform team members of the need to continue pre-admission therapies for underlying sleep disorders. Sleep-promoting protocols often designate a dedicated nocturnal sleep time. During these specified hours, efforts should be made to reduce the presence and perception of environmental disturbances such as noise, light, and patient care interactions. To reduce bothersome noises, patient doors should be closed with attention to avoiding staff/visitor conversations within proximity to the patient. Volumes on medical equipment should be reduced and alarms silenced when possible. Ear plugs and eye masks can be offered. Regarding light, bright daytime light and minimal overnight light is recommended to promote circadian alignment. Patient care interactions should also be minimized during the designated sleep time. Non-urgent care should be performed outside of this timeframe, while time-sensitive matters should be clustered. The sleep and circadian-related impacts of acute illness and critical care therapies should be considered and minimized when possible. Current practice guidelines recommend protocolized daily sedation interruptions and using minimal effective doses of such medications. Best practice also includes promoting early mobility with physical therapy and rehabilitation, though sleep-related benefits have yet to be demonstrated.

6　Future Directions

Knowledge about effective non-pharmacologic strategies to promote sleep and circadian alignment in ICU patients continues to expand. Significant challenges must be dealt with to facilitate successful advancement of research in this field. Key challenges include more precisely defining sleep deficiency among patients admitted to the ICU and defining reliable, feasible sleep and circadian outcome measures that will allow the rigorous testing of sleep promotion interventions. Sleep metrics should likely include both subjective measures, such as validated patient-reported perceived symptom scales, as well as objective sleep and circadian parameters. Additionally, outcomes might be expanded to include relevant critical care patient outcomes, such as delirium, length of stay and mortality. Finally, many or most non-pharmacologic sleep promotion interventions are complex, multicomponent bundles, therefore advancement of the implementation science required to create and sustain such interventions is a key next step in developing and providing evidence for non-pharmacologic ICU sleep promotion.

7   Conclusions

Adequate sleep and maintenance of circadian rhythms are essential, yet often elusive elements in critical illness recovery. Various non-pharmacologic strategies exist to address the diverse entities contributing to sleep and circadian disruption in critically ill patients. These include protocols focused on improving patient factors; optimizing the ICU environment to both provide a sleep opportunity and promote circadian alignment; and minimizing acute illness and treatment-related sequalae. Though existing data is sparse and overall low quality, there is growing evidence that these interventions provide subjective improvement in patients' perception of sleep and improve clinically important outcomes such as delirium. Thus, there are many steps that critical care providers can take at this time to improve sleep in the ICU. Further research is needed to evaluate objective effects of non-pharmacologic interventions on sleep and circadian outcomes in the critically ill population, as this area shows tremendous potential to provide a wide-reaching benefit to critically ill patients.

References

1. Freedman NS, Gazendam J, Levan L, Pack AI, Schwab RJ. Abnormal sleep/wake cycles and the effect of environmental noise on sleep disruption in the intensive care unit. Am J Respir Crit Care Med. 2001;163(2):451–7.
2. Elliott R, McKinley S, Cistulli P, Fien M. Characterisation of sleep in intensive care using 24-hour polysomnography: an observational study. Crit Care. 2013;17(2):R46.
3. Knauert MP, Malik V, Kamdar BB. Sleep and sleep disordered breathing in hospitalized patients. Semin Respir Crit Care Med. 2014;35(5):582–92.
4. Krachman SL, D'Alonzo GE, Criner GJ. Sleep in the intensive care unit. Chest. 1995;107(6):1713–20.
5. Pisani MA, Friese RS, Gehlbach BK, Schwab RJ, Weinhouse GL, Jones SF. Sleep in the intensive care unit. Am J Respir Crit Care Med. 2015;191(7):731–8.
6. Thille AW, Reynaud F, Marie D, Barrau S, Rousseau L, Rault C, et al. Impact of sleep alterations on weaning duration in mechanically ventilated patients: a prospective study. Eur Respir J. 2018;51(4):1702465.
7. Dijk DJ, Czeisler CA. Contribution of the circadian pacemaker and the sleep homeostat to sleep propensity, sleep structure, electroencephalographic slow waves, and sleep spindle activity in humans. J Neurosci. 1995;15(5 Pt 1):3526–38.
8. Shilo L, Dagan Y, Smorjik Y, Weinberg U, Dolev S, Komptel B, et al. Patients in the intensive care unit suffer from severe lack of sleep associated with loss of normal melatonin secretion pattern. Am J Med Sci. 1999;317(5):278–81.
9. Mundigler G, Delle-Karth G, Koreny M, Zehetgruber M, Steindl-Munda P, Marktl W, et al. Impaired circadian rhythm of melatonin secretion in sedated critically ill patients with severe sepsis. Crit Care Med. 2002;30(3):536–40.
10. Gehlbach BK, Chapotot F, Leproult R, Whitmore H, Poston J, Pohlman M, et al. Temporal disorganization of circadian rhythmicity and sleep-wake regulation in mechanically ventilated patients receiving continuous intravenous sedation. Sleep. 2012;35(8):1105–14.

11. Olofsson K, Alling C, Lundberg D, Malmros C. Abolished circadian rhythm of melatonin secretion in sedated and artificially ventilated intensive care patients. Acta Anaesthesiol Scand. 2004;48(6):679–84.

12. Verceles AC, Silhan L, Terrin M, Netzer G, Shanholtz C, Scharf SM. Circadian rhythm disruption in severe sepsis: the effect of ambient light on urinary 6-sulfatoxymelatonin secretion. Intensive Care Med. 2012;38(5):804–10.

13. Maas MB, Lizza BD, Abbott SM, Liotta EM, Gendy M, Eed J, et al. Factors disrupting melatonin secretion rhythms during critical illness. Crit Care Med. 2020;48(6):854–61.

14. Roche Campo F, Drouot X, Thille AW, Galia F, Cabello B, d'Ortho MP, et al. Poor sleep quality is associated with late noninvasive ventilation failure in patients with acute hypercapnic respiratory failure. Crit Care Med. 2010;38(2):477–85.

15. DePietro RH, Knutson KL, Spampinato L, Anderson SL, Meltzer DO, Van Cauter E, et al. Association between inpatient sleep loss and hyperglycemia of hospitalization. Diabetes Care. 2017;40(2):188–93.

16. Brown R, Pang G, Husband AJ, King MG. Suppression of immunity to influenza virus infection in the respiratory tract following sleep disturbance. Reg Immunol. 1989;2(5):321–5.

17. Irwin M, McClintick J, Costlow C, Fortner M, White J, Gillin JC. Partial night sleep deprivation reduces natural killer and cellular immune responses in humans. FASEB J. 1996;10(5):643–53.

18. Angeles-Castellanos M, Ramirez-Gonzalez F, Ubaldo-Reyes L, Rodriguez-Mayoral O, Escobar C. Loss of melatonin daily rhythmicity is asociated with delirium development in hospitalized older adults. Sleep Sci. 2016;9(4):285–8.

19. Knauert MP, Gilmore EJ, Murphy TE, Yaggi HK, Van Ness PH, Han L, et al. Association between death and loss of stage N2 sleep features among critically ill patients with delirium. J Crit Care. 2018;48:124–9.

20. Honarmand K, Rafay H, Le J, Mohan S, Rochwerg B, Devlin JW, et al. A systematic review of risk factors for sleep disruption in critically ill adults. Crit Care Med. 2020;48(7):1066–74.

21. Sunderram J, Sofou S, Kamisoglu K, Karantza V, Androulakis IP. Time-restricted feeding and the realignment of biological rhythms: translational opportunities and challenges. J Transl Med. 2014;12:79.

22. Devlin JW, Skrobik Y, Gelinas C, Needham DM, Slooter AJC, Pandharipande PP, et al. Clinical practice guidelines for the prevention and Management of Pain, agitation/sedation, delirium, immobility, and sleep disruption in adult patients in the ICU. Crit Care Med. 2018;46(9):e825–e73.

23. Ding Q, Redeker NS, Pisani MA, Yaggi HK, Knauert MP. Factors influencing Patients' sleep in the intensive care unit: perceptions of patients and clinical staff. Am J Crit Care. 2017;26(4):278–86.

24. Wade DF, Moon Z, Windgassen SS, Harrison AM, Morris L, Weinman JA. Non-pharmacological interventions to reduce ICU-related psychological distress: a systematic review. Minerva Anestesiol. 2016;82(4):465–78.

25. Umbrello M, Sorrenti T, Mistraletti G, Formenti P, Chiumello D, Terzoni S. Music therapy reduces stress and anxiety in critically ill patients: a systematic review of randomized clinical trials. Minerva Anestesiol. 2019;85(8):886–98.

26. Chlan LL, Weinert CR, Heiderscheit A, Tracy MF, Skaar DJ, Guttormson JL, et al. Effects of patient-directed music intervention on anxiety and sedative exposure in critically ill patients receiving mechanical Ventilatory support a randomized clinical trial. Jama-J Am Med Assoc. 2013;309(22):2335–44.

27. Su CP, Lai HL, Chang ET, Yiin LM, Perng SJ, Chen PW. A randomized controlled trial of the effects of listening to non-commercial music on quality of nocturnal sleep and relaxation indices in patients in medical intensive care unit. J Adv Nurs. 2013;69(6):1377–89.

28. Jaber S, Bahloul H, Guetin S, Chanques G, Sebbane M, Eledjam JJ. Effects of music therapy in intensive care unit without sedation in weaning patients versus non-ventilated patients. Ann Fr Anesth Reanim. 2007;26(1):30–8.

29. Gimenez S, Romero S, Alonso JF, Mananas MA, Pujol A, Baxarias P, et al. Monitoring sleep depth: analysis of bispectral index (BIS) based on polysomnographic recordings and sleep deprivation. J Clin Monit Comput. 2017;31(1):103–10.
30. Richardson S. Effects of relaxation and imagery on the sleep of critically ill adults. Dimens Crit Care Nurs. 2003;22(4):182–90.
31. Wang YLWY. Effect of foot massage combined with the use of a Chinese herbal sleep pillow on sleep in coronary care unit patients. J Qual Nursing. 2012;18(1):38–9.
32. Chen JH, Chao YH, Lu SF, Shiung TF, Chao YF. The effectiveness of valerian acupressure on the sleep of ICU patients: a randomized clinical trial. Int J Nurs Stud. 2012;49(8):913–20.
33. Barczi SR, Juergens TM. Comorbidities: psychiatric, medical, medications, and substances. Sleep Med Clin. 2006;1(2):231–45.
34. Finan PH, Goodin BR, Smith MT. The association of sleep and pain: an update and a path forward. J Pain. 2013;14(12)
35. Lautenbacher S, Kundermann B, Krieg JC. Sleep deprivation and pain perception. Sleep Med Rev. 2006;10(5)
36. Sandvik RK, Olsen BF, Rygh LJ, Moi AL. Pain relief from nonpharmacological interventions in the intensive care unit: a scoping review. J Clin Nurs. 2020;29(9–10):1488–98.
37. Duprey MS, Dijkstra-Kersten SMA, Zaal IJ, Briesacher BA, Saczynski JS, Griffith JL, et al. Opioid use increases the risk of delirium in critically ill adults independently of pain. Am J Respir Crit Care Med. 2021;204(5):566–72.
38. Peppard PE, Young T, Barnet JH, Palta M, Hagen EW, Hla KM. Increased prevalence of sleep-disordered breathing in adults. Am J Epidemiol 2013;177(9):1006–14.
39. Sanner BM, Konermann M, Doberauer C, Weiss T, Zidek W. Sleep-Disordered breathing in patients referred for angina evaluation–association with left ventricular dysfunction. Clin Cardiol. 2001;24(2):146–50.
40. Schober AK, Neurath MF, Harsch IA. Prevalence of sleep apnoea in diabetic patients. Clin Respir J. 2011;5(3):165–72.
41. Motamedi KK, McClary AC, Amedee RG. Obstructive sleep apnea: a growing problem. Ochsner J 2009;9(3).
42. Spurr K, Morrison DL, Graven MA, Webber A, Gilbert RW. Analysis of hospital discharge data to characterize obstructive sleep apnea and its management in adult patients hospitalized. in Canada: 2006 to 2007. Can Respir J 2010;17(5).
43. Leiter JC, Knuth SL, Bartlett D. The effect of sleep deprivation on activity of the genioglossus muscle. Am Rev Respir Dis 1985;132(6).
44. Goldstein C. Management of Restless Legs Syndrome/Willis-Ekbom disease in hospitalized and perioperative patients. Sleep Med Clin. 2015;10(3)
45. Hening WA. Current guidelines and standards of practice for restless legs syndrome. Am J Med. 2007;120(1 Suppl 1):S22–7.
46. Ewing R. The rest project: how penn medicine is helping patients sleep better in the hospital. https://www.pennmedicine.org/news/news-blog/2018/april/the-rest-project-how-penn-medicine-is-helping-patients-sleep-better-in-the-hospital https://www.pennmedicine.org/news/news-blog/2018/april/the-rest-project-how-penn-medicine-is-helping-patients-sleep-better-in-the-hospital: Penn Medicine News; 2018.
47. Konkani A, Oakley B. Noise in hospital intensive care units–a critical review of a critical topic. J Crit Care. 2012;27(5):522. e1–9
48. Gabor JY, Cooper AB, Crombach SA, Lee B, Kadikar N, Bettger HE, et al. Contribution of the intensive care unit environment to sleep disruption in mechanically ventilated patients and healthy subjects. Am J Respir Crit Care Med. 2003;167(5):708–15.
49. Altman MT, Pulaski C, Mburu F, Pisani MA, Knauert MP. Non-circadian signals in the intensive care unit: point prevalence morning, noon and night. Heart Lung. 2018;47(6):610–5.
50. Fan EP, Abbott SM, Reid KJ, Zee PC, Maas MB. Abnormal environmental light exposure in the intensive care environment. J Crit Care. 2017;40:11–4.

51. Knauert MP, Pisani M, Redeker N, et al. Pilot study: an intensive care unit sleep promotion protocol. BMJ Open Respir Res. 2019;6(1):e000411.
52. Lusczek ER, Knauert MP. Light levels in ICU patient rooms: dimming of daytime light in occupied rooms. J Patient Exp. 2021;8:23743735211033104.
53. Gao CA, Knauert MP. Circadian biology and its importance to intensive care unit care and outcomes. Semin Respir Crit Care Med. 2019;40(5):629–37.
54. Tamburri LM, DiBrienza R, Zozula R, Redeker NS. Nocturnal care interactions with patients in critical care units. Am J Crit Care. 2004;13(2):102–13.
55. Le A, Friese RS, Hsu CH, Wynne JL, Rhee P, O'Keeffe T. Sleep disruptions and nocturnal nursing interactions in the intensive care unit. J Surg Res. 2012;177(2):310–4.
56. Knauert MP, Pisani M, Redeker N, Murphy T, Araujo K, Jeon S, et al. Pilot study: an intensive care unit sleep promotion protocol. BMJ Open Respir Res. 2019;6(1):e000411.
57. Hu RF, Jiang X, Chen J, Zeng Z, Chen X, Li Y, et al. Non-pharmacological interventions for sleep promotion in the intensive care unit. Cochrane Database Syst Rev 2018.
58. Delaney L, Litton E, Van Haren F. The effectiveness of noise interventions in the ICU. Curr Opin Anaesthesiol. 2019;32(2):144–9.
59. van de Pol I, van Iterson M, Maaskant J. Effect of nocturnal sound reduction on the incidence of delirium in intensive care unit patients: an interrupted time series analysis. Intensive Crit Care Nurs. 2017;41:18–25.
60. Knauert MP, Redeker NS, Yaggi HK, Bennick M, Pisani MA. Creating naptime: an overnight, nonpharmacologic intensive care unit sleep promotion protocol. J Patient Exp. 2018;5(3):180–7.
61. Kahn DM, Cook TE, Carlisle CC, Nelson DL, Kramer NR, Millman RP. Identification and modification of environmental noise in an ICU setting. Chest J. 1998;114(2):535–40.
62. Olson DM, Borel CO, Laskowitz DT, Moore DT, McConnell ES. Quiet time: a nursing intervention to promote sleep in neurocritical care units. Am J Crit Care. 2001;10(2):74–8.
63. Boyko Y, Jennum P, Nikolic M, Holst R, Oerding H, Toft P. Sleep in intensive care unit: the role of environment. J Crit Care. 2017;37:99–105.
64. Kamdar BB, King LM, Collop NA, Sakamuri S, Colantuoni E, Neufeld KJ, et al. The effect of a quality improvement intervention on perceived sleep quality and cognition in a medical ICU. Crit Care Med. 2013;41(3):800–9.
65. Tonna JE, Dalton A, Presson AP, Zhang C, Colantuoni E, Lander K, et al. The effect of a quality improvement intervention on sleep and delirium in critically ill patients in a surgical ICU. Chest. 2021;
66. Demoule A, Carreira S, Lavault S, Pallanca O, Morawiec E, Mayaux J, et al. Impact of earplugs and eye mask on sleep in critically ill patients: a prospective randomized study. Crit Care. 2017;21(1):284.
67. Hu RF, Jiang XY, Chen J, Zeng Z, Chen XY, Li Y, et al. Non-pharmacological interventions for sleep promotion in the intensive care unit. Cochrane Database Syst Rev. 2015;10:CD008808.
68. Litton E, Carnegie V, Elliott R, Webb SA. The efficacy of earplugs as a sleep hygiene strategy for reducing delirium in the ICU: a systematic review and meta-analysis. Crit Care Med. 2016;44(5):992–9.
69. Fang CS, Wang HH, Wang RH, Chou FH, Chang SL, Fang CJ. Effect of earplugs and eye masks on the sleep quality of intensive care unit patients: a systematic review and meta-analysis. J Adv Nurs 2021.
70. Gallacher S, Enki D, Stevens S, Bennett MJ. An experimental model to measure the ability of headphones with active noise control to reduce patient's exposure to noise in an intensive care unit. Intensive Care Med Exp. 2017;5(1):47.
71. Vetter C, Pattison PM, Houser K, Herf M, Phillips AJK, Wright KP, et al. A review of human physiological responses to light: implications for the development of integrative lighting solutions. Leukos 2021.
72. Brown T, Brainard G, Cajochen C, Czeisler C, Hanifin J, Lockley S, et al. Recommendations for healthy daytime, evening, and night-time indoor light exposure. Preprints 2020. 2020.

73. Engwall M, Fridh I, Johansson L, Bergbom I, Lindahl B. Lighting, sleep and circadian rhythm: an intervention study in the intensive care unit. Intensive Crit Care Nurs. 2015;31(6):325–35.
74. Taguchi T, Yano M, Kido Y. Influence of bright light therapy on postoperative patients: a pilot study. Intensive Crit Care Nurs. 2007;23(5):289–97.
75. Ono H, Taguchi T, Kido Y, Fujino Y, Doki Y. The usefulness of bright light therapy for patients after oesophagectomy. Intensive Crit Care Nurs. 2011;27(3):158–66.
76. Taguchi T. Bright light treatment for prevention of perioperative delirium in elderly patients. J Nurs Educ Pract. 2013;3:10–8.
77. Gehlbach BK, Patel SB, Van Cauter E, Pohlman AS, Hall JB, Zabner J. The effects of timed light exposure in critically ill patients: a randomized controlled pilot clinical trial. Am J Respir Crit Care Med. 2018;198(2):275–8.
78. Simons KS, Laheij RJ, van den Boogaard M, Moviat MA, Paling AJ, Polderman FN, et al. Dynamic light application therapy to reduce the incidence and duration of delirium in intensive-care patients: a randomised controlled trial. Lancet Respir Med. 2016;4(3):194–202.
79. Zhang KS, Pelleg T, Hussain S, Kollipara V, Loschner A, Foroozesh MB, et al. Prospective randomized controlled pilot study of high-intensity Lightbox phototherapy to prevent ICU-acquired delirium incidence. Cureus. 2021;13(4):e14246.
80. Hardin KA. Sleep in the ICU: potential mechanisms and clinical implications. Chest. 2009;136(1):284–94.
81. Alexopoulou C, Kondili E, Diamantaki E, Psarologakis C, Kokkini S, Bolaki M, et al. Effects of dexmedetomidine on sleep quality in critically ill patients: a pilot study. Anesthesiology. 2014;121(4):801–7.
82. Zaal IJ, Devlin JW, Hazelbag M, Klouwenberg PMCK, van der Kooi AW, Ong DSY, et al. Benzodiazepine-associated delirium in critically ill adults. Intensive Care Med. 2015;41(12):2130–7.
83. Hager DN, Dinglas VD, Subhas S, Rowden AM, Neufeld KJ, Bienvenu OJ, et al. Reducing deep sedation and delirium in acute lung injury patients: a quality improvement project. Crit Care Med. 2013;41(6):1435–42.
84. Depner CM, Stothard ER, Wright KP Jr. Metabolic consequences of sleep and circadian disorders. Curr Diab Rep. 2014;14(7):507.
85. Depner CM, Melanson EL, McHill AW, Wright KP Jr. Mistimed food intake and sleep alters 24-hour time-of-day patterns of the human plasma proteome. Proc Natl Acad Sci U S A. 2018;115(23):E5390–E9.
86. Van Dyck L, Vanhorebeek I, Wilmer A, Schrijvers A, Derese I, Mebis L, et al. Towards a fasting-mimicking diet for critically ill patients: the pilot randomized crossover ICU-FM-1 study. Crit Care. 2020;24(1):249.
87. Korwin A, Honiden S, Intihar T, Wasden K, Heard A, Powierza C, et al., editors. A Pilot Protocol for Intermittent Feeding in Mechanically Ventilated Medical Intensive Care Unit Patients. American Thoracic Society; 2021.
88. Korwin A, Honiden S, Intihar T, Wasden K, Powierza C, Knauert M, editors. Intermittent feeding in mechanically ventilated medical intensive care unit patients: preliminary outcomes. American Thoracic Society; 2021.
89. Morrison SA, Mirnik D, Korsic S, Eiken O, Mekjavic IB, Dolenc-Groselj L. Bed rest and hypoxic exposure affect sleep architecture and breathing stability. Front Physiol. 2017;8:410.
90. Rohr J. Benefits of early mobility on sleep in the intensive care unit. Crit Care Nurs Clin North Am. 2021;33(2):193–201.
91. Axelsson J, Ingre M, Kecklund G, Lekander M, Wright KP, Sundelin T. Sleepiness as motivation: a potential mechanism for how sleep deprivation affects behavior. Sleep 2020;43(6).
92. Pun BT, Balas MC, Barnes-Daly MA, Thompson JL, Aldrich JM, Barr J, et al. Caring for critically ill patients with the ABCDEF bundle: results of the ICU liberation collaborative in over 15,000 adults. Crit Care Med. 2019;47(1):3–14.
93. Kamdar BB, Combs MP, Colantuoni E, King LM, Niessen T, Neufeld KJ, et al. The association of sleep quality, delirium, and sedation status with daily participation in physical therapy in the ICU. Crit Care. 2016;19:261.

94. Mantua J, Spencer RMC. Exploring the nap paradox: are mid-day sleep bouts a friend or foe? Sleep Med. 2017;37:88–97.
95. Louzon PR, Heavner MS, Herod K, Wu TT, Devlin JW. Sleep-promotion bundle development, implementation, and evaluation in critically ill adults: roles for pharmacists. Ann Pharmacother. 2022;56(7):839–49.

Best Practices for Improving Sleep in the ICU: Part II: Pharmacologic

Caitlin S. Brown, Alejandro A. Rabinstein, and Gilles L. Fraser

1 Introduction

Sleep disruption in the intensive care unit (ICU) is common with over 60% of critically ill patients reporting poor sleep during their ICU stay [1, 2]. After appropriate implementation of non-pharmacologic strategies, as discussed in chapter "Best Practices for Improving Sleep in the ICU. Part I: Non-pharmacologic", clinicians may look to pharmacological strategies to improve sleep in their critically ill patients. In this chapter we seek to identify optimal sleep agents in critically ill adults.

1.1 Methodologic Considerations when Evaluating ICU Pharmacologic Sleep Agents

Prospective, randomized controlled trials (RCTs) are the preferred approach for evaluating the efficacy and safety of pharmacologic sleep agents in the ICU. A number of methodological factors are important to consider when reviewing published RCTs or designing a new trial. Realizing a RCT with high external validity better

C. S. Brown (✉)
Department of Pharmacy, Mayo Clinic, Rochester, MN, USA
e-mail: Brown.caitlin1@mayo.edu

A. A. Rabinstein
Division of Neurology, Mayo Clinic, Rochester, MN, USA
e-mail: Rabinstein.alejandro@mayo.edu

G. L. Fraser
(Ret.) Professor of Medicine, Tufts University, Boston, MA, USA

© The Author(s), under exclusive license to Springer Nature Switzerland AG 2022
G. L. Weinhouse, J. W. Devlin (eds.), *Sleep in Critical Illness*,
https://doi.org/10.1007/978-3-031-06447-0_15

informs sleep medication prescribing decisions, risk factors for disrupted sleep vary considerably (as highlighted in chapter "Risk Factors for Disrupted Sleep in the ICU") between different ICU populations [e.g., medical (vs. surgical), mechanically ventilated (vs. non ventilated), higher (vs. lower) severity of illness]. Given the potential inter-relationship between sleep quality and delirium (chapters "Sleep Disruption and Its Relationship with Delirium: Electrophysiologic Perspectives" and "Sleep Disruption and Its Relationship with Delirium: Clinical Perspectives"), the way in which delirium is handled in any medication-based, sleep improvement RCT is important. If delirium occurrence is a trial outcome, then enrollment of delirium-free patients in the RCT may be important. As noted in chapters "Sleep Disruption and Its Relationship with Delirium: Electrophysiologic Perspectives" and "Recommended Method(s) for Routine Sleep Assessment and Monitoring", delirium may affect polysomnography (PSG) assessments and the ability of ICU patients to self-report their sleep quality. As discussed in chapter "Recommended Method(s) for Routine Sleep Assessment and Monitoring", the ability to rigorously assess sleep in the ICU is complex. As a result, trials evaluating sleep-promoting agents have used various assessment methods, which further complicate an already complex issue. PSG remains the gold standard objective method to evaluate sleep, but in an ICU setting, it still may not be feasible to perform, even in the research context.

Common ICU medications affect sleep quality (chapter "Effects of Common ICU Medications on Sleep"); whether the use of these medications are prospectively controlled for may affect study results. Non-pharmacologic sleep improvement strategies (e.g., noise reduction, light modulation) remain the foundation for sleep improvement efforts in the ICU (chapter "Best Practices for Improving Sleep in the ICU. Part I: Non-pharmacologic"); their use should be standardized in any medication trial. Current knowledge of the many ICU (chapter "ICU Sleep Disruption and Its Relationship with ICU outcomes") and post-ICU (chapter "Long-Term Outcomes: Sleep in Survivors of Critical Illness") outcomes affected by disrupted sleep should be considered when defining the study outcomes evaluated in any ICU sleep medication trial. An evaluation of circadian rhythm disruption may be important for specific medications (chapter "Characteristics of Sleep in Critically Ill Patients. Part II: Circadian Rhythm Disruption"). As reviewed in chapter "Effects of Common ICU Medications on Sleep", medication administration at night may interrupt sleep.

Realizing the neuroactive medications evaluated for ICU sleep improvement may have additional pharmacologic properties (e.g., analgesia, anxiety, delirium reduction, sedation), this chapter will primarily focus on the pharmacologic properties of medications postulated to improve sleep and sleep-related outcomes. Figure 1 shows proposed pharmacologic targets that will be discussed in this chapter.

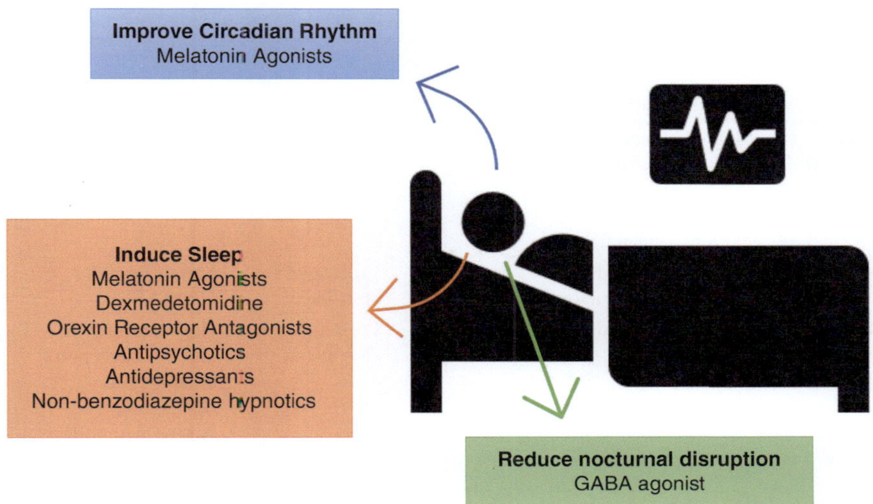

Fig. 1 Proposed pharmacologic targets to improve sleep

2 Dexmedetomidine

2.1 Sleep-Related Pharmacology

Dexmedetomidine is a selective α_2-adrenergic agonist commonly utilized as a sedative and analgesic agent in the ICU [3]. The pharmacology of dexmedetomidine is highlighted in Table 1. Hypotheses for the mechanisms by which dexmedetomidine may induce sleep are complex. Animal models have shown that dexmedetomidine reduces the neuronal firing in the locus coeruleus [4–6]. This decrease in adrenergic activity results in initiation and maintenance of a sleep-like state [3, 7]. Small studies in healthy humans have shown that dexmedetomidine promotes biomimetic non-rapid eye movement (NREM) stages 2 (N2) and 3 (N3) sleep [7–9]. The relationship between sleep and altered consciousness under sedation is discussed in greater detail in chapter "Normal Sleep Compared to Altered Consciousness During Sedation". Side effects of dexmedetomidine are related to its α_2 adrenergic agonism, and include hypotension and bradycardia [3]. Additionally, recent reports have shown potential for dexmedetomidine induced-hyperthermia [10, 11].

Table 1 Pharmacologic agents studied for their effects on sleep in critically Ill adults

Drug	Mechanism of Action for Sleep	Dosing	Side Effects	Considerations
Dexmedetomidine [3, 7, 10, 11]	α2 adrenergic agonist, resulting in decreased neuron firing	0.2–1.5 mcg/kg/hr	Hypotension, bradycardia, fever	Can be used in non-mechanically ventilated patients
Melatonin [16, 27]	MT1 and MT2 receptor agonist	3–10 mg at bedtime	Prolonged sleepiness	Metabolized by CYP1A2
Ramelteon [19, 20, 28]	MT1 and MT2 receptor agonist	8 mg at bedtime	Prolonged sleepiness	Higher affinity to MT1 and MT2 receptors compared to melatonin. Active metabolite
Propofol [32, 52]	GABA agonist	5–50 mcg/kg/min	Respiratory depression, hypotension, PRIS	Lipid emulsion
Benzodiazepines [33, 52]	GABA agonist	Varies by specific medication	Respiratory depression	Midazolam: Active metabolite renally cleared Lorazepam: Propylene glycol excipient

GABA γ-Aminobutyric acid, *PRIS* Propofol related infusion syndrome

2.2 Comparative Trials Evaluating a Sleep Outcome

Based on evidence in animals and healthy human subjects, several studies have investigated dexmedetomidine for sleep in critically ill adults (Table 2). Oto and colleagues evaluated the use of nighttime (2100 to 0600 h) dexmedetomidine in 10 adults receiving mechanical ventilation and as needed (PRN) midazolam and fentanyl (or morphine) to maintain a Richmond Agitation Sedation Scale (RASS) goal of −1 to −4 compared to the daytime (0600 to 2100 h) use of PRN midazolam and fentanyl (or morphine) alone. Sleep was monitored continuously for 24 h with PSG [12]. In the nighttime (vs. daytime) period median (IQR) total sleep time (TST) (i.e., total time spent in any sleep stage) was more than twice as high [4.7 (4.2, 8.1) vs 1.7 (0.8, 2.0)] and the Sleep Efficiency (SE) (i.e., TST in proportion to a defined period) was nearly five-times higher (11.3% vs. 52.3%). The time spent in each stage of sleep was similar between the day and night periods; patients spent no time in REM sleep during either period [12]. The study found no statistically significant correlations between the dexmedetomidine infusion dose and any of the PSG outcomes [12]. This investigation was limited by the lack of a control group, no washout period for nocturnal midazolam and fentanyl/morphine use, a small sample size, a short 24-h study period, and the lack of protocolization of non-pharmacologic sleep interventions. Despite these limitations, this trial supports the hypothesis that dexmedetomidine increases sleep time and efficiency when administered at night to critically ill mechanically ventilated adults.

A pilot study by Alexopoulou and colleagues studied 13 adults, mechanically ventilated ≥48 h, who were not receiving vasoactive or sedative medications [13]. Patients were evaluated with PSG over three consecutive nights (from 2100 h on night 1 to 0600 h on day 3). On night 2 each patient was administered dexmedetomidine (0.5 mcg/kg bolus × 1 followed by continuous infusion of 0.2 to 0.7 mcg/kg/ hr. titrated to RASS of −1 to −2). PSG data from night 2 (vs night 1 and 3) revealed dexmedetomidine to be associated with improved sleep efficiency (P < 0.002), a reduced sleep fragmentation index (sum of arousals and awakenings per hour of sleep) (P = 0.02), and greater TST (P = 0.03) (Table 2) [13]. Alexopoulou et al. attempted to mitigate the potential confounding effects of non-dexmedetomidine sedation on their results by ensuring no patients had detectable serum concentrations of benzodiazepines or propofol at the time of enrollment, however 3 of the 13 patients received opioids for pain during the study period. Patients who received antipsychotics during the study period were withdrawn from the study. A major limitation of these data is that patients who did not sleep during the night were excluded from the analysis. Nonetheless, this small observational study also supports the conclusion dexmedetomidine may have a role as a sleep-improving agent in critically ill adults [13].

In another pilot study, Wu X, et al. randomized 61 adults ≥65 years, admitted to the ICU after non-cardiac surgery, who were not requiring mechanical ventilation [14] to receive 15 h of a dexmedetomidine 1 mcg/kg/h infusion (from 1700 h the night of surgery until the next morning at 0800 h) or placebo. Based on continuous PSG assessment the dexmedetomidine (vs. placebo) groups spent nearly three times as long with stage N2 sleep (43.5 vs. 15.8%, P = 0.05) and both greater TST (213 vs 130 min, P = 0.03) and sleep efficiency (22.4 vs 15.0%, p = 0.03) [14] (Table 2). In the morning after the study infusion was stopped, patients administered dexmedetomidine (vs placebo) rated their median (IRQ) sleep quality (using an 11 point scale where 0 indicated best possible sleep and 10 indicated worst possible sleep) to be better [1 (0,3) vs. 3 (2,7); P = 0.005] [14]. Hypotension, bradycardia, tachycardia, respiratory depression, and desaturations requiring interventions were not different between the two groups [14]. Although perioperatively-administered sedatives and analgesics may have influenced ICU sleep, the use of these medications was similar between the two groups. Non-pharmacologic interventions to improve sleep were not standardized and the number of sleep interruptions was not collected. This study provides hypothesis-generating findings supporting the usefulness of dexmedetomidine to improve sleep in the ICU in older adults after major surgery in the immediate postoperative period.

Lastly, a double-blind, placebo-controlled study by Skrobik and colleagues found that nocturnal, continuous, low-dose nocturnal dexmedetomidine in critically ill adults free of delirium requiring continuous sedation reduced incident ICU delirium occurrence by 44% (Table 2) [15]. A secondary outcome was sleep quality based on daily (09:00 h) administration of the Leeds Sleep Evaluation Questionnaire (LSEQ) score by the bedside nurse to patients with a RASS > −1 and who remained delirium-free. The average LSEQ score was similar between the dexmedetomidine

Table 2 Summary of trials of Dexmedetomidine for improving sleep

Dexmedetomidine (DEX)

Study	Patient population	N	Study drug & dosing	Results				P value
				Outcome	Intervention group	Control group		
Oto 2012 [12]	Adults receiving sedation & mechanical ventilation >48 h	10	• *0600–2100:* Received midazolam, morphine, fentanyl PRN for pain or agitation • *2100–0600:* DEX loading dose of 1 mcg/kg, followed by 0.2–0.7 mcg/kg/h to RASS -1 to −4, PRN midazolam, morphine, fentanyl		2100–0600	0600–2100		
				Total sleep time (h)	4.7 (4.2,8.1)	1.7 (0.8,2)		
				Sleep efficiency (%)	52.3 (47,89.7)	11.3 (5,13.7)		
				Arousal/ awakening index (n/h)	9.3 (3, 19.5)	20.2 (11.3,34.2)		
				Total sleep in each stage (min)	1:76 (32,145)	1: 46 (13,57)		
					2:188 (136,449)	2: 54 (16, 67)		
					3 & 4: 0 (0,1.3)	3 & 4: 0 (0,0)		
					REM: 0 (0,0)	REM: 0 (0,0)		
Alexopoulou 2014 [13]	Adults mechanically ventilated ≥48 h and anticipated ICU stay ≥5 days without vasoactive or sedatives	13	• During a 3 night study period on night 2 patients received DEX 0.5 mcg/kg bolus followed by 0.2 to 0.7 mcg/kg/hr. titrated to RASS -1 to −2		Night 1	Night 2 (DEX)	Night 3	
				Sleep efficiency (%)	9.7 (1.6, 45.1)	64.8 (51.4, 79.9)	6.9 (0.0, 17.1)	<0.002
				Sleep fragmentation index (events/h of sleep)		2.7 (1.6, 4.9)	*Night 1 & 3* 7.6 (4.8, 14.2)	0.023
				Percentage of total sleep at night (%)	48 (32, 71)	79 (66, 87)	N/A	0.032
				Total sleep in each stage (%)	*1*: 56.2 (24.7,79.3)	*1*: 16.1 (6.2, 21.3)	*1*: 45.2 (29.5,58.7)	
					2: 39.2 (20.7,66.4)	2: 78.7 (69.2, 92.5)	2: 47.5 (41.3, 70.5)	
					*3:*0 (0,0)	*3:*0 (0,0)	*3:* 0 (0,0)	
					REM: 0(0,0)	*REM:* 0 (0,0)	*REM:* 0 (0,0)	

Wu 2016 [14]	≥ 65 years of age admitted to ICU after noncardiac surgery & not requiring mechanical ventilation	61	• 1 mcg/kg/h DEX for 15 h on the night of surgery (1700–0800) • Placebo	Percentage of N2 sleep	43.5 (16.6, 80.2)	15.8 (1.3, 62.8)	0.048
				Total sleep time (min)	213 (124, 324)	130 (72, 220)	0.028
				Sleep efficiency (%)	22.4 (14.2, 37.1)	15 (7.9,-26.3)	0.033
				Total sleep in each stage (min)	*1:* 92 (9, 169)	*1:*77 (35,103)	0.462
					2: 89 (37,142)	*2:* 17 (0,131)	0.019
					3: 0 (0)	*3:* 0 (0,0)	0.314
					REM: 0 (0,0)	*REM:* 0, (0,0)	1.00
Skrobik 2018 [15]	Adults admitted to ICU And receiving intermittent or continuous Sedatives, Expected to require ≥48 h of ICU care & delirium free	64	• At 21:30 sedatives were halved and DEX was initiated at 2 mcg/kg/h to a goal RASS -1 (max 0.7 mcg/kg/h) • Placebo	LSEQ	n = 34	n = 30	Mean diff 0.02 (95% CI 0.42–1.92)

h hour, *ICU* Intensive care unit, *RASS* Richmond Agitation Sedation Scale, *PRN* As needed, *REM* Rapid Eye Movement, *N/A* Not available, *LSEQ* Leeds Sleep Evaluation Questionnaire

Data represented as median (IQR) unless specified

and placebo groups [15]. Among the 10 individual LSEQ domains, only domain 9 (degree of tiredness) was significantly improved in the dexmedetomidine (vs placebo) group (mean difference 2, p < 0.05) [15]. Bradycardia and hypotension was similar between the two groups. It remains unclear if reductions in delirium occurrence and LSEQ domain 9 observed in the dexmedetomidine group was a result of nocturnal dexmedetomidine use or the reduced use of medications known to increase delirium and disrupt sleep (e.g., benzodiazepines, propofol).

In conclusion, several small, hypothesis-generating, studies suggest dexmedetomidine, particularly when it is administered overnight, may improve sleep in critically ill adults; however, larger, randomized trials are needed to determine whether dexmedetomidine can be routinely used as a sleep aid in critically ill adults.

3　Melatonin Agonists

3.1　Melatonin

3.1.1　Sleep-Related Pharmacology

Melatonin is primarily synthesized and released from the pineal gland, but can also be synthesized and released from extrapineal sources, including the gastrointestinal tract [16]. As highlighted in chapter "Characteristics of Sleep in Critically Ill Patients. Part II: Circadian Rhythm Disruption", endogenous melatonin synthesis is inhibited by light and enhanced by darkness, emphasizing the potential benefit of interventions that modulate light in the ICU to improve sleep (chapter "Best Practices for Improving Sleep in the ICU. Part I: Non-pharmacologic") [16]. The suprachiasmatic nucleus of the hypothalamus controls the sleep-wake cycle, and activation of the MT1 and MT2 receptors in the suprachiasmatic nucleus decrease neuronal firing and lead to sleep-wake cycle phase shifting [17–19]. Ongoing research seeks to identify the precise mechanism of MT1 and MT2 receptors and their effect on the sleep-wake cycle and different sleep stages [20]. Melatonin, when administered as an oral medication, is well tolerated, and side effects, including fatigue and daytime sleepiness, are usually minimal [16]. Melatonin should be administered approximately one hour before its intended effects. Of note, melatonin, as an over-the-counter, non-pharmaceutical product is not regulated by the FDA and thus product strength may vary.

3.1.2　Comparative Trials Evaluating a Sleep Outcome

The first placebo-controlled study assessing melatonin in critically ill adults compared sleep duration and awakenings after the administration of 3 mg of controlled release melatonin at 22:30 h in 8 critically ill adults with the use of a placebo in 6 general medical ward patients and found each outcome not to be statistically different between the two groups (Table 3) [21]. This investigation was limited by a very small sample size (and potential type-II error) and a control group who was not critically ill.

Table 3 Summary of trials of melatonin agonists for improving sleep

Melatonin

Study	Patient population	N	Study drug & dosing	Outcome	Results		P value
					Intervention group	Control group	
Shilo 2000 [21]	Patients in pulmonary ICU, stable, not receiving BZD or opioids Control were general hospital ward patients	14	• 3 mg controlled release melatonin at 22:00 • Placebo	Duration of sleep from 22:30–06:30 (h) (mean ± SD)	6.3 ± 1.1	7.4 ± 2.1	
				Sleep awakenings (n) (mean ± SD)	1.4 ± 3.7	1.8 ± 6.3	NS
Ibrahim 2006 [22]	ICU patients with tracheostomy not receiving sedation	32	• 3 mg melatonin at 22:00 for at least 48 h of ICU discharge • Placebo	Observed sleep at night (min)	243.4 (0, 344.1)	240 (75, 331.3)	0.98
				Observed sleep during the day (min)	138.7 (50, 230)	104 (0, 485)	0.42
Bourne 2008 [24]	ICU patients with acute respiratory failure and tracheostomy not receiving sedation	24	• 10 mg melatonin at 21:00 for 4 nights • Placebo	SEI—BIS (ratio)[b]	0.39 (0.27, 0.51)	0.26 (0.17, 0.36)	0.09
				SEI—Actinography (ratio)	0.73 (0.53, 0.93)	0.75 (0.67, 0.83)	0.84
				SEI—Nurse assessment (ratio)[c]	0.45 (0.26, 0.64)	0.51 (0.35, 0.68)	0.58
				SEI—Patient assessment (ratio)[d]	0.41 (0.24, 0.59)	0.50 (0.43, 0.58)	0.32

(continued)

Table 3 (continued)

Melatonin

Study	Patient population	N	Study drug & dosing	Results			
				Outcome	Intervention group	Control group	P value
Gandolfi 2020 [25]	Adult patients with at least 1 ICU night stay	203	• 10 mg melatonin at 20:00 for 7 days • Placebo	RCSQ overall (mean ± SD)	69.7 ± 21.2	60.7 ± 26.3	0.029
				RCSQ in ICU (mean ± SD)	69.7 ± 21.4	60.7 ± 26.3	0.027
				RCSQ in ICU Very poor sleep (0–25 mm), (n (%))	3(3.1)	14 (14.6)	RR (95% CI) 0.21 (0.06–0.72)
				RCSQ in ICU Poor sleep (26–50 mm), (n (%))	17 (17.7)	15 (15.6)	RR (95% CI) 1.13 (0.60–2.14)
				RCSQ in ICU Good sleep (51–75 mm), (n (%))	32 (33.3)	34 (35.4)	RR (95% CI) 0.94 (0.64–1.39)
				RCSQ in ICU Very good sleep (76–100 mm), (n (%))	44 (45.8)	33 (34.4)	RR (95% CI) 1.33 (0.94–1.89)
				Delirium (intensive Care delirium screening checklist (ICDSC)), (%)	2.3%	1.7%	0.666

Table 3 (continued)

Melatonin

Study	Patient population	N	Study drug & dosing	Results			
				Outcome	Intervention group	Control group	P value

Ramelteon

Study	Patient population	N	Study drug & dosing	Results			
				Outcome	Intervention group	Control group	P value
Hatta 2014 [29]	65 to 89 years of age and admitted to the hospital with medical condition	67 (24 ICU)	• Ramelteon 8 mg nightly until delirium or 7 days • Placebo	Awakenings per night (mean (SD))[a]	1.3 (1.6)	1.6 (1.2)	0.28
				Sleep duration (h) (mean (SD))[a]	6.3 (1.6)	6.3 (1.6)	0.67
				Difficulty falling asleep (n (%))	10 (30)	14 (41)	0.45
				Difficulty staying asleep (n (%))	14 (42)	14 (41)	>0.99
				Waking too early (n (%))	7 (21)	5 (15)	0.54
				Poor sleep quality (n (%))	21 (64)	19 (56)	0.62
				Disturbance of natural sleep-wake cycle (n (%))	7 (21)	3 (9)	0.19
Nishikimi 2018 [30]	Adults (age ≥ 20) admitted to ICU	88	• Ramelteon 8 mg at 20:00 until ICU discharge • Placebo	Awakenings per night (n/ night)	0.80	1.31	0.045
				Nights without awakening (%)	51	30	0.048
				Hours of sleep (mean)	7.29	6.78	0.252

h hour, *ICU* Intensive care unit, *NS* Not significant, *SD* Standard Deviation, *SEI* Sleep efficiency index, *RCSQ* Richards Campbell Sleep Questionnaire, *RR* Relative risk, *BIS* Bispectral index

Data represented as median (IQR) unless otherwise specified

[a]Based on patient report, nursing observations/records, and rater observations

[b]Sleep defined as BIS < 80

[c]Direct nurse observation using hourly epochs

[d]RCSQ

Ibrahim and colleagues conducted a 2006, double-blind, randomized, placebo-controlled pilot study in 32 ICU patients with tracheostomy [22]. Sedatives were stopped for >12 h in all patients and melatonin 3 mg (or placebo) was administered nightly at 22:00 h for a minimum of 48 h. The duration of nurse-observed nighttime or daytime sleep was similar between the two groups (Table 3) [22]. Unsurprisingly, post-treatment median (IQR) melatonin levels were significantly higher in the melatonin (vs. placebo) group [3543 (1533, 8100) vs. 3 (1.6, 9.3) pg/mL, p < 0.0001] [22]. The study did collect median number of nighttime procedures performed in each group and while similar between the groups (melatonin 3.7, placebo 4.6) they were high. With reduced nighttime procedures/interruptions being an important part of ICU sleep improvement bundles [23], non-pharmacologic interventions to improve sleep should be optimized in all ICU sleep medication studies (chapter "Best Practices for Improving Sleep in the ICU. Part I: Non-pharmacologic") [22]. The investigation had several limitations, most notably that sleep was assessed using nursing observation. The results of this trial do not support the routine use of melatonin in critically ill patients to improve sleep.

Another small randomized, double-blind placebo-controlled trial by Bourne et al. included 24 ICU adults with acute respiratory failure and tracheostomy who were not receiving sedation. Patients were randomized to oral melatonin 10 mg or placebo at 2100 for four nights [24]. The primary outcome was sleep efficiency index (SEI) and was measured using bispectral index (BIS), actigraphy, nurse assessment and patient self-assessment. None of the SEI outcomes were different between the two groups (Table 3) [24]. Pharmacokinetic monitoring revealed supratherapeutic concentrations of melatonin in the morning suggesting a lower nighttime dose in the ICU population may help reduce daytime sleepiness [24]. Like the prior study, this investigation also did not find a benefit with the use of melatonin in critically ill adults.

A more recent, double-blind, randomized, placebo-controlled trial by Gandolfi et al. randomized 203 critically ill adults to receive melatonin 10 mg or placebo at 20:00 for 7 consecutive nights [25]. Patient-perceived sleep quality as evaluated using the validated, 10-domain, 100-point, Richards Campbell Sleep Questionnaire (RCSQ) was found to be significantly better in the melatonin (vs. placebo) group (69.7 ± 21.2 vs 60.7 ± 26.3; P = 0.029) [25]. The incidence of delirium was similar between groups (Table 3) [25]. The study was potentially limited most by patients receiving concomitant sedative and/or opioid therapy, which may impact sleep although use was similar between the two groups. Melatonin concentrations (collected in 6 melatonin patients and 3 placebo patients) group were significantly higher in the melatonin group at 02:00 h, 06:00 h, and 12:00 h [25]. While the study was large and thus adequately powered, sleep outcomes were evaluated solely using patient self-report (vs. an objective assessment method like PSG or actigraphy). Additionally, non-pharmacological interventions were not standardized or measured. Consistent with the recommendations from the PADIS 2018 guideline panel, current evidence does not support the routine use of melatonin in critically ill adults to improve sleep [26]. Future randomized controlled trials are required that evaluate ICU sleep using objective assessment methods.

The ideal dose of melatonin that should be used to improve sleep in critically ill adults remains unclear. Extensive variation in pharmacokinetic variables exists after melatonin administration in the ICU that are probably related to the study population, dose, administration route, formulation, and type of blood concentration assay used [27]. While melatonin has an average T_{max} of 50 min and bioavailability 15%, these vary widely in critically ill adults [27]. However, C_{max} is increased in patients during a fed state (compared to fasting); elimination is decreased in patients with liver and kidney injury [27]. The results from the Bourne et al. and Gandolfi et al. studies, where 10 mg nighttime dose of melatonin was administered, suggests the elevated daytime melatonin concentrations resulting from this dose may worsen daytime drowsiness [24, 25]. The effect of end organ dysfunction and gut function abnormalities, both common in the ICU, on the pharmacokinetics and pharmacodynamics of melatonin in this population requires further research.

3.2 Ramelteon

3.2.1 Sleep-Related Pharmacology

Ramelteon is a synthetic melatonin agonist with a similar mechanism of action to melatonin (MT1 and MT2 agonist), but with a higher affinity for MT1 and MT2 receptors (Table 1) [19, 28]. Agonist activity at the MT1 and MT2 receptors leads to phase shifting of the circadian clock, though additional research is needed to fully understand the role of MT1 and MT2 receptors in sleep [19, 20]. Similar to melatonin, ramelteon is well tolerated and side effects are minimal and include daytime somnolence, nausea, and fatigue [19].

3.2.2 Comparative Trials Evaluating a Sleep Outcome

The DELIRA-J study group sought to identify if ramelteon improved rates of delirium in a multicenter, rater-blinded, randomized, placebo-controlled trial [29]. Hospitalized patients 65–89 years of age (n = 67) were randomized to ramelteon 8 mg at bedtime or placebo, although only 24 (36%) of the enrolled patients were admitted to an ICU [29]. A secondary outcome of this study evaluated sleep metrics as measured by patient reports, nursing observations and records, and rater (trained site coordinators) observations. No differences between the two groups for any sleep-related outcome were found (Table 3) [29]. The specific characteristics of the ICU subgroup including mechanical ventilation status and sedatives/analgesic use were not reported. Given the small number of ICU patients, and subjective evaluation of sleep, no definitive conclusions can be drawn from this trial.

Nishikimi et al. conducted a single-center, randomized, placebo-controlled trial of ramelteon 8 mg or placebo at 20:00 every night until ICU discharge in 88 critically ill adults admitted to a ten-bed emergency and medical ICU [30]. The primary outcome of the study was duration of ICU stay; secondary outcomes included awakenings per night, nights without awakenings and mean hours of sleep in a subset of non-intubated patients. Sleep metrics were evaluated via retrospective chart review. While ICU duration was not different between the two groups, the ramelteon (vs. placebo) group experienced fewer awakenings per night (0.80 vs.1.31; p = 0.045) and a higher proportion of nights without awakenings (51 vs. 30%; p = 0.048) (Table 3). Mean hours of sleep were similar (7.29 vs 6.78 h; p = 0.252) [30]. Important limitations of this study include sleep assessments were only performed in the subset of patients not intubated and was based on retrospective chart review. Sedation and analgesic practices were not reported, and it is unclear if this could have impacted study results.

Lastly a randomized, double-blind trial evaluated ramelteon versus placebo in patients undergoing elective pulmonary thromboendarterectomy. No sleep outcomes were evaluated, but ramelteon did not reduce delirium incidence (relative risk, 0.8; 95% CI, 0.5–1.4; p = 0.516) or duration of delirium (placebo median 2 days vs. ramelteon 3 days; p = 0.181) [31].

In summary, there is currently a lack of evidence to support the routine use of ramelteon to improve sleep in critically ill adults. While the results from the study by Nishikimi et al. suggest that ramelteon may have a potential role as a sleep aid, larger and more rigorous studies are needed to confirm these findings.

4   Gabaminergic Agents

4.1   Sleep-Related Pharmacology

Many critically ill mechanically ventilated patients require sedation and analgesia. Gabaminergic agents, including propofol and benzodiazepines, are two frequently used sedatives that have also been studied for sleep. As described in chapter "Effects of Common ICU Medications on Sleep", both propofol and benzodiazepines potentiate the inhibitory neurotransmitter γ-Aminobutyric acid (GABA) (which has been shown to increase NREM, but not REM sleep) (Table 1) [32, 33]. Despite having similar mechanism of actions, the pharmacokinetic and pharmacodynamic characteristics of propofol and benzodiazepines differ substantially (e.g., onset, duration of action, metabolism, elimination, etc).

4.2   Comparative Trials Evaluating a Sleep Outcome

To study the effects of midazolam and propofol on sleep in the ICU, Treggiari-Venzi and colleagues randomized 40 non-intubated ICU patients following trauma, elective orthopedic, thoracic, or abdominal surgery to midazolam or propofol for 5 nights from 22:00 to 06:00 [34]. At noon each day patients completed the Hospital

Anxiety and Depression Scale (HAD), which also measures quality of sleep, the degree of restlessness, dreams or nightmares and memories about the nighttime [34]. The study found no differences in quality of sleep between the two groups (Table 4). Limitations of this study include a small sample size, being restricted to trauma/surgical patients, and lack of placebo control group.

The effectiveness of propofol on sleep was further studied by McLeod and colleagues. Twenty-nine ICU patients expected to require sedation for >50 h were randomized to light sedation (Ramsay score 2–3) with propofol and morphine on a 24-h basis or light sedation during the day and deeper sedation with propofol and morphine at night (Ramsay score 4–5 from 22:00–06:00). The presence or absence of diurnal sedation was assessed by blinded investigators via visual assessment of sedation scores and propofol infusion rates plotted against time on graphs [35]. Nine out of 15 patients in the additional night sedation group had diurnal sedation compared to three out of 14 patients in the constant light sedation group (Table 4) [35]. It is important to note that sedation scales do not measure sleep in critically ill patients. This small study provides insights that propofol can be titrated to different depths of sedation; but, given the complexity of measuring sleep in the ICU, it does not provide evidence that deeper sedation leads to improved sleep.

Kondili and colleagues conducted a randomized crossover physiological study and objectively measured sleep with PSG in 13 critically ill mechanically ventilated adults not receiving sedation or analgesia [36]. Patients received propofol from 22:00 to 07:00 targeting a Ramsay score of 3 (patient responds to commands only) for one night. The study was protocolized and patients' sleep efficiency, sleep fragmentation, and sleep stage were compared to a night in which they did not receive propofol. There were no statistically significant differences between sleep outcomes on the nights patients received propofol compared to the nights they did not receive propofol, except for a reduction REM sleep associated with propofol administration (Table 4) [36]. The strengths of this study include PSG monitoring in patients not receiving sedation and analgesia. The results of this small study showed propofol did not improve sleep in critically ill patients; however only 13 patients were included.

Lastly, a study by Engelmann et al. compared propofol versus flunitrazepam for inducing and maintaining sleep in critically ill adults [37]. This randomized, double-blind trial included 66 ICU patients without mechanical ventilation or sedation admitted to ICU after surgical intervention. Patients were randomized to flunitrazepam (0.015 mg/kg bolus over 2 min) or propofol (2 mg/kg/h over 7 h) starting at 23:00. Sleep was assessed by an amended version of Pittsburgh sleep diary (PghSD) and BIS [37]. The results of the PghSD found statistically significant differences favoring propofol in regards to the median frequency of awakening (6 vs 3, P < 0.001), median duration of awakenings (0 vs. 15 min, p < 0.001), and sleep quality (2 vs 3, P < 0.001) (Table 4). There were no statistically significant differences for sleep duration based on the PghSD. Additionally, median BIS was significantly lower in propofol (vs flunitrazepam) group (74.05 vs. 78.7, P = 0.016). Strengths of this study include use of a standardized protocol to decrease interventions and sounds at night and attempts by the investigators to eliminate the

Table 4 Summary of trials of gabaminergic agonists for improving sleep

Gabinergic Agents

Study	Patient population	N	Study drug & dosing	Results			
				Outcome	Intervention group	Control group	P value
Treggiari-Venzi 1996 [34]	Non-intubated ICU patients with LOS ≥ 5 days	40	• Midazolam (bolus 0.01–0.07 mg/kg & continuous infusion 0.03–0.2 mg/kg/h from 22:00–0600 • Propofol bolus 0.2–0.3 mg/kg & continuous infusion of 0.3–3 mg/kg/h from 22:00–06:00		Midazolam	Propofol	
				Quality of sleep day 1—HAD score (mean ± SD)	6.3 + 3.4	6.5 ± 3.3	NS
				Quality of sleep day 3—HAD score (mean ± SD)	6.3 ± 3.2	6.6 ± 2.9	NS
				Quality of sleep day 5—HAD score (mean ± SD)	7.2 ± 2.9	7.2 ± 2.3	NS
McLeod 1997 [35]	ICU patients expected to require sedation >50 h	29	• Constant light sedation (morphine and propofol) for Ramsay score of 2–3 • Constant light sedation (morphine and propofol) between 0600 h and 2200 h and additional night sedation between 2200 h and 0600 h for goal Ramsay score of 4–5		Constant light sedation	Increased night sedation	
				Sedation rhythmicity (cosinor analysis) (r%)	8 (0–56)	27 (6–35)	p < 0.01
				Diurnal sedation (n (%))	3 (21.4)	9 (60)	

					With Propofol	Without Propofol	
Kondili 2012 [36]	ICU patients mechanically ventilated and not receiving sedation or analgesia	13	• Propofol 22:00 to 07:00: Bolus of 0.01–0.05 mg/kg followed by continuous infusion to goal Ramsay 3 • No propofol	TST (min)	260 (113, 417)	214 (40, 285)	0.37
				SEI (%)	76.3 (28.4, 96.9)	62.6 (13.1, 85.9)	0.37
				Stage 1 (% TST)	20.8 (5.6, 80.6)	30.7 (4.6, 66.7)	1.00
				Stage 2 (% TST)	48.9 (4.8, 84.0)	46.1 (3.0, 80.4)	0.66
				SWS (% TST)	0 (0, 5.8)	0 (0, 0)	0.75
				REM (% TST)	0 (0, 0)	1.4 (0, 13.0)	0.04
				TSFI (events/hour)	4.8 (1.3, 14.6)	8.1 (2.9, 16.2)	0.33
				Stage shifts (n)	22 (11, 28)	21 (7, 48)	0.69
				Intersleep awake (% TST)	6.8 (1.2, 43.5)	11.4 (3.1, 42.9)	0.79
					Propofol	Flunitrazepam	
Engelman 2014 [37]	Patients with surgical intervention admitted to anesthesiological ICU without mechanical ventilation or sedation	66	• Propofol 2 mg/kg/hr. for 7 h starting at 23:00 • Flunitrazepam 0.015 mg/kg at bolus dose at 23:00	Awakenings per sleep diary (n) [a]	0	3	<0.001
				Duration of awakenings per sleep diary (mins)[a]	0	15	<0.001
				Total sleep time per sleep diary (h)[a]	6	5	0.623
				Sleep quality per sleep diary[a]	2	3	<0.001
				Quality of falling asleep[a]	2	2	0.341
				BIS	74.05	78.7	0.016

h hour, *ICU* Intensive care unit, *NS* Not significant, *REM* Rapid Eye Movement, *LOS* Length of stay, *HAD* Hospital Anxiety and Depression Scale, *SWS* Slow wave sleep, *TST* Total sleep time, *TSFI* Total sleep fragmentation index, *PghSD* Pittsburgh Sleep Diary, *BIS* Bispectral index

All results reported as median (Interquartile range (IQR)) unless specified

[a]Amended version of the PghSD

Sleep efficiency index: Patient's total sleep time over the time available for sleep (ratio or %)

Total sleep fragmentation index: Sum of arousals and awakenings per hour of sleep confounding effects of other sedatives and analgesics. Limitations of this study include the different pharmacokinetics of the two agents, and lack of a placebo group.

In conclusion, there is no strong evidence to support the use of gabaminergic agents as sleep aids in critically ill adults. The 2018 SCCM guidelines recommend against the use of propofol to improve sleep in the ICU [26]. Also, gabaminergic agents are respiratory depressants and may not be safe in patients without a secured airway, thus limiting their applicability to many ICU adults.

5 Additional Agents: Antipsychotics, Antidepressants, and Non-benzodiazepine Hypnotics

Numerous other agents including antipsychotics, antidepressants, and non-benzodiazepine hypnotics are also often prescribed as sleep drugs in the ICU. A recent study found that approximately 10% of critically ill patients are prescribed a new nocturnal neuroactive agent(s) during their ICU stay [38]. Of these agents, antipsychotics accounted for 36.7% and antidepressants for 8.6% [38]. Despite these agents being prescribed for sleep, literature supporting their efficacy in the ICU does not exist.

Chapter "Effects of Common ICU Medications on Sleep (Table 1)" highlights the impact of antidepressants and antipsychotics and their effect on sleep. Many antidepressants decrease REM sleep and are not routinely recommended as a sleep agent unless underlying depression is thought to contribute to altered sleep [39]. In spite of these shortcomings, potentially promising sleep alterations have been shown for mirtazapine and trazodone (chapter "Effects of Common ICU Medications on Sleep"—Table 1). Unfortunately, there is a lack of clinical trials evaluating these agents in critically ill adults. A systematic review and meta-analysis evaluated trazodone compared to placebo in a largely outpatient setting, and found trazodone improved perceived sleep quality (mean difference − 0.41, 95% CI -0.82 to −0.00, P < 0.05) and decreased night time awakenings (mean difference − 0.51, 95% CI -0.97 to −0.05, P = 0.03), but there were no differences in sleep efficiency (mean difference 0.09, 95% CI -0.19 to 0.38, P > 0.05) [40]. There is a paucity of literature evaluating mirtazapine as a sleep agent; however two small studies in healthy adults found mirtazapine improved sleep and decreased sleep awakenings [41, 42]. However, mirtazapine also led to increased daytime drowsiness and slower reaction time [41]. In patients previously on mirtazapine and trazodone as outpatients, these agents can be continued or reinitiated in the ICU; however in the absence of literature new initiation of these agents is not recommended.

Chapter "Effects of Common ICU Medications on Sleep—Table 1" also highlights the effects of antipsychotics on sleep. A survey from 2013 found quetiapine to be the most prescribed antipsychotic for sleep and sedation [43]. A small study (n = 13) compared quetiapine versus placebo in outpatients and found no improvement in sleep outcomes [44]. However, a study in healthy individuals found that quetiapine improved total sleep time and decreased nighttime awakenings, but led to increased daytime fatigue [41]. Due to the lack of evidence for benefit and the potential for adverse reactions seen in healthy patients and outpatients, quetiapine is not routinely recommended as a sleep agent in critically ill adults. If patients require atypical antipsychotics for other indications, quetiapine may improve the underlying cause for lack of sleep and could be utilized.

As previously mentioned, there is also a lack of evidence to support the use of non-benzodiazepine hypnotics for sleep in critically ill patients. A systematic review of treatment of insomnia in the community setting found statistically significant, but minimal clinical improvement in sleep with non-benzodiazepine hypnotics compared to placebo (decreased PSG sleep latency by 22 min) [39]. Due to the minimal clinical improvement and lack of data in critically ill adults, non-benzodiazepine hypnotics are not routinely recommended for use in the ICU.

Newer sleep agents include the orexin receptor antagonists (Suvorexant and Lemborexant). These agents work by promoting sleep inhibiting orexin A and B, neuropeptides that promote wakefulness [45, 46]. A number of studies have evaluated suvorexant in the treatment of ICU delirium and sleep [45, 47, 48]. Suvorexant did not improve sleep parameters in one study [49], but delirium outcomes were improved [45, 47, 48]. Suvorexant may be a promising new agent to improve delirium in critically ill patients, and transiently improve their sleep; however adequately powered RCTs are needed. An ongoing RCT is comparing placebo vs suvorexant in critically ill post coronary artery bypass graft surgery adults. The primary outcome is evaluating nighttime wakefulness after persistent sleep onset as determined by electroencephalogram (EEG) between placebo and suvorexant [50].

6 Continuation of Sleep Agents from Home

Many patients who are regularly take a sleep agent at home will be admitted to the ICU. A survey from 2005–2010 found that 4% of adults over the age of 20 had taken a prescription sleep aid in the previous month [51]. Therefore the question often arises whether to continue their home sleep agents or hold the medication during the ICU stay. In the absence of data for guidance, patient specific factors including need for sedation, neurologic exam, risk for medication withdrawal, and patient interaction should be considered when deciding whether to continue a home sleep aid in the ICU.

7   Recommendations for Best Practices

There is much to learn regarding sleep disturbances, sleep monitoring, and pharmacological sleep management in critically ill adults. Many pharmacologic options to treat sleep in the ICU seem biologically plausible; however, literature is lacking to support the routine use of any agent. Therapeutic and non-pharmacologic interventions should be directed at the cause of sleep disturbances (eg pain, delirium, noise), and more research is needed to determine which pharmacological agents actually improve sleep in the ICU [26]. Figure 2 shows recommendations for utilization of sleep agents in critically ill adults.

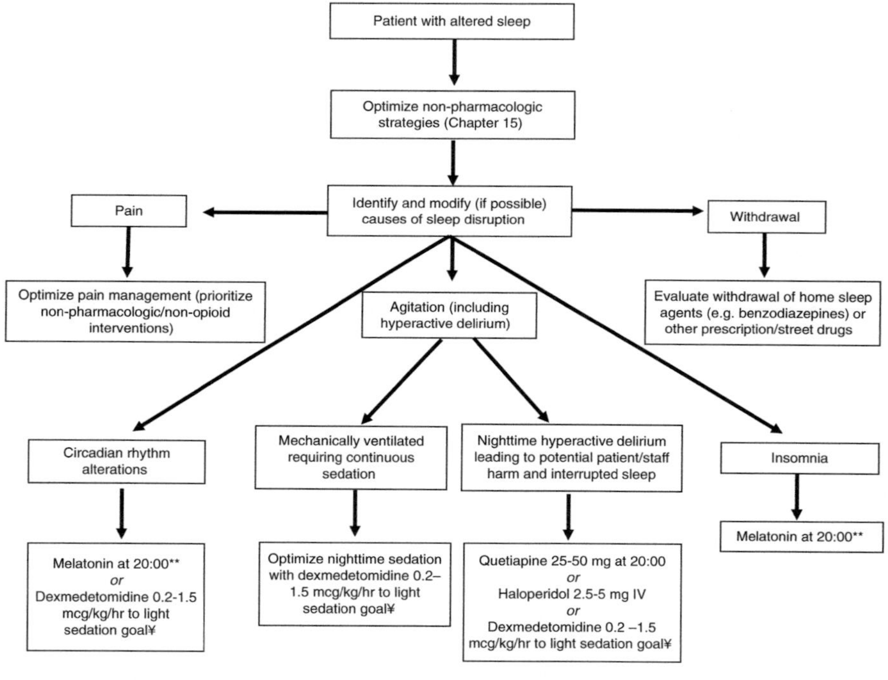

Fig. 2 Pharmacologic treatment algorithm for sleep in critically ill adults*

8 Future Areas of Research

Sleep in critically ill patients is complex. To study the efficacy of pharmacological agents for sleep in the ICU we must first determine the optimal way to measure sleep. The studies outlined in this chapter highlight the heterogeneity in efficacy outcomes for sleep agents. PSG is an objective measure of sleep, and the ideal tool to acquire the primary endpoint of future studies. The application of PSG in the ICU is not simple, but several pilot studies have demonstrated that it is feasible for research purposes. Patient reported sleep quality may be a desirable endpoint, but many critically ill patients may be unable to communicate such information reliably or at all. As previously mentioned, there are also many confounders to be considered when studying sleep in the ICU, most notably encephalopathy, sedation and analgesia. Future studies should include a rigorous protocol to optimize non-pharmacological measures, include a non-pharmacological arm (ideally with administration of placebo), and use a double-blind design. Newer sleep-promoting agents, such as lemborexant and suvorexant, should be tested more in the ICU setting. Once we learn how best to measure sleep in the ICU and what metrics impact outcomes, we can begin to have a better understanding of the role pharmacological agents play in promoting sleep in critically ill adults.

9 Conclusion

There is currently a lack of high-quality evidence for the recommendation of sleep agents in critically ill adults. Optimization of non-pharmacologic strategies is paramount, and addition of pharmacologic strategies should be patient specific and weigh the risk versus benefit. Future studies are needed to identify pharmacologic treatment strategies as sleep agents in critically ill adults.

References

1. Freedman NS, Kotzer N, Schwab RJ. Patient perception of sleep quality and etiology of sleep disruption in the intensive care unit. Am J Respir Crit Care Med. 1999;159(4 I):1155–62.
2. Simini B. Patients' perceptions of intensive care. Lancet. 1999;354(9178):571–2.
3. Weerink MAS, Struys MMRF, Hannivoort LN, Barends CRM, Absalom AR, Colin P. Clinical pharmacokinetics and pharmacodynamics of Dexmedetomidine. Clin Pharmacokinet. 2017;56(8):893–913.
4. Nacif-Coelho C, Correa-Sales C, Chang LL, Maze M. Perturbation of Ion Channel conductance alters the hypnotic response to the $\alpha2$-adrenergic agonist Dexmedetomidine in the locus Coeruleus of the rat. Anesthesiology. 1994;81:1527–34.
5. Correa-Sales C, Rabin BC, Maze M. A hypnotic response to dexmedetomidine, an $\alpha2$ agonist is mediated in the locus coeruleus in rats. Anesthesiology. 1992;76:948–52.

6. Nelson LE, Lu J, Guo T, Saper CB, Franks NP, Maze M. The α2-adrenoceptor agonist dexmedetomidine converges on an endogenous sleep-promoting pathway to exert its sedative effects. Anesthesiology. 2003;98(2):428–36.

7. Akeju O, Hobbs LE, Gao L, et al. Dexmedetomidine promotes biomimetic non-rapid eye movement stage 3 sleep in humans: a pilot study. Clin Neurophysiol. 2018;129(1):69–78.

8. Akeju O, Kim SE, Vazquez R, et al. Spatiotemporal dynamics of dexmedetomidine-induced electroencephalogram oscillations. PLoS One. 2016;11(10):1–18.

9. Huupponen E, Maksimow A, Lapinlampi P, et al. Electroencephalogram spindle activity during dexmedetomidine sedation and physiological sleep. Acta Anaesthesiol Scand. 2008;52(2):289–94.

10. Schurr JW, Ambrosi L, Lastra JL, McLaughlin KC, Hacobian G, Szumita PM. Fever associated with Dexmedetomidine in adult acute care patients: a systematic review of the literature. J Clin Pharmacol. 2021;61(7):848–56.

11. Grayson KE, Bailey M, Balachandran M, et al. The effect of early sedation with Dexmedetomidine on body temperature in critically ill patients. Crit Care Med. 2021;49(7):1118–28.

12. Oto J, Yamamoto K, Koike S, Onodera M, Imanaka H, Nishimura M. Sleep quality of mechanically ventilated patients sedated with dexmedetomidine. Intensive Care Med. 2012;38(12):1982–9.

13. Alexopoulou C, Kondili E, Diamantaki E, et al. Effects of dexmedetomidine on sleep quality in critically ill patients: a pilot study. Anesthesiology. 2014;121(4):801–7.

14. Wu XH, Cui F, Zhang C, et al. Low-dose Dexmedetomidine improves sleep quality pattern in elderly patients after noncardiac surgery in the intensive care unit: a pilot randomized controlled trial. Anesthesiology. 2016;125(5):979–91.

15. Skrobik Y, Duprey MS, Hill NS, Devlin JW. Low-dose nocturnal dexmedetomidine prevents ICU delirium a randomized, placebo-controlled trial. Am J Respir Crit Care Med. 2018;197(9):1147–56.

16. Tordjman S, Chokron S, Delorme R, et al. Melatonin: pharmacology, functions, and therapeutic benefits. Curr Neuropharmacol. 2017;15:434–43.

17. Dubocovich ML, Markowska M. Functional MT1 and MT2 melatonin receptors in mammals. Endocrine. 2005;27(2):101–10.

18. Liu J, Clough S, Hutchinson A, Adamah-Biassi E, Popovska-Gorevski M, Dubocovich M. MT1 and MT2 melatonin receptors: a therapeutic perspective. Annu Rev Pharmcol Toxicol. 2016;56:361–83.

19. Williams WPT, McLin DE, Dressman MA, Neubauer DN. Comparative review of approved melatonin agonists for the treatment of circadian rhythm sleep-wake disorders. Pharmacotherapy. 2016;36(9):1028–41.

20. Gobbi G, Comai S. Differential function of melatonin MT1 and MT2 receptors in REM and NREM sleep. Front Endocrinol (Lausanne). 2019;10(87):1–12.

21. Shilo L, Daga Y, Smorjik Y, et al. Effect of melatonin on sleep quality of COPD intensive care patients: a pilot study. Chronobiol Int. 2000;17(1):71–6.

22. Ibrahim MG, Bellomo R, Hart GK, et al. A double-blind placebo-controlled randomised pilot study of nocturnal melatonin in tracheostomised patients. Crit Care Resusc. 2006;8(3):187–91.

23. Louzon PR, Heavner MS, Herod K, Wu TT, Devlin JW. Sleep-promotion bundle development, implementation, and evaluation in critically ill adults: roles for pharmacists. Ann Pharmacother. 2022;56(7):839–49.

24. Bourne RS, Mills GH, Minelli C. Melatonin therapy to improve nocturnal sleep in critically ill patients: encouraging results from a small randomised controlled trial. Crit Care. 2008;12(2):1–9.

25. Gandolfi JV, Di Bernardo APA, Chanes DAV, et al. The effects of melatonin supplementation on sleep quality and assessment of the serum melatonin in ICU patients: a randomized controlled trial. Crit Care Med. 2020;48(12):e1286–93.

26. Devlin JW, Skrobik Y, Gélinas C, et al. Clinical practice guidelines for the prevention and Management of Pain, agitation/sedation, delirium, immobility, and sleep disruption in adult patients in the ICU. Crit Care Med. 2018;46(9):e825–73.
27. Harpsoe N, Andersen L, Gogenur I, Rosenberg J. Clinical pharmacokinetics of melatonin: a systematic review. Eur J Clin Pharmacol. 2015;71:901–9.
28. Kato K, Hirai K, Nishiyama K, et al. Neurochemical properties of ramelteon (TAK-375), a selective MT 1/MT2 receptor agonist. Neuropharmacology. 2005;48(2):301–10.
29. Hatta K, Kishi Y, Wada K, et al. Preventive effects of ramelteon on delirium: a randomized placebo-controlled trial. JAMA Psychiat. 2014;71(4):397–403.
30. Nishikimi M, Numaguchi A, Takahashi K, et al. Effect of administration of ramelteon, a melatonin receptor agonist, on the duration of stay in the ICU: a single-center randomized placebo-controlled trial. Crit Care Med. 2018;46(7):1099–105.
31. Jaiswal SJ, Vyas AD, Heisel AJ, et al. Ramelteon for prevention of postoperative delirium: a randomized controlled trial in patients undergoing elective pulmonary Thromboendarterectomy*. Crit Care Med. 2019;47(12):1751–8.
32. Sahinovic MM, Struys MMRF, Absalom AR. Clinical pharmacokinetics and pharmacodynamics of Propofol. Clin Pharmacokinet. 2018;57(12):1539–58.
33. Lancel M. Role of GABA(a) receptors in the regulation of sleep: initial sleep responses to peripherally administered modulators and agonists. Sleep. 1999;22(1):33–42.
34. Treggiari-Venzi M, Borgeat A, Fuchs-Buder T, et al. Overnight sedation with midazolam or propofol in the ICU: effects on sleep quality, anxiety and depression. Intensive Care Med. 1996;22:1186–90.
35. McLeod G, Wallis C, Dick J, Cox C, Patterson A, Colvin J. Use of 2% propofol to produce diurnal sedation in critically ill patients. Intensive Care Med. 1997;23(4):428–34.
36. Kondili E, Alexopoulou C, Xirouchaki N, Georgopoulos D. Effects of propofol on sleep quality in mechanically ventilated critically ill patients: a physiological study. Intensive Care Med. 2012;38(10):1640–6.
37. Engelmann C, Wallenborn J, Olthoff D, Kaisers UX, Rüffert H. Propofol versus flunitrazepam for inducing and maintaining sleep in postoperative ICU patients. Indian J Crit Care Med. 2014;18(4):212–9.
38. Hamidi A, Roberts RJ, Weinhouse GL, et al. Characterization of nocturnal neuroactive medication use and related sleep documentation in critically ill adults. Crit Care Explor. 2021;3(3):e0367.
39. Huedo-Medina TB, Kirsch I, Middlemass J, Klonizakis M, Siriwardena AN. Effectiveness of non-benzodiazepine hypnotics in treatment of adult insomnia: meta-analysis of data submitted to the Food and Drug Administration. BMJ. 2013;346(7889):1–13.
40. Yi X-Y, Ni S-F, Ghadami MR, et al. Trazodone for the treatment of insomnia: a meta-analysis of randomized placebo-controlled trials. Sleep Med. 2018;45:25–32.
41. Karsten J, Hagenauw LA, Kamphuis J, Lancel M. Low doses of mirtazapine or quetiapine for transient insomnia: a randomised, double-blind, cross-over, placebo-controlled trial. J Psychopharmacol. 2017;31(3):327–37.
42. Aslan S, Isik E, Cosar B. The effects of mirtazapine on sleep: a placebo controlled, double-blind study in young healthy volunteers. Sleep. 2002;25(6):677–9.
43. Hermes EDA, Sernyak M, Rosenheck R. Use of second-generation antipsychotic agents for sleep and sedation: a provider survey. Sleep. 2013;36(4):597–600.
44. Thompson W, Quay TAW, Rojas-Fernandez C, Farrell B, Bjerre LM. Atypical antipsychotics for insomnia: a systematic review. Sleep Med. 2016;22:13–7.
45. Hatta K, Kishi Y, Wada K, et al. Preventive effects of Suvorexant on delirium. J Clin Psychiatry. 2017;78(8):e970–9.
46. Janto K, Prichard RJ, Pusalavidyasagar S. An Update on Dual Orexin Receptor Antagonists and Their Potential Role in Insomnia Therapeutics. Journal of Clinical Sleep Medicine. 2018:14(08);1399–1408.

47. Masuyama T, Sanui M, Yoshida N, et al. Suvorexant is associated with a low incidence of delirium in critically ill patients: a retrospective cohort study. Psychogeriatrics. 2018;18(3):209–15.
48. Izuhara M, Izuhara HK, Tsuchie K, et al. Real-world preventive effects of Suvorexant in intensive care delirium: a retrospective cohort study. J Clin Psychiatry. 2020;81(6)
49. Bennett T, Bray D, Neville MW. Suvorexant, a dual orexin receptor antagonist for the management of insomnia. P T. 2014;39(4):264–6.
50. Eikermann M. Suvorexant and Sleep/Delirium in ICU Patients [Internet]. Clinicaltirals.gov. 2020 [cited 2021 Nov 19];Available from: https://clinicaltrials.gov/ct2/show/NCT04092894?term=suvorexant&cond=sleep+intensive+care&draw=2&rank=1
51. Chong Y, Fryer CD, Gu Q. Prescription sleep aid use among adults: United States, 2005-2010. NCHS Data Brief. 2013;127:1–8.
52. Barr J, Fraser GL, Puntillo K, et al. Clinical practice guidelines for the management of pain, agitation, and delirium in adult patients in the intensive care unit. Crit Care Med. 2013;41(1):263–306.

Sleep Considerations in Critically Ill Children

Mallory A. Perry and Sapna R. Kudchadkar

1 Introduction

Critical illness can severely disrupt and impact sleep in infants, children, and adolescents during an important phase of human neurodevelopment. In addition to critical illness itself, the pediatric intensive care unit (PICU) is a unique environment that further contributes to sleep architecture dysregulation [1–3]. The PICU specializes in the management of critically ill children with both acute and chronic illnesses. The heterogeneity of the PICU patient population is profound in several ways; in fact the PICU is the hospital unit with the greatest diversity of patients and diagnoses. Aside from diagnoses, heterogeneity in chronological and developmental age, length of stay, baseline functional status, and genetic and familial influence make the PICU population unique [4]. The sleep needs of children constantly change, thus a comprehensive understanding of the neurodevelopmental needs of children across the age spectrum is vital to understanding the impact of critical illness and PICU admission on sleep in this setting and the potential long-term implications of disrupted sleep in this population.

In this chapter, we provide a comprehensive overview of pediatric sleep development and the PICU-specific factors which may negatively impact sleep. The specific chapter objectives are to provide an in-depth overview of: (1) the neurobiological considerations of sleep in the developing child; (2) the appropriate tools for

M. A. Perry
Children's Hospital of Philadelphia Research Institute, Philadelphia, PA, USA
e-mail: perrym2@chop.edu

S. R. Kudchadkar (✉)
Departments of Anesthesiology & Critical Care Medicine, Pediatrics, and Physical Medicine and Rehabilitation, Johns Hopkins University School of Medicine, Baltimore, MD, USA
e-mail: sapna@jhmi.edu

G. L. Weinhouse, J. W. Devlin (eds.), *Sleep in Critical Illness*,
https://doi.org/10.1007/978-3-031-06447-0_16

assessing sleep in critically ill children; (3) PICU and patient -specific risk factors for poor sleep; and (4) potential strategies to mitigate risk factors for poor sleep in an effort to promote sleep restoration,

2 Neurobiological Considerations

To understand and evaluate sleep in children, it is imperative to have an understanding of the underlying neurobiological and neurodevelopmental mechanisms of sleep from infancy through adolescence. Throughout this crucial period of development, sleep evolves with neurologic maturation [5]. Children's sleep-wake patterns develop and change as they age. Initially, they are reliant on their mother in utero and deeply influenced by environmental factors. Sleep is integral to homeostasis and normal sleep-wake patterns are essential to critical illness healing given its effect on thermoregulation, inflammation, and immunity [6]. The following sections provide an overview of circadian rhythm as it applies to children from newborn to adolescence, including recommendations for those sleep requirements known to promote and optimize health at various ages and developmental stages.

2.1 Circadian Rhythms

Our circadian rhythm (CR) is the endogenously- driven, yet externally influenced intrinsic rhythm which cycles over an estimated 24-h period [7]. As outlined in chapter "Characteristics of Sleep in Critically Ill Patients. Part II: Circadian Rhythm Disruption", it is influenced by a complex interplay of hormones, intrinsic circuitry, temperature and established routines [1, 7]. Of note, the neuroplasticity of children throughout their lifespan is a hallmark of pediatric sleep research. In the pediatric critical care setting, neuroplasticity has important implications on CR and how both clinicians and researchers assess and manage sleep. In order to fully understand the impact of critical illness on CR and sleep in children, one must consider all developmental stages and normal sleep patterns.

A newborn infant's CR is developed in utero, and through hypothalamic regulation in the suprachiasmatic nuclei (SCN), modulates sleep patterns and acts as the central "clock". The SCN is the master CR pacemaker, regulating melatonin production through direct input from the eyes, including light [7–9]. Newborns are born with an immature circadian system; their sleep-wake rhythm is weak and inherited from the mother's sleep-wake patterns during pregnancy [10]. Early postnatal sleep development is affected not only by the mother's sleep-wake pattern but also though light exposure during early development [9, 10]. Postnatally, light is detected in the retina and transmitted along the retinohypothalamic tract to the SCN [11]. While neonates are born with the overall components of circadian rhythm, it remains immature and develops over time.

There is also a neuroendocrine basis for CR regulation. The endogenous bio-markers melatonin, cortisol, body temperature, movement, blood pressure, digestion, and consolidated sleep are all a part of the CR [12]. Within the first 2-months of postnatal development, CR begins to change and develop. Cortisol and melatonin production and increased sleep efficiency begin at approximately 8 weeks of age, followed by body temperature rhythm and circadian gene development by 11 weeks [11, 12]. Overall, CR becomes more consistent at 3 to 6 months of age. The early development of CR highlights the important role of attention to environmental stimuli (e.g., light and sound) and how they impact a child's overall health. Specifically, cycled day-night lighting throughout early development, especially in the setting of critical illness, is imperative to promote healing [13]. It is important to note, however, that low light exposure in infancy may be just as deleterious to long-term health as high light exposure. Animal studies have shown that low light during infancy may lead to long-lasting psychological behaviors including anxiety and avoidance behaviors, which are carried into adulthood. The mice in this study also experienced stunted growth, which did eventually normalize in adolescence [14]. This aligns with a large, international study of infants exposed to low light exposure throughout the newborn period, leading to the potential onset of bipolar disorder [15]. In addition, prolonged light exposure in mice postnatally demonstrated long-term effects on peripheral circadian clock genes, affecting heart, lung, and splenic function in adulthood. Such changes have been linked to effects on blood pressure, inflammation, and dysregulated immune responses in animal studies [16].

Important CR-related mechanisms effect sleep during adolescence and young adulthood. Sleep deprivation during adolescence is epidemic; half of American adolescents receive inadequate sleep. Hormonal changes during adolescence may alter CR [17]. Timing of sleep development in adolescence is affected by external factors such as school and/or work, in addition to intrinsic biological factors including sex [17]. While the effect of gonadal sex hormones on sleep throughout adolescence is believed to be important, a definitive association between sex hormones and sleep has not yet been established. Research demonstrates adolescent biological females have a delay in the timing of sleep a year earlier than males, which is in line with females' earlier and younger pubertal onset. Similarly, there is an observed correlation between sleep and secondary sex development between adolescent females and males [18–20]. This earlier sleep pattern in females is observed across both cultures and different mammalian species [17]. Understanding sex-dependent and hormonal changes is vital to understanding the overall development of sleep patterns and CR in children and adolescents.

2.2 Sleep Recommendations

American Academy of Pediatrics (AAP) guidelines provide recommendations for the number of hours required in children to promote optimal health [21]. Table 1 outlines the number of recommended hours of sleep at each chronological age to

Table 1 Recommended hours of sleep per age of child

Age	Recommended hours of sleep (per 24 hours)[a]
Infants: 4–12 months	12–16
Toddler: 1–2 years	11–14
Preschool: 3–5 years	10–13
School age: 6–12 years	9–12
Adolescent: 13–18 years	8–10

[a]includes naps throughout the day

best support neurodevelopment and promote healing. Of note, the AAP does not include recommendations for newborns less than 4 months of age, due to the wide variability in their sleep patterns (i.e. frequent feedings) and duration and the limited evidence demonstrating an association between sleep and health outcomes at this age. However, the National Science Foundation recommends children less than 4 months old should sleep between 14–17 h per day [22].

Appropriate sleep has been shown to positively improve attention, behavior, learning/memory, emotional regulation, quality of life and mental and physical health [21]. Despite the importance of sleep for optimal critical care recovery, sleep is often disturbed in the PICU setting: frequent awakenings are common and sleep duration is reduced. Disrupted sleep occurs most often during high-stress periods when lifesaving interventions are being delivered and painful procedures are required.

3 Sleep Assessment

Similar to critically ill adults (please refer to chapter "Methods for Routine Sleep Assessment and Monitoring"), the evaluation and study of sleep patterns in the PICU setting is important. However, multiple PICU-specific factors affect the ability to rigorously evaluate sleep in this setting including the heterogeneity of patient age, developmental level, and disease processes present. The following sections propose both quantitative and qualitative sleep measures for sleep researchers and ICU clinicians interested in investigating the sleep patterns of critically ill children, disruption in sleep-wake cycles in the PICU, and their impact on health.

3.1 Quantitive Sleep Assessment

3.1.1 Electroencephalographic (EEG) Monitoring

Polysomnography, the gold standard for sleep assessment which includes EEG, electrooculogram (EOG) and electromyography (EMG) is infrequently utilized in PICUs due to challenges they bring in patients requiring other invasive devices and the easy displacement of leads. However, EEG monitoring is widely used in the PICU to evaluate brain function and recognize seizure occurrence. Pediatric studies demonstrate EEG sleep slow-wave activity is associated with high levels of synaptic density – a vital component of neurologic maturation [23–25]. While EEG sleep monitoring in the PICU is feasible across age groups, and may provide insight into sleep-wake patterns, EEG patterns may be confounded by critical illness, delirium, and the use of sedative medications and neuromuscular blockade. These variables can render EEG difficult to interpret [6, 26]. When evaluating sleep in the PICU with EEG it is recommended that monitoring occur for at least 24-h so that all sleep episodes, including naps are captured and sleep-wake patterns are temporally characterized [27]. When Kudchadkar et al. [27]. compared sleep with EEG between critically ill and healthy children, the critically ill children failed to exhibit day-night sleep organization and exhibited decreased slow-wave sleep activity-an essential component of neurodevelopment and homeostasis. The critically ill children also had reduced rapid eye movement (REM) sleep despite REM sleep over the lifespan being at its highest during infancy and early childhood [28].

Methods for assessing sleep via EEG are often impractical in critically ill patients given normal sleep is hard to differentiate from disorganized sleep in the sedated state [29]. Studies of EEG use in the PICU have concluded children receiving continuous opioid and benzodiazepine infusions experience severe disruptions from their baseline normal sleep including decreased variability in slow-wave activity [27]. In recent years, goal-driven sedation protocols have been emphasized in PICUs to reduce over-sedation, promote sleep architecture and decrease delirium [30, 31]. (see also chapters "Effects of Common ICU Medications on Sleep" and "Best Practices for Improving Sleep in the ICU. Part I: Non-pharmacologic").

3.1.2 Actigraphy

Actigraphy, that monitors changes in motion as a surrogate for sleep, is an easily accessible quantitative measure that can be rapidly deployed in the PICU. Actigraphy is quick and simple to apply/remove and in contrast to EEG does not require specialized equipment and technicians. Actigraphs can also assess sleep longitudinally over several days without interfering with daily ICU care. Actigraphy should be placed on either an unrestricted, preferably non-dominant, hand and/or ankle based on the child's age and the bedside team's clinical judgment. While polysomnography is the gold standard for sleep research, actigraphy may be more useful clinically in the PICU setting. Though actigraphy is convenient for obtaining sleep data in the PICU, it is limited by a lack of standardization. Non-standardized devices, inconsistent reporting, and lack of reference standards for analysis make it difficult to compare results between clinical studies. Actigraphy may overestimate sleep quality in critically ill children due to factors including worsening critical illness, immobility/bedrest, and the use of sedation and/or neuromuscular blockade.

In otherwise healthy children, activity is consolidated to the waking (daytime) hours, therefore the rest-activity cycle often serves as a proxy to assess sleep-wake cycles in children. The Daytime Activity Ratio Estimate (DARE) acknowledges this principle by utilizing minute level data in critically ill children to calculate the ratio between mean daytime (08:00–20:00) activity and the mean 24-h (00:00–24:00) activity [6]. DARE is easily obtainable and reproducible, allowing results from various studies to be compared and explored. Compared to traditional actigraphy algorithms, it also does not overestimate wake-sleep times. A study by Kudchadkar et al. [6]. examined the applicability of actigraphy and DARE analysis in the PICU. Only about half (56%) of activity occurred during predefined daytime hours (08:00–20:00) confirming a lack of consolidation of the rest-activity cycle. These findings are also consistent with those from the adult literature, where rest-activity consolidation only occurred in 46.6% of all hospital days [6, 32]. In the DARE-analyzed patients, there was also a trend towards sleep improvement after ICU discharge [6, 32].

3.1.3 Melatonin

Alterations of melatonin production may negatively impact sleep in critically ill children [33]. Melatonin primarily works to regulate CR that promotes neuroprotection, antiinflammation and overall immunity via its important antioxidant effects [33, 34]. It is endogenously produced via the pineal gland from serotonin, a neurotransmitter hormone responsible for mood stabilization and sleep promotion [35]. Melatonin production occurs cyclically; spurred by an endogenous CR clock, which is primarily influenced by light/dark cycling throughout a 24-h period [34]. As such, melatonin secretion patterns follow a day-night diurnal pattern; melatonin secretion is highest during nighttime (i.e., dark) hours, peaks in the middle of the night, and is lowest during the waking (i.e., light) hours [36].

While several studies have evaluated melatonin levels in critically ill adults in the context of CR, [37–40] research on melatonin levels in pediatric ICU patients remains limited. Under normal circumstances, melatonin production in children begins around 21:00 and peaks between the hours of 01:00 and 04:00. Baseline levels are reached between 06:00 and 09:00, which follows a light/dark pattern. In utero, melatonin is produced but decreases with gestational age [41]. Postnatally, concentrations of serum melatonin rise in concordance with CR development 4 to 12 weeks postpartum. Daily and total melatonin levels stabilize throughout childhood and nocturnal serum melatonin peaks between the ages of 1 and 3 years [33]. In critical illness, several factors may negatively impact diurnal melatonin production and secretion (see below).

3.2 Qualitative Sleep Assessment

Qualitative sleep assessment, including patient and/or family assessment of the child's sleep quality, can strengthen the results of quantitative sleep data. Although validated sleep quality scales are available across different age groups, use of these scales may not be feasible in children who are sedated or have delirium. As such, a proxy may be necessary. These instruments are also useful in assessing baseline sleep and post-critical illness sleep once a child's intensive therapies start to de-escalate.

3.2.1 Age-Appropriate Sleep Scales

The characteristics of pediatric sleep scales most frequently used in PICU practice are described in Table 2. The scale chosen for use should match the age and developmental appropriateness of the child being evaluated. These questionnaires can also be used at the time of PICU admission to characterize a child's baseline sleep

Table 2 Age-appropriate sleep scales for critically Ill children

Scale	Age range/Items	Domains	Language
Children's Sleep Habits Questionnaire (CSHQ, [42])	Parent report 4–10 years (school age) 45 items	– Bedtime resistance – Sleep onset delay – Sleep duration – Sleep anxiety – Night awakenings – Parasomnias – Sleep disordered breathing – Daytime sleepiness	– English
Patient Reported Outcomes Measurement Information System (PROMIS [43])	Self-report 8–17 years Parent report 5–17 years Short forms: 4 and 8 items	– Sleep disturbance – Sleep impairment	– English
PedsQL Multidimensional Fatigue Scale [44]	Self-report 5–7, 8–12, and 13–18 years Parent report 2–4 (toddler), 5–7 (young child) and 8–18 (adolescent) 18 items	– General fatigue – Sleep/rest fatigue – Cognitive fatigue	– English
Brief Infant Sleep Questionnaire (BISQ) [45]	Parent report 0–29 months 33 items	– Nocturnal sleep duration – Night awakenings – Method of falling asleep	– English – Chinese – Nepali – Portuguese – Turkish – Spanish

(continued)

Table 2 (continued)

Scale	Age range/Items	Domains	Language
Children's Sleep Habits Questionnaire (CHSQ [46])	Parent report 4–10 years 35 items	– Bedtime resistance – Sleep onset delay – Sleep duration – Sleep anxiety – Night wakings – Parasomnias – Sleep disordered breathing – Daytime sleepiness	– English – Chinese – Dutch – Hebrew – Portuguese – Spanish
Paediatric Sleep Questionnaire (PSQ [47])	Parent report 2–18 years 22 items	– Sleepiness – Snoring – Attention/ hyperactivity	– English – Portuguese – Chinese – Spanish – Turkish – Malay
Tayside Children's Sleep Questionnaire (TCSQ [48])	Parent report 1–5 years 10 items	– Initial settling of child – Night-time disruption – Early morning arousal	– English

Key: *PedsQL Pediatric Qualify of Life*

habits for both clinical and research purposes (i.e. Children's Sleep Habits Questionnaire, Brief Infant Sleep Questionnaire). In contrast, the PROMIS and PedsQL scales are typically used in the research setting after PICU discharge.

3.2.2 Sleep Diaries

While EEG and actigraphy can provide quantitative data regarding sleep duration, sleep quality is best measured qualitatively. Quantitatively collected sleep data can simultaneously complement qualitative sleep data found in sleep diaries. Similar to sleep scales, sleep diaries may be best used once PICU care is de-escalated and the child has recovered from their imminent life-threatening illness. Parents can serve as proxies to compare the baseline sleep habits of their child to those observed during and after critical illness. Sleep diaries provide a longitudinal, comprehensive assessment of a child's sleep-wake patterns.

In healthy children and infants, sleep diaries have been used to assess sleep-wake patterns. One healthy infant study noted discrepancies between sleep diaries and actigraphy measures, which may indicate actigraphy is useful in assessing movement but not sleep patterns [49]. Pediatric sleep researchers and clinicians conclude that subjective sleep diaries and actigraphy may be used in a complementary fashion to estimate sleep start, end, and duration, but may not be beneficial in accurately assessing nighttime awakenings [50].

The fragmented sleep patterns of the PICU patient may persist after PICU discharge. Despite the normalization of sleep patterns in the post-PICU period, as indicated by improvements in sleep questionnaires and scales, parents of critically ill child survivors often still perceive sleep fragmentation in their child after PICU discharge [51, 52].

4 Risk Factors for Poor Sleep

The PICU environment and the therapies delivered in this setting, coupled with a child's critical illness, pose a unique threat to sleep quality and overall circadian rhythm. Similar to adults (and as outlined in chapter "Risk Factors for Disrupted Sleep in the ICU"), the ICU environment can be stressful and hostile to healthy sleep [53]. Figure 1 outlines PICU-specific risk factors for poor sleep. Many of these factors are similar to those seen in adult ICUs.

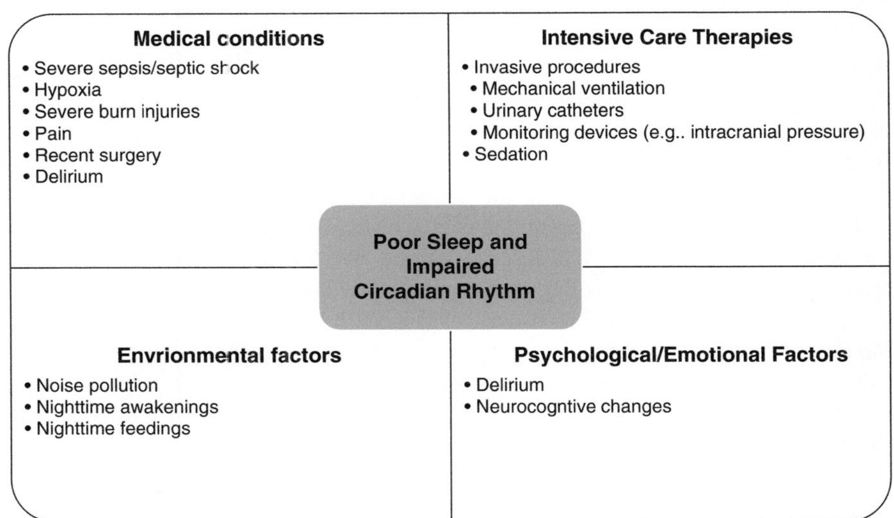

Fig. 1 PICU specific risk factors for poor sleep and impaired circadian rhythm

4.1 Medical Conditions

Critical illness itself poses a threat to sleep in the PICU. Animal studies demonstrate conditions leading to organ dysfunction and/or failure increase the risk for worse sleep architecture [54]. In particular, sepsis, which leads to overwhelming systemic inflammation and often multiorgan failure, is highly associated with sleep disruption in children [55–58]. Adult studies of sepsis and melatonin levels have found that sepsis negatively impacts melatonin production and thereby disrupts CR [59]. There are limited PICU-specific studies investigating sepsis and melatonin concentrations. One study conducted by Bagci et al. evaluated CR-related outcomes in a small cohort (n = 40) of critically ill children, with and without sepsis, and found sepsis did not affect nocturnal melatonin serum concentrations [60]. Melatonin has immune-related properties including anti-inflammatory and antioxidant effects and has been postulated to be a potential sepsis therapy due to its protective effect in adults and newborns [61–66]. In addition to sepsis, hypoxia may also perturb CR and overall sleep. Hypoxia has been associated with sleep fragmentation and malaise [67],which may also affect sleep architecture in this population.

4.2 Co-Administered Therapies

While nearly all ICU interventions have the potential to negatively-impact sleep and CR in the PICU setting, mechanical ventilation (both invasive and non-invasive) is of particular interest to disrupted sleep although this relationship is complex (see chapter "Mechanical Ventilation and Sleep") [68–70]. Some children are unable to communicate their needs or understand the rationale for interventions that are delivered. This lack of understanding on the part of critically ill children may necessitate use of sedation [2, 71–73]. While sedatives and anxiolytics are often necessary to main safety and promote healing, the profiles of sedatives vary in their effects on sleep architecture (see chapter "Effects of Common ICU Medications on Sleep"). Most commonly, a combination of opioids, benzodiazepines, ketamine, barbiturates, and alpha-2 agonists (e.g., clonidine and dexmedetomidine) are used [2]. Additionally, neuromuscular blockade may be used to facilitate ventilator synchrony which may further complicate sleep assessment and restoration [73, 74]. PICU-specific studies including the *RESTORE* (Randomized Evaluation of Sedation Titration for Respiratory Failure) clinical trial [31] and the SANDWICH (Sedation and Weaning in Children) trial [30] investigated the effects of protocolized sedation on mechanical ventilation outcomes. While neither study's primary endpoint was sleep, they confirmed that children requiring mechanical ventilation could be safely managed in more awake states with less sedation. As with adults, the reduced use of benzodiazepines, known to potentiate poor sleep architecture and increase ICU delirium, is recommended [75].

Other care-related factors, which may impact CR and sleep include continuous enteral feeding, patient care activities, and restraints [13, 53, 76, 77]. There is ambiguity on how nutrition should be optimally delivered (ie., continuous vs. bolus; 12 h vs 24 h) in the pediatric setting despite that the timing and duration of feeding has been shown to affect CR in adults (chapter "Best Practice for Improving Sleep in the ICU. Part I: Non-pharmacologic"). To preserve sleep in the ICU, it is imperative to mimic a child's pre-PICU routine. While newborns and infants may feed nocturnally, toddlers, school-aged children, and adolescents generally do not. Bolus feeding, as opposed to continuous 24-h feeding, is physiologically aligned with day-to-day routines and provides the child freedom to move and participate in rehabilitation therapies [77]. This is vital considering that early rehabilitation minimizes the risk of poor post-PICU outcomes, including delirium, PICU-acquired weakness, muscle atrophy, and prolonged PICU length of stay; all while improving functional outcomes [78, 79]. Point prevalence studies, however have demonstrated that overall, there are inconsistent practices of early mobilization in critically ill children [80], illustrating the increased need for standardized programs to promote healing through mobilization [76, 80].

In addition to immobility and nutrition, disruptions in sleep-wake patterns with patient care activities are also detrimental to CR and sleep. As such, care should be clustered at night whenever possible, and similar to nutrition, should be synchronized to the child's pre-PICU routine (e.g. daily sleep requirements, timing of naps). All hands-on care should emulate their routine to provide neurodevelopmental appropriate care and restorative healing.

4.3 Environmental Factors

Given the neurobiological influence of day-night light cycling on CR, decreased exposure to sunlight during the day with prolonged artificial lighting at night are risk factors for CR dysregulation. Sound also plays a crucial role. Noise pollution is a serious concern for recovery and has been acknowledged for its negative effects as early as the 1800s [81]. In response to the negative effects of high levels of noise on restorative healing, the World Health Organization (WHO) introduced guidelines for varying industries regarding appropriate noise levels. Specifically in the hospital, the WHO recommends that overall average noise levels should not exceed 35 decibels (dB) with a maximum of 40 dB overnight [82]. Specific to the PICU, a multi-site study surveyed PICUs' light and sound levels. Results indicated that, in general, PICUs are not conducive to sleep. On average, sound levels always exceeded 45 dB, with peaks above 85 dB at all sites [83].

4.4 Psychological/Emotional Factors

An ICU admission is usually frightening for children given they often cannot adequately express their fear and concerns. In several studies examining sleep in children admitted to the PICU with severe burns who frequently experience severe pain, fear and anxiety are closely related to poor sleep [84, 85]. Notably, this psychological distress may last for months after the injury and subsequent PICU discharge. While PICU and post-PICU psychological distress is likely greatest in severely burned children, it should be considered in all critically ill children. A child's stress may be increased if they witness their family members' anxiety and stress related to their child's hospitalization. The absence of family at the bedside may also increase patient stress.

5 Sleep Restoration and Promotion

Compared to adults, unique challenges exist with sleep improvement in critically ill children. The greater variability in chronological and developmental age of children makes sleep promotion protocols difficult to create and enforce. Similar strategies used for critically ill adults (see chapters "Best Practices for Improving Sleep in the ICU. Part I: Non-pharmacologic" and "Best Practices for Improving Sleep in the ICU. Part II: Pharmacologic") can be employed in in the PICU, as long as they are appropriately adapted for age and baseline physical function [86]. PICU Liberation bundles are an interdisciplinary collaborative effort created to offset the harmful effects of excessive and prolonged sedation, immobilization, sleep disruption, and delirium [86–88]. While ICU liberation bundles focus on five distinct elements each of these can be appropriately tailored to the PICU setting. The five elements of the ICU Liberation Bundle as promoted by the Society of Critical Care Medicine [89] are as follows:

- A: Assess, manage and treat pain
- B: Both spontaneous awakenings and breathing trials
- C: Choice of sedation and analgesia
- D: Delirium, assessment, management, and treatment
- E: Early mobility and exercise
- F: Family engagement and empowerment

Adherence to the ICU Liberation Bundle may reasonably be expected to improve sleep by enforcing better sleep hygiene, stress reduction, and minimizing iatrogenic harm [86].

A comprehensive PICU baseline sleep evaluation is vital to emulate the child's home sleep pattern and nonpharmacologic approaches should be prioritized given the lack of rigorous data to support the use of pharmacologic sleep improvement strategies with melatonin, antipsychotics and antidepressants in critically ill children. Table 3 outlines both non-pharmacological and pharmacological approaches through which sleep can be optimized in the high-risk PICU population to promote CR and overall healing.

Table 3 Pharmacological and non-pharmacological sleep restoration therapies

Pharmacological Therapies
• *Choice of sedation*   – Sparing use of benzodiazepines as first-line agents
• *Sleep aids*   – Melatonin
Non-pharmacological therapies

• *Environmental interventions*
  – Earplugs
  – Headphone
  – White noise
  – Music
  – Decreased noise/alarms
  – Controlled day/night light cycling

• *Behavioral interventions*
  – Skin to skin contact
  – Guided imagery

• *Physical therapy*   – Early progressive mobility

• *Complementary therapies*
  – Massage
  – Acupuncture
  – Aromatherapy
  – Modified yoga

6 Conclusion

The PICU environment paired with the developmental changes that occur through-out childhood and adolescence may lead to disrupted sleep and CR rhythm dysregu-lation in critically ill children. It is imperative for sleep researchers and clinicians to understand the neurobiological considerations of sleep and sleep requirements in children and how these needs change throughout the lifespan. Chronological and developmental age-appropriate scales for sleep assessment are imperative to use not only to quantify sleep, but also to qualitatively assess sleep and its impact on the child's overall function during the PICU stay and beyond. The implementation of both quantitative (i.e. melatonin, actigraphy, EEG) and qualitative assessments (i.e. sleep diaries) may provide complementary information for researchers and clini-cians to have comprehensive picture of the child's sleep and CR. Considering the PICU environment is often not conducive to maintaining CR and/or pre-critical ill-ness sleep patterns, clinicians must be aware of the environmental, intrinsic and disease-specific factors which may induce sleep dysfunction and/or CR dysregula-tion in critically ill children. Once identified, appropriate measures to either main-tain and/or restore CR and sleep using multimodal approaches – including pharmacologic and nonpharmacological complementary therapies are necessary to promote healing.

References

1. Berger J, Zaidi M, Halferty I, et al. Sleep in the hospitalized child: a contemporary review. Chest. 2021;160(3):1064–74.
2. Kudchadkar SR, Aljohani OA, Punjabi NM. Sleep of critically ill children in the pediatric intensive care unit: a systematic review. Sleep Med Rev. 2014;18(2):103–10.
3. Kudchadkar SR, Yaster M, Punjabi NM. Sedation, sleep promotion, and delirium screening practices in the care of mechanically ventilated children: a wake-up call for the pediatric critical care community*. Crit Care Med. 2014;42(7):1592–600.
4. Herrup EA, Wieczorek B, Kudchadkar SR. Feasibility and perceptions of PICU diaries*. Pediatr Crit Care Med. 2019;20(2):e83–90.
5. Curcio G, Ferrara M, De Gennaro L. Sleep loss, learning capacity and academic performance. Sleep Med Rev. 2006;10(5):323–37.
6. Kudchadkar SR, Aljohani O, Johns J, et al. Day-night activity in hospitalized children after major surgery: an analysis of 2271 hospital days. J Pediatr. 2019;209:190–197.e191.
7. NIGMS. Circadian Rhythms. 2021 [cited August 2, 2021] Available from: https://www.nigms.nih.gov/education/fact-sheets/Pages/circadian-rhythms.aspx
8. Moore RY. Suprachiasmatic nucleus in sleep-wake regulation. Sleep Med. 2007;8(Suppl 3):27–33.
9. Rivkees SA. The development of circadian rhythms: from animals to humans. Sleep Med Clin. 2007;2(3):331–41.
10. Brooks E, Canal MM. Development of circadian rhythms: role of postnatal light environment. Neurosci Biobehav Rev. 2013;37(4):551–60.
11. Yates J. Perspective: the long-term effects of light exposure on establishment of newborn circadian rhythm. J Clin Sleep Med. 2018;14(10):1829–30.
12. Joseph D, Chong NW, Shanks ME, et al. Getting rhythm: how do babies do it? Arch Dis Child Fetal Neonatal Ed. 2015;100(1):F50–4.
13. Perry M, Dawkins-Henry O, Awojoodu R, et al. Study protocol for a two-center test of a nurse-implemented chronotherapeutic restoring bundle in critically ill children: Restore Resilience (R 2). Contemporary Clinical Trials. 2021;A19;23:100840.
14. Borniger JC, McHenry ZD, Abi Salloum BA, et al. Exposure to dim light at night during early development increases adult anxiety-like responses. Physiol Behav. 2014;133:99–106.
15. Bauer M, Glenn T, Alda M, et al. Influence of light exposure during early life on the age of onset of bipolar disorder. J Psychiatr Res. 2015;64:1–8.
16. Brooks E, Patel D, Canal MM. Programming of mice circadian photic responses by postnatal light environment. PLoS One. 2014;9(5):e97160.
17. Hagenauer MH, Perryman JI, Lee TM, et al. Adolescent changes in the homeostatic and circadian regulation of sleep. Dev Neurosci. 2009;31(4):276–84.
18. Carskadon MA, Vieira C, Acebo C. Association between puberty and delayed phase preference. Sleep. 1993;16(3):258–62.
19. Carskadon MA, Acebo C, Richardson GS, et al. An approach to studying circadian rhythms of adolescent humans. J Biol Rhythm. 1997;12(3):278–89.
20. Carskadon M. Maturation of processes regulating sleep in adolescents. In: Marcus C, Carroll J, Donnelly D, Loughlin G, editors. Sleep in Children: Developmental Changes in Sleep Patterns. 2nd ed. Informa Healthcare; 2008. p. 95–109.
21. Paruthi S, Brooks LJ, D'Ambrosio C, et al. Recommended amount of sleep for pediatric populations: a consensus statement of the American Academy of sleep medicine. J Clin Sleep Med. 2016;12(6):785–6.
22. Hirshkowitz M, Whiton K, Albert SM, et al. National Sleep Foundation's sleep time duration recommendations: methodology and results summary. Sleep Health. 2015;1(1):40–3.
23. Tarokh L, Van Reen E, LeBourgeois M, et al. Sleep EEG provides evidence that cortical changes persist into late adolescence. Sleep. 2011;34(10):1385–93.

24. Feinberg I, Campbell IG. Sleep EEG changes during adolescence: an index of a fundamental brain reorganization. Brain Cogn. 2010;72(1):56–65.
25. Kurth S, Jenni OG, Riedner BA, et al. Characteristics of sleep slow waves in children and adolescents. Sleep. 2010;33(4):475–80.
26. Watson PL, Pandharipande P, Gehlbach BK, et al. Atypical sleep in ventilated patients: empirical electroencephalography findings and the path toward revised ICU sleep scoring criteria. Crit Care Med. 2013;41(8):1958–67.
27. Kudchadkar SR, Yaster M, Punjabi AN, et al. Temporal characteristics of the sleep EEG power Spectrum in critically ill children. Journal of clinical sleep medicine: JCSM: official publication of the American Academy of Sleep Medicine. 2015;11(12):1449–54.
28. El Shakankiry HM. Sleep physiology and sleep disorders in childhood. Nat Sci Sleep. 2011;3:101–14.
29. Calandriello A, Tylka JC, Patwari PP. Sleep and delirium in pediatric critical illness: what is the relationship? Med Sci (Basel). 2018;6(4)
30. Blackwood B, Tume LN, Morris KP, et al. Effect of a sedation and ventilator liberation protocol vs usual care on duration of invasive mechanical ventilation in pediatric intensive care units: a randomized clinical trial. JAMA. 2021;326(5):401–10.
31. Curley MAQ, Wypij D, Watson RS, et al. Protocolized sedation vs usual care in pediatric patients mechanically ventilated for acute respiratory failure: a randomized clinical trial. JAMA. 2015;313(4):379–89.
32. Duclos C, Dumont M, Blais H, et al. Rest-activity cycle disturbances in the acute phase of moderate to severe traumatic brain injury. Neurorehabil Neural Repair. 2014;28(5):472–82.
33. Foster JR. Melatonin in critically ill children. J Pediatr Intensive Care. 2016;5(4):172–81.
34. Marseglia L, Aversa S, Barberi I, et al. High endogenous melatonin levels in critically ill children: a pilot study. J Pediatr. 2013;162(2):357–60.
35. Reiter RJ, Paredes SD, Manchester LC, et al. Reducing oxidative/nitrosative stress: a newly-discovered genre for melatonin. Crit Rev Biochem Mol Biol. 2009;44(4):175–200.
36. Pisani MA, Friese RS, Gehlbach BK, et al. Sleep in the intensive care unit. Am J Respir Crit Care Med. 2015;191(7):731–8.
37. Shilo L, Dagan Y, Smorjik Y, et al. Patients in the intensive care unit suffer from severe lack of sleep associated with loss of normal melatonin secretion pattern. Am J Med Sci. 1999;317(5):278–81.
38. Frisk U, Olsson J, Nylén P, et al. Low melatonin excretion during mechanical ventilation in the intensive care unit. Clin Sci (Lond). 2004;107(1):47–53.
39. Olofsson K, Alling C, Lundberg D, et al. Abolished circadian rhythm of melatonin secretion in sedated and artificially ventilated intensive care patients. Acta Anaesthesiol Scand. 2004;48(6):679–84.
40. Mistraletti G, Sabbatini G, Taverna M, et al. Pharmacokinetics of orally administered melatonin in critically ill patients. J Pineal Res. 2010;48(2):142–7.
41. Commentz JC, Henke A, Dammann O, et al. Decreasing melatonin and 6-hydroxymelatonin sulfate excretion with advancing gestational age in preterm and term newborn male infants. Eur J Endocrinol. 1996;135(2):184–7.
42. Owens JA, Spirito A, McGuinn M. The Children's Sleep Habits Questionnaire (CSHQ): psychometric properties of a survey instrument for school-aged children. Sleep. 2000 Dec 15;23(8):1043–51. PMID: 11145319.
43. Forrest CB, Meltzer LJ, Marcus CL, de la Motte A, Kratchman A, Buysse DJ, Pilkonis PA, Becker BD, Bevans KB. Development and validation of the PROMIS pediatric sleep disturbance and sleep-related impairment item banks. Sleep. 2018;41(6):zsy054. https://doi.org/10.1093/sleep/zsy054.
44. Varni JW, Limbers CA, Bryant WP, Wilson DP. The PedsQL multidimensional fatigue scale in pediatric obesity: feasibility, reliability and validity. Int J Pediatr Obes. 2010;5(1):34–42. https://doi.org/10.3109/17477160903111706.

45. Sadeh A. A brief screening questionnaire for infant sleep problems: validation and findings for an Internet sample. Pediatrics. 2004 Jun;113(6):e570-7. https://doi.org/10.1542/peds.113.6.e570. PMID: 15173539.
46. Owens JA, Spirito A, McGuinn M. The children's sleep habits questionnaire (CSHQ): psychometric properties of a survey instrument for school-aged children. Sleep. 2000, Dec 15;23(8):1043–51.
47. Chervin RD, Hedger K, Dillon JE, Pituch KJ. Pediatric sleep questionnaire (PSQ): validity and reliability of scales for sleep-disordered breathing, snoring, sleepiness, and behavioral problems. Sleep Med. 2000 Feb 1;1(1):21–32.
48. McGreavey JA, Donnan PT, Pagliari HC, Sullivan FM. The Tayside Children's sleep questionnaire: a simple tool to evaluate sleep problems in young children. Child Care Health Dev. 2005;31(5):539–44.
49. Hall WA, Liva S, Moynihan M, et al. A comparison of actigraphy and sleep diaries for infants' sleep behavior. Front Psych. 2015;6:19.
50. Werner H, Molinari L, Guyer C, et al. Agreement rates between actigraphy, diary, and questionnaire for children's sleep patterns. Arch Pediatr Adolesc Med. 2008;162(4):350–8.
51. Corser N. Sleep of 1- and 2-year-old children in intensive care. Issues Compr Pediatr Nurs. 2009;19:17–31.
52. Pollack MM, Holubkov R, Funai T, et al. Pediatric intensive care outcomes: development of new morbidities during pediatric critical care. Pediatr Crit Care Med. 2014;15(9):821–7.
53. Telias I, Wilcox ME. Sleep and circadian rhythm in critical illness. Crit Care. 2019;23(1):82.
54. Baracchi F, Ingiosi AM, Raymond RM, et al. Sepsis-induced alterations in sleep of rats. Am J Physiol Regul Integr Comp Physiol. 2011;301(5):R1467–78.
55. Shankar-Hari M, Phillips GS, Levy ML, et al. Developing a new definition and assessing new clinical criteria for septic shock: for the third international consensus definitions for sepsis and septic shock (Sepsis-3). JAMA. 2016;315(8):775–87.
56. Seymour CW, Liu VX, Iwashyna TJ, et al. Assessment of clinical criteria for sepsis: for the third international consensus definitions for sepsis and septic shock (Sepsis-3). JAMA. 2016;315(8):762–74.
57. Singer M. The new sepsis consensus definitions (Sepsis-3): the good, the not-so-bad, and the actually-quite-pretty. Intensive Care Med. 2016;42(12):2027–9.
58. Weiss SL, Peters MJ, Alhazzani W, et al. Surviving sepsis campaign international guidelines for the Management of Septic Shock and Sepsis-Associated Organ Dysfunction in children. Pediatr Crit Care Med. 2020;21(2):e52–e106.
59. Sertaridou EN, Chouvarda IG, Arvanitidis KI, et al. Melatonin and cortisol exhibit different circadian rhythm profiles during septic shock depending on timing of onset: a prospective observational study. Ann Intensive Care. 2018;8(1):118.
60. Bagci S, Horoz Ö, Yildizdas D, et al. Melatonin status in pediatric intensive care patients with sepsis. Pediatr Crit Care Med. 2012;13(2):e120–3.
61. Haimovich B, Calvano J, Haimovich AD, et al. In vivo endotoxin synchronizes and suppresses clock gene expression in human peripheral blood leukocytes. Crit Care Med. 2010;38(3):751–8.
62. Mundigler G, Delle-Karth G, Koreny M, et al. Impaired circadian rhythm of melatonin secretion in sedated critically ill patients with severe sepsis. Crit Care Med. 2002;30(3):536–40.
63. Li CX, Liang DD, Xie GH, et al. Altered melatonin secretion and circadian gene expression with increased proinflammatory cytokine expression in early-stage sepsis patients. Mol Med Rep. 2013;7(4):1117–22.
64. Gitto E, Karbownik M, Reiter RJ, et al. Effects of melatonin treatment in septic newborns. Pediatr Res. 2001;50(6):756–60.
65. Henderson R, Kim S, Lee E. Use of melatonin as adjunctive therapy in neonatal sepsis: a systematic review and meta-analysis. Complement Ther Med. 2018;39:131–6.
66. Galley HF, Lowes DA, Allen L, et al. Melatonin as a potential therapy for sepsis: a phase I dose escalation study and an ex vivo whole blood model under conditions of sepsis. J Pineal Res. 2014;56(4):427–38.

67. Mortola JP. Hypoxia and circadian patterns. Respir Physiol Neurobiol. 2007;158(2–3):274–9.
68. Ozsancak A, D'Ambrosio C, Garpestad E, et al. Sleep and mechanical ventilation. Crit Care Clin. 2008;24(3):517–31.
69. Parthasarathy S, Tobin MJ. Effect of ventilator mode on sleep quality in critically ill patients. Am J Respir Crit Care Med. 2002;166(11):1423–9.
70. Parthasarathy S. Sleep during mechanical ventilation. Curr Opin Pulm Med. 2004;10(6):489–94.
71. Al-Samsam RH, Cullen P. Sleep and adverse environmental factors in sedated mechanically ventilated pediatric intensive care patients. Pediatr Crit Care Med. 2005;6(5):562–7.
72. Carno MA, Connolly HV. Sleep and sedation in the pediatric intensive care unit. Crit Care Nurs Clin North Am. 2005;17(3):239–44.
73. Carno MA, Hoffman LA, Henker R, et al. Sleep monitoring in children during neuromuscular blockade in the pediatric intensive care unit: a pilot study. Pediatr Crit Care Med. 2004;5(3):224–9.
74. Johnson KL, Cheung RB, Johnson SB, et al. Therapeutic paralysis of critically ill trauma patients: perceptions of patients and their family members. Am J Crit Care. 1999;8(1):490–8.
75. Barnes SS, Kudchadkar SR. Sedative choice and ventilator-associated patient outcomes: don't sleep on delirium. Ann Transl Med. 2016;4(2):34.
76. Ista E, Scholefield BR, Manning JC, et al. Mobilization practices in critically ill children: a European point prevalence study (EU PARK-PICU). Crit Care. 2020;24(1):368.
77. Ichimaru S, Amagai T. Intermittent and bolus methods of feeding in critical care. In; 2014. pp 1–17.
78. Walsh CJ, Batt J, Herridge MS, et al. Muscle wasting and early mobilization in acute respiratory distress syndrome. Clin Chest Med. 2014;35(4):811–26.
79. Needham DM, Korupolu R, Zanni JM, et al. Early physical medicine and rehabilitation for patients with acute respiratory failure: a quality improvement project. Arch Phys Med Rehabil. 2010;91(4):536–42.
80. Kudchadkar SR, Nelliot A, Awojoodu R, et al. Physical rehabilitation in critically ill children: a multicenter point prevalence study in the United States. Crit Care Med. 2020;48(5):634–44.
81. Nightingale F. Notes on nursing: what it is, and what it is not. London: Harrison; 1860.
82. Berglund B, Lindvall T, Schwela DH. Guidelines for community noise. In ed. Geneva, Switzerland: World Health Organization; 1999.
83. Darbyshire JL, Young JD. An investigation of sound levels on intensive care units with reference to the WHO guidelines. Crit Care. 2013;17(5):R187.
84. Cureton-Lane RA, Fontaine DK. Sleep in the pediatric ICU: an empirical investigation. Am J Crit Care. 1997;6(1):56–63.
85. Stoddard FJ, Ronfeldt H, Kagan J, et al. Young burned children: the course of acute stress and physiological and behavioral responses. Am J Psychiatry. 2006;163(6):1084–90.
86. Choong K, Abu-Sultaneh S. Applying the ICU Liberation Bundle to Critically Ill Children. 2020 [cited 2021 August 11, 2021] Available from: https://www.sccm.org/Communications/Critical-Connections/Archives/2020/Applying-the-ICU-Liberation-Bundle-to-Critically-I
87. Marra A, Ely EW, Pandharipande PP, et al. The ABCDEF bundle in critical care. Crit Care Clin. 2017;33(2):225–43.
88. Ely EW. The ABCDEF bundle: science and philosophy of how ICU liberation serves patients and families. Crit Care Med. 2017;45(2):321–30.
89. SCCM. [cited Available from: https://www.sccm.org/Clinical-Resources/ICULiberation-Home/ABCDEF-Bundles
90. Wieczorek B, Ascenzi J, Kim Y, et al. PICU up!: impact of a quality improvement intervention to promote early mobilization in critically ill children. Pediatr Crit Care Med. 2016;17(12):e559–66.

Sleep in Critical Illness: Future Directions

Melissa P. Knauert and Sairam Parthasarathy

1   Introduction

Sleep is critically important to human health. This has been demonstrated in acute, sub-acute and chronic sleep deprivation and restriction models [1]. Even short-term sleep loss negatively influences cognition [2], alertness [3, 4], mood [5, 6], glucose control [7–9], cardiovascular health [10–14], immune system function [15, 16], and respiratory physiology [17–20] (chapter "Biologic Effects of Disrupted Sleep"). Moreover, chronic, or habitual short sleep duration and poor sleep quality are associated with increased morbidity and mortality and pose global health threats [21–24].

This crisis has extended into the hospital and intensive care unit (ICU) but with a less proven impact. To date, it has been demonstrated that ICU patients have a high prevalence of abnormal sleep features: sleep is short, fragmented, poorly timed, and perceived to be of poor quality by patients (chapter "Characteristics of Sleep in Critically Ill Patients. Part I: Sleep Fragmentation and Sleep Stage Disruption") [25–28]. Beyond the physiologic consequences of poor sleep, it is a major complaint and source of distress among patients that persists even after hospitalization [29]. The severe sleep disruption seen in the ICU is, not surprisingly, accompanied by abnormal circadian alignment and amplitude [30, 31]. Because sleep is of the longest duration and highest quality when it is aligned with the

M. P. Knauert (✉)
Department of Internal Medicine, Section of Pulmonary, Critical Care and Sleep Medicine, Yale School of Medicine, New Haven, CT, USA
e-mail: Melissa.Knauert@yale.edu

S. Parthasarathy
Division of Pulmonary, Allergy, Critical Care & Sleep Medicine, University of Arizona College of Medicine, Tucson, AZ, USA
e-mail: spartha1@arizona.edu

G. L. Weinhouse, J. W. Devlin (eds.), *Sleep in Critical Illness*, https://doi.org/10.1007/978-3-031-06447-0_17

291

biologic (i.e., circadian) night, misalignment or loss of circadian rhythm in ICU patients will significantly worsen their sleep [32, 33]. Circadian misalignment has additional consequences throughout the body as the central clock, peripheral clocks, and human behaviors become dyssynchronous, a condition termed internal dyssynchrony (chapter "Characteristics of Sleep in Critically Ill Patients. Part II: Circadian Rhythm Disruption"). The consequences of internal dyssynchrony are just starting to be understood in non-ICU populations [33, 34].

ICU sleep disruption is likely a complex multi-domain syndrome that changes over the trajectory of critical illness and recovery and includes elements of sleep duration, timing, architecture, fragmentation, patient perception, and encompasses the field of circadian rhythms with both circadian alignment and amplitude being of potential importance. Furthermore, there is acknowledgement that sleep derangements in ICU patients are caused by a wide range of heterogeneous factors such as patient sleep history, discomfort, anxiety, severity of illness, type of illness, medications, and environmental conditions and that susceptibility could vary dependent on various factors such as age, sex, race and ethnicity [35, 36] (chapter "Risk Factors for Disrupted Sleep in the ICU"). It remains unclear how these key biological variables impact ICU sleep disruption and how ICU sleep disruption varies among different sub-populations [37].

There is expanding interest in investigating and leveraging ICU sleep to improve patient outcomes [38], but many unanswered questions exist in the field (chapters "ICU Sleep Disruption and Its Relationship with ICU Outcomes" and "Long-Term Outcomes: Sleep in Survivors of Critical Illness"). Although recommended by the Society of Critical Care Medicine's Pain, Agitation, Delirium, Immobility, and Sleep (PADIS) guideline panel [39], key issues currently preclude the wide-spread use of multicomponent ICU sleep promotion interventions in the ICU. Small studies and heterogenous study elements (i.e., varied patient populations, sleep measures, intervention type, et cetera) have limited the quality of evidence to-date and made meta-analysis challenging. However, advances in sleep measurement technology and growing interprofessional, multi-site collaboration may help overcome these methodological challenges and strengthen the evidence to support use of these protocols. Herein we will discuss future directions for ICU sleep disruption methods, measures, risk factors, interventions, and outcomes. Though much of the discussion centers on gaps in research, addressing these gaps is intended to lead directly to implementation of sleep promotion strategies at the bedside and thus benefit ICU patients.

2 Measures of Sleep in the Intensive Care Unit

The methodological challenges of measuring sleep and circadian rhythms in the ICU have posed a major barrier to scientific understanding in this field. The barriers include the prolonged duration and intensity of monitoring, need for expert staff to apply and maintain equipment and interpret data, high cost, and patient burden and tolerance. These limitations have led to studies with small sample sizes and short measurement windows of what is likely a process that evolves from pre-ICU illness onset until weeks to months after recovery [29].

2.1 Objective Sleep Measures

As noted in polysomnography (PSG) monitoring in ICU patients remains informative, but extraordinarily resource intensive [26, 28, 40–44]. Additionally, conventional EEG scoring rules are unreliable in this population [42, 45–48]; although alternate rules have been proposed, universal agreement on these scoring methods does not exist and significant expertise to apply them to ICU patients is required [46, 47] (chapter "Methods for Routine Sleep Assessment and Monitoring"). These scoring challenges further intensify PSG resource issues. It is, in fact, critical that we delineate the full trajectory of ICU sleep disruption; therefore, longitudinal monitoring that is feasible and tolerable is a critical next step in moving ICU sleep disruption investigations forward.

Automated EEG algorithms have been studied as a strategy to alleviate PSG-related challenges. Although feasible and familiar, the Bispectral Index does not provide detailed sleep architecture data [49, 50] and thus its utility is limited. However, the concept of automated, real-time algorithms is important, and alternative EEG algorithms such as spectral power and the odds ratio product have been studied in a small number of ICU patients [48, 51, 52]. These techniques are promising and may provide both research and clinical staff an objective method to evaluate sleep that is both rigorous, feasible, and acceptable to patients. The automated, real-time nature of these algorithms will improve study quality and bring us closer to longitudinal clinical monitoring of sleep by ICU providers rather than sleep experts. This creates an essential bridge between research and clinical measurement needs and thus allows widespread implementation of sleep monitoring and promotion. In the future, it may be that sleep can be feasibly monitored in the ICU as a standard part of care allowing clinicians to respond in real time when it found to be disrupted.

2.2 Measures of Patients' Sleep Perception

Patients' perception of sleep, when evaluated using the validated the Richards-Campbell Sleep Questionnaire (RCSQ), is an important additional domain of ICU sleep disruption over and above objective sleep measurement data [53]. However, many critically ill adults cannot participate in sleep questionnaires due to limitations in consciousness (e.g., sedation), cognition (e.g., delirium) and communication (e.g., intubation) and thus subjective measures of sleep cannot be reliably collected for many ICU patients. Nevertheless, if we reframe ICU sleep disruption as a longitudinal syndrome, this low risk, low cost, easy to implement sleep measure may be useful in tracking sleep during illness recovery or in patients who are able to communicate. Furthermore, the RCSQ could be readily implemented by ICU care providers with minimal training and interpreted in real-time to allow for immediate response to poor sleep. As noted above, real-time, provider-based (e.g., without specialized sleep measurement training), bedside monitoring is key to improving ICU patient outcomes via sleep promotion.

2.3 Circadian Measures

Measures of circadian alignment and amplitude have also been a challenge in ICU patients. Melatonin and its metabolite 6-sulfatoxymelatonin are the gold standard indicators of central clock alignment and circadian amplitude; however, in the critically ill population which has unpredictable alignment, sampling of blood (melatonin) or urine (6-sulfatoxymelatonin) to assess circadian phase must be frequent (i.e., every 1 or 2 h) and around the clock. This is highly cumbersome and thus limits study sample size. Alternative physiologic signals that reflect circadian phase such as core body temperature, blood pressure, and heart rate have been used [54–56]; among these, heart rate stands out as readily available and continuously monitored in essentially all ICU patients. Rapid, automated data management and assessment of heart rate could provide metrics of circadian phase that reflect alignment over the prior 24-h on a rolling basis. As with automated EEG tools, this would facilitate investigation and clinical practices vis a vis the circadian domains of ICU sleep disruption.

Novel biomarkers of circadian phase that use RNA expression analysis to estimate melatonin onset have been developed recently in non-critically ill human populations and require only 1 or 2 blood samples per 24 h period [57, 58]; however preliminary studies suggest that these measures cannot estimate phase in ICU patients [59]. Further development of these tools may ultimately allow use in ICU patients, but they are less likely to be adopted as standard bedside tools.

2.4 Measurement Conclusions

In summary, limitations in readily available, reliable, and feasible ICU sleep measurement methods have hindered progress in the field. Although we know severe sleep and circadian rhythm derangements exist in the ICU, results from ICU studies are variable and likely attributable to differing measurement approaches. We do not understand the natural history of the ICU sleep disruption, if elements of ICU sleep disruption are adaptive, and what aspects of ICU sleep disruption are iatrogenic versus inherent to acute illness. Knowledge in these areas would contribute to a more robust definition of ICU sleep disruption and allow us to understand which

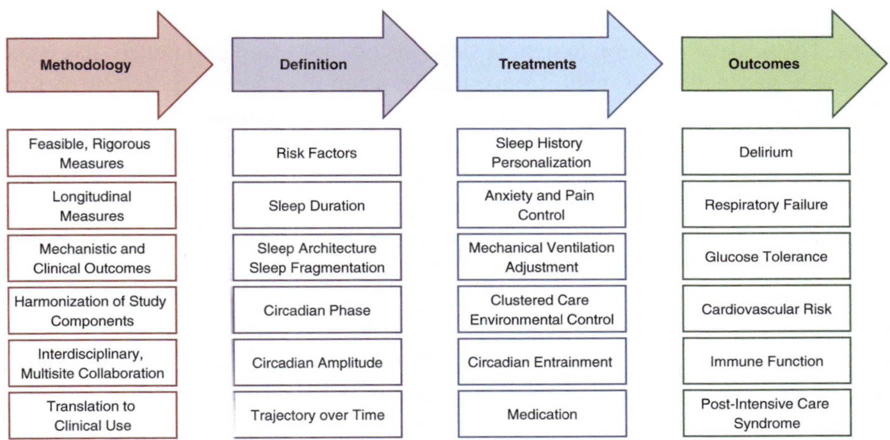

Fig. 1 Model of how improved methodology will promote understanding of intensive care unit sleep and circadian disruption, support the development of efficacious and effective interventions and lead to improved critical illness outcomes

sleep disruption domains are most closely linked to outcomes and thus intervene in a targeted manner. Key future directions are highlighted in Fig. 1.

3 Prevalence and Risk Factors for ICU Sleep Disruption

3.1 *Prevalence*

Sleep disruption affects most ICU patients [25, 26, 28, 44, 45, 60]. However, the downstream consequences of sleep disruption in the ICU need further study. Methodologic variability has contributed to crucial gaps in defining both ICU sleep disruption and how risk factors, outcomes, and interventions are defined and evaluated. The tremendously high prevalence of sleep disruption in the ICU has also fostered debate regarding whether sleep disruption is a de facto problem for all ICU patients or for only certain subpopulations.

3.2 *Patient Risk Factors*

A history of sleep deficiency and use of sleep aids prior to ICU admission are established risk factors for poor ICU sleep [39]. Notably, chronic short sleep is a widespread societal health problem, and the use of sleep aids is common in the general adult population [61]. Furthermore, formal assessment of sleep comorbidities, sleep preferences, sleep schedule and quality are not standard aspects of ICU intake, nor have these elements been commonly included in ICU sleep disruption investigations. This lack of attention to patient sleep history and sleep preferences has been a notable gap within the field. Concerningly, sleep disorders such as obstructive sleep apnea [62–64], restless leg syndrome [65], and insomnia [66] are common, can be exacerbated during critical illness, and often go both unrecognized and untreated during hospitalization. Personalization of sleep promotion, currently untested but likely to be highly important, requires engagement with patients to better understand individual reasons for sleep disruption (chapter "Best Practices for Improving Sleep in the ICU. Part I: Non-pharmacologic").

Psychologic factors such as pain, anxiety, lack of privacy and loss of patients' preferred sleep routines can also impact sleep in the ICU [37, 67, 68] (chapter "Risk Factors for Disrupted Sleep in the ICU"). These risk factors for ICU sleep disruption are often overlooked by care teams and should be considered and included in pharmacologic and non-pharmacologic sleep promotion bundles [68, 69] (chapters "Best Practices for Improving Sleep in the ICU. Part I: Non-pharmacologic" and "Best Practices for Improving Sleep in the ICU. Part II: Pharmacologic"). Similarly physiologic factors such as toileting needs, nausea, cough, and restriction of mobility [37, 68] can limit sleep and should also be appreciated as potentially modifiable risk factors. Patients interviewed about their sleep while admitted to the ICU described anxiety over the severity of their illness and an expectation that they be closely monitored for safety reasons [67]. Thus, when leaving ICU patients undisturbed to provide a period of rest, it is important to reassure patients that they are being remotely monitored and provide for basic needs such as toileting.

Severity of illness and mechanical ventilation have each been explored as risk factors for ICU sleep disruption; however, studies evaluating either factor have not shown a consistent relationship with disrupted sleep (chapter "Risk Factors for Disrupted Sleep in the ICU"). These inconsistent findings may relate to variations among studies and/or weaknesses in study methodology (e.g., heterogenous study populations, varied methods of sleep measurement, varied ventilator modes, small sample sizes) [37, 40, 44, 70, 71]. Future work can clarify the importance of putative risk factors by leveraging new sleep measurement technologies as discussed above. It is likely pre-hospital, psychologic, physiologic, illness-related and iatrogenic factors exist that can be modified, perhaps in a personalized manner, to mitigate ICU sleep disruption and improve critical illness outcomes (chapters "ICU Sleep Disruption and Its Relationship with ICU Outcomes" and "Long-Term Outcomes: Sleep in Survivors of Critical Illness").

3.3 ICU Environment

The ICU environment has been a major target of ICU sleep disruption investigations. The environment is a risk factor, a challenge to measure, and a target of intervention. Environmental control interventions do reduce disturbances including noise, light, and care interruptions [72–75]. However, key issues remain. Sound in most ICUs continues to exceed all recommendations [76–78], and it is not clear that modern buildings can achieve recommended sound levels due to air handlers, medical devices, monitors, and machine hum [76, 77, 79]. Furthermore, it is unclear what elements of sound are most disruptive to sleep (e.g., variability, average, peaks, source of sound). Notably, sound peaks account for approximately 20% of sleep arousals [80–82] which highlights the importance of sound as an ICU sleep disruption risk factor, but also highlights that other concomitant factors are contributing to arousals.

Light has also been noted to be abnormal in the ICU. Recent attention has focused on the lack of sufficient light during the day [83, 84] which may be as important as abnormally high light levels overnight. This shift reflects a growing understanding of the significant contribution of circadian processes to ICU sleep disruption [85]. Finally, care interruptions, frequent in the ICU [75, 86, 87], are a complex source of sleep disruption bringing sound, light, anxiety, and pain into the intended sleep period. Although multi-component interventions have addressed care interruptions and shown benefits [68, 88], additional research to better understand these interventions on a more granular level is required. Inclusion of the environment and care processes remains necessary but not sufficient for ICU sleep promotion.

4 Sleep Promotion

4.1 Addressing Patient Risk Factors

As noted above, the ability to initiate or maintain sleep in the ICU is hampered by multiple patient factors that are variably addressed in published sleep promotion bundles. These factors include, but are not limited to, pre-existing or undiagnosed sleep disorders, sleep history, anxiety, pain, and mechanical ventilation (chapters "Risk Factors for Disrupted Sleep in the ICU" and "Effects of Common ICU Medications on Sleep").

It seems clear that patients with pre-existing sleep disorders should generally continue their outpatient treatment during hospitalization if a contraindication does not exist; however, the benefit of this approach has not been proven. Similarly, while the incorporation of patient sleep preferences including timing, bedding, lighting, and room temperature is a low-risk intervention that could be considered, evidence to support this practice is just emerging [89]. Personalization of ICU sleep promotion is a logical next step in the design of sleep promotion interventions.

Although relaxation techniques (e.g. massage) have been associated with improved subjective sleep quality and an increase in total sleep [90–92], a paucity of published evidence precluded the 2018 PADIS guidelines from being able to make recommendations for their routine use [39]. Music therapy is one of the most frequently tested interventions and may be particularly promising. A systemic review of eleven studies demonstrated consistent associations between music therapy and reduced anxiety or stress in ICU patients [93]; as with multicomponent bundles discussed below, data supporting music's direct impact on sleep is more limited [94, 95]. Additionally, patient musical preferences and expertise in music therapy are needed for such interventions to be successful and this may ultimately prove a barrier to widespread implementation.

For patients with respiratory failure requiring mechanical ventilation, adjustment of ventilator support has been shown to improve sleep in small studies (chapter "Mechanical Ventilation and Sleep"). Increased support can improve sleep during acute respiratory failure [70, 71]; however, there is a risk of over-assistance which can disrupt sleep via hyperventilation and resultant central apneas [44, 96–98]. Proportional assist ventilation which delivers pressure proportional to the patient's instantaneous efforts may improve efforts to walk this delicate balance and thus improve sleep [40, 99] (See below Respiratory Outcomes).

4.2 Reducing Environmental and Care Interruptions

Control of the ICU environment and ICU care patterns have historically been a major focus for ICU sleep promotion interventions. Multicomponent, sleep promotion bundles are guideline recommended for ICU patients [39] and, as noted above, interventions have been able to reduce disturbances including noise, light and care interruptions [72–75]. Improvements in sleep outcomes have been more difficult to demonstrate [100, 101], but this lack of demonstrable change in sleep may be due to limitations in sleep measurement and intervention complexity leading to implementation challenges rather than true lack of effect. Next steps in developing bundled sleep promotion interventions should include the additional elements noted above but also may benefit from inclusion of an implementation framework in the testing and expanded use of such interventions [68, 102, 103].

More recently circadian principals have been applied to ICU sleep promotion interventions; this is a key a step forward in ICU sleep improvement. Light is the most influential circadian cue, and circadian entrainment depends on exposure to light that has sufficient intensity and duration and has the correct spectral characteristics (i.e., mimicking natural sunlight) [104, 105]. Though sample sizes are small, daytime light interventions have demonstrated improved patient satisfaction with their sleep [106], fostered earlier postoperative mobility [107], and reduced postoperative delirium [107–109]. Among studies that did not show benefit, abnormally high lighting levels in the control group [110] and inappropriate timing, duration, and spectral characteristics of the light intervention [111] may have limited findings. These missteps in the design of light interventions highlight the importance of understanding the aspects of light that are most impactful on the human circadian system [104, 105]. Additionally, comprehensive circadian-related light recommendations are just emerging and will need to be tracked carefully by the ICU sleep disruption research community [104, 105]. There are further gaps in investigation of non-photic circadian cues notably feeding schedule and exercise (i.e., mobility, physical therapy, and rehabilitation). Time-restricted daytime feeding and increased daytime mobility in concert with bright daytime light are likely to improve synchrony among the central clock and peripheral clocks, establish a predictable circadian night, and thus improve sleep [32]; however, this remains to be tested in the ICU setting.

4.3 Pharmacologic Interventions

There is no guideline recommended pharmacologic intervention to promote sleep in the ICU [39], yet neuroactive medications are prescribed nocturnally to promote sleepiness or treat nocturnal agitation at a tremendously high frequency (chapter "Best Practices for Improving Sleep in the ICU. Part II: Pharmacologic"). In one study, 10% of ICU patients were newly prescribed a scheduled sleep aid and more than 80% had this therapy continued beyond the ICU [112]. Melatonin agonists, alpha-2-agonists, and orexin antagonists are the most extensively tested agents with mixed results regarding whether they improve sleep or reduce delirium [113–116]. Though these agents may hold future promise, current studies have small samples, have included patients with a relatively low severity of illness (i.e., potentially at lower risk for disrupted sleep and/or delirium), and have relied on patient self-reports to characterize sleep quality. In the future, adequately powered multicenter randomized controlled trials involving ICU patients with a higher severity of illness and implementing objective sleep measurement methods combined with non-pharmacologic sleep promotion interventions are warranted [36]. Furthermore, in the vulnerable, often older, ICU population, all sleep aid medications convey risk, especially when continued beyond the ICU. Thus, while this may be a future intervention for a select patient group, extreme caution should be taken to minimize the dose and duration of their use.

4.4 Treatment Conclusions

ICU sleep disruption has multiple domains and diverse causes. Interventions have needed to include multiple components which raise challenges in implementation and sustainability of sleep promotion bundles. Furthermore, the call to personalize sleep promotion adds another component of complexity to intervention design. To effectively test and demonstrate improved outcomes for ICU patients, there needs to be a further evolution of bundled approaches to include patient, environmental, and acute illness factors linked to ICU sleep disruption. This requires multi-disciplinary stakeholder buy-in, monitoring processes, mechanisms to adapt to changes in the ICU, and implementation expertise to assure best testing and application of complex sleep promotion protocols. Finally, there needs to be a feasible way forward to adopt these interventions across critical care settings and thus provide broad benefit for ICU patients.

The best way forward may be leveraging entities such as the ICU ABCDEF bundle [117] which has proven benefit vis a vis delirium reduction and already contains established (e.g., pain and anxiety treatment) and proposed (e.g., early mobilization) elements of sleep promotion interventions. Adding more specific sleep and circadian promotion strategies (e.g., environmental control, clustering of care, daytime bright light) to the existing bundle may be an efficient means of moving ICU sleep promotion forward and further improving key, related outcomes such as delirium. Interestingly, the ABCDEF bundle may also promote daytime wake and daytime function which are likely important components of ICU sleep promotion despite limited evidence at this time.

5 Outcomes

Sleep and circadian rhythms play an important role in recovery from injury and illness. This has been demonstrated in acute, sub-acute and chronic sleep deprivation and restriction models [1]. As noted in the opening of this chapter short-term sleep loss negatively influences multiple essential organ systems with high relevance to critical illness recovery. This includes cognitive [2–6], respiratory [17–20], metabolic (7–9, cardiovascular [10–14], and immune [15, 16] function (chapter "Sleep Disruption and Its Relationship with ICU Outcomes"). Furthermore, in line with data demonstrating that habitual sleep quality and quantity is linked to mortality in the general population [118–120], emerging data suggests that acute sleep and circadian disruption may be linked to mortality in the ICU as well [55, 121]. As noted above, there is also concern that sleep disturbance in the ICU is part of longer-term sleep disturbance that starts with the onset of acute illness and continues during recovery (chapter "Long-Term Outcomes: Sleep in Survivors of Critical Illness"). Therefore, improving or protecting sleep and circadian function throughout the trajectory of critical illness may be beneficial in terms of a long list of critical illness outcomes.

5.1 Delirium

For many years, ICU sleep disruption has been hypothesized to be a modifiable risk factor for ICU delirium. Indeed, there have been some successes in reducing delirium via sleep promotion interventions [122]; the failure to demonstrate sleep improvement in these studies is hypothesized to be most likely due to measurement limitations although this remains to be proven. More recently, the relationship between sleep deficiency and delirium has been shown to be bidirectional [123, 124] and there may be synergy in designing interventions that address ICU sleep disruption and delirium concurrently (see also chapters "Sleep Disruption and Its Relationship with Delirium: Electroencephalographic Perspectives" and "Sleep

Disruption and Its Relationship with Delirium: Clinical Perspectives") as noted in the ABCDEF bundle discussion above.

5.2 Respiratory Failure

Improved sleep may also contribute to better respiratory outcomes while decrements in sleep may lead to poor respiratory outcomes. Studies in healthy volunteers have shown that sleep deprivation reduces respiratory and peripheral muscle endurance [17–20]. Studies have also shown that sleep disturbances are associated with failure to liberate from non-invasive [42] and invasive mechanical ventilation [125]. Interestingly, a recent study highlighted the relevance of having normal wakefulness patterns (closely related to sleep quality and quantity) at the time of liberation from mechanical ventilation [126]. Thus, adjusting ventilator modes within the constructs of lung protective ventilation strategies may improve sleep and respiratory outcomes. However, to date, studies are limited. Multiple open and closed loop ventilator modes have been used to achieve sleep relevant goals such as ventilator synchrony; however, it remains unclear if there is an optimal mode of ventilation vis a vis sleep promotion or if any mode which achieves physiologic goals (e.g., ventilator synchrony) is beneficial to sleep. Larger studies are needed before these modes can be implemented for sleep promotion.

5.3 Other Outcomes

Other outcomes of interest include metabolic, cardiovascular, and immune function. Nutritional intake in the setting of sleep deprivation and/or circadian misalignment are associated with glucose intolerance, an important critical care issue [7, 127]. Similarly, cardiovascular events due to acute sleep deprivation have been suggested by studies that show increased arrythmia risk and risk of cardiac death following sleep interruption [10, 11, 128]. Studies of immune function and sleep reveal that short sleep is associated with a higher risk of clinical illness and decreased vaccine response [129, 130]. These outcomes related to sleep and circadian disruption in alternate populations remain to be explored in ICU cohorts.

5.4 Long Term Outcomes

Finally, more than half of ICU survivors report sleep disturbance 6 months following ICU admission [131]. Given sleep's close association with the three domains of post intensive care syndrome (PICS) [132], cognition [2–4], mood [5, 6], and skeletal muscle strength [133], the interaction of poor sleep and PICS is likely to be significant. However, this critically important area remains relatively unexplored [134]. As noted above feasible, tolerable, rigorous longitudinal monitoring of sleep would be necessary to support such investigation (chapter "Methods for Routine Sleep Assessment and Monitoring").

6 Conclusions

Sleep and circadian rhythm disruption are pervasive in patients admitted to the ICU. Risk factors for and causes of ICU sleep and circadian disruption are numerous and include broad categories of patient, environmental, and acute illness factors. Based on studies in non-critically ill patients, there is tremendous potential for sleep promotion to improve critical care outcomes via improvements in cognitive, respiratory, cardiovascular, immune, and metabolic function. Though the lack of feasible, tolerable, rigorous objective methods to evaluate ICU sleep has slowed research progress, new technologies may soon overcome this barrier. Many unanswered questions remain regarding the natural history of sleep and circadian rhythm disruption during the acute and recovery phases of critical illness, yet there is hope that robust evidence supporting the use of multicomponent sleep promotion interventions is on the horizon. Moreover, well designed research into pharmacological interventions and long-term outcomes are needed. For more discussion on ICU sleep research priorities please refer to a recent research working group paper [135] and new sleep funding priorities from the National Institutes of Health [136].

References

1. Watson NF, Badr MS, Belenky G, Bliwise DL, Buxton OM, Buysse D, et al. Recommended amount of sleep for a healthy adult: a joint consensus statement of the American Academy of sleep medicine and Sleep Research Society. Sleep. 2015;38(6):843–4.
2. Killgore WD. Effects of sleep deprivation on cognition. Prog Brain Res. 2010;185:105–29.
3. Dinges DF, Pack F, Williams K, Gillen KA, Powell JW, Ott GE, et al. Cumulative sleepiness, mood disturbance, and psychomotor vigilance performance decrements during a week of sleep restricted to 4-5 hours per night. Sleep. 1997;20(4):267–77.
4. Lim J, Dinges DF. Sleep deprivation and vigilant attention. Ann N Y Acad Sci. 2008;1129:305–22.
5. Banks S, Dinges DF. Behavioral and physiological consequences of sleep restriction. J Clin Sleep Med. 2007;3(5):519–28.
6. Goldstein AN, Walker MP. The role of sleep in emotional brain function. Annu Rev Clin Psychol. 2014;10:679–708.
7. Spiegel K, Leproult R, Van Cauter E. Impact of sleep debt on metabolic and endocrine function. Lancet. 1999;354(9188):1435–9.

8. Spiegel K, Tasali E, Leproult R, Van Cauter E. Effects of poor and short sleep on glucose metabolism and obesity risk. Nat Rev Endocrinol. 2009;5(5):253–61.
9. Broussard JL, Ehrmann DA, Van Cauter E, Tasali E, Brady MJ. Impaired insulin signaling in human adipocytes after experimental sleep restriction: a randomized, crossover study. Ann Intern Med. 2012;157(8):549–57.
10. Miner SE, Pahal D, Nichols L, Darwood A, Nield LE, Wulffhart Z. Sleep disruption is associated with increased ventricular ectopy and cardiac arrest in hospitalized adults. Sleep. 2016;39(4):927–35.
11. Jiddou MR, Pica M, Boura J, Qu L, Franklin BA. Incidence of myocardial infarction with shifts to and from daylight savings time. Am J Cardiol. 2013;111(5):631–5.
12. Roenneberg T, Wirz-Justice A, Skene DJ, Ancoli-Israel S, Wright KP, Dijk DJ, et al. Why should we abolish daylight saving time? J Biol Rhythm. 2019;34(3):227–30.
13. Faraut B, Boudjeltia KZ, Vanhamme L, Kerkhofs M. Immune, inflammatory and cardiovascular consequences of sleep restriction and recovery. Sleep Med Rev. 2012;16(2):137–49.
14. Tobaldini E, Fiorelli EM, Solbiati M, Costantino G, Nobili L, Montano N. Short sleep duration and cardiometabolic risk: from pathophysiology to clinical evidence. Nat Rev Cardiol. 2019;16(4):213–24.
15. Spiegel K, Sheridan JF, Van Cauter E. Effect of sleep deprivation on response to immunization. JAMA. 2002;288(12):1471–2.
16. Prather AA, Janicki-Deverts D, Hall MH, Cohen S. Behaviorally assessed sleep and susceptibility to the common cold. Sleep. 2015;38(9):1353–9.
17. Chen HI, Tang YR. Sleep loss impairs inspiratory muscle endurance. Am Rev Respir Dis. 1989;140(4):907–9.
18. Cooper KR, Phillips BA. Effect of short-term sleep loss on breathing. J Appl Physiol Respir Environ Exerc Physiol. 1982;53(4):855–8.
19. Martin BJ. Effect of sleep deprivation on tolerance of prolonged exercise. Eur J Appl Physiol Occup Physiol. 1981;47(4):345–54.
20. Rault C, Sangare A, Diaz V, Ragot S, Frat JP, Raux M, et al. Impact of sleep deprivation on respiratory motor output and endurance. A physiological study. Am J Respir Crit Care Med. 2020;201(8):976–83.
21. Cappuccio FP, D'Elia L, Strazzullo P, Miller MA. Sleep duration and all-cause mortality: a systematic review and meta-analysis of prospective studies. Sleep. 2010;33(5):585–92.
22. Parthasarathy S, Vasquez MM, Halonen M, Bootzin R, Quan SF, Martinez FD, et al. Persistent insomnia is associated with mortality risk. Am J Med. 2015;128(3):268–75 e2.
23. Basner M, Dinges DF. Sleep duration in the United States 2003-2016: first signs of success in the fight against sleep deficiency? Sleep 2018;41(4).
24. Chattu VK, Manzar MD, Kumary S, Burman D, Spence DW, Pandi-Perumal SR. The global problem of insufficient sleep and its serious public health implications. Healthcare-Basel 2018;7(1).
25. Freedman NS, Kotzer N, Schwab RJ. Patient perception of sleep quality and etiology of sleep disruption in the intensive care unit. Am J Respir Crit Care Med. 1999;159(4):1155–62.
26. Elliott R, McKinley S, Cistulli P, Fien M. Characterisation of sleep in intensive care using 24-hour polysomnography: an observational study. Crit Care. 2013;17(2):R46.
27. Elliott R, Rai T, McKinley S. Factors affecting sleep in the critically ill: an observational study. J Crit Care. 2014;29(5):859–63.
28. Knauert MP, Yaggi HK, Redeker NS, Murphy TE, Araujo KL, Pisani MA. Feasibility study of unattended polysomnography in medical intensive care unit patients. Heart Lung. 2014;43(5):445–52.
29. Altman MT, Knauert MP, Pisani MA. Sleep disturbance after hospitalization and critical illness: a systematic review. Ann Am Thorac Soc. 2017;14(9):1457–68.
30. Gehlbach BK, Chapotot F, Leproult R, Whitmore H, Poston J, Pohlman M, et al. Temporal disorganization of circadian rhythmicity and sleep-wake regulation in mechanically ventilated patients receiving continuous intravenous sedation. Sleep. 2012;35(8):1105–14.

31. Maas MB, Lizza BD, Abbott SM, Liotta EM, Gendy M, Eed J, et al. Factors disrupting melatonin secretion rhythms during critical illness. Crit Care Med. 2020;48(6):854–61.
32. Dijk DJ, Czeisler CA. Contribution of the circadian pacemaker and the sleep homeostat to sleep propensity, sleep structure, electroencephalographic slow waves, and sleep spindle activity in humans. J Neurosci. 1995;15(5 Pt 1):3526–38.
33. Depner CM, Melanson EL, McHill AW, Wright KP Jr. Mistimed food intake and sleep alters 24-hour time-of-day patterns of the human plasma proteome. Proc Natl Acad Sci U S A. 2018;115(23):E5390–E9.
34. Allada R, Bass J. Circadian mechanisms in medicine. N Engl J Med. 2021;384(6):550–61.
35. Parthasarathy S, Tobin MJ. Sleep in the intensive care unit. Intensive Care Med. 2004;30(2):197–206.
36. Poongkunran C, John SG, Kannan AS, Shetty S, Bime C, Parthasarathy S. A meta-analysis of sleep-promoting interventions during critical illness. Am J Med. 2015;128(10):1126–37 e1.
37. Honarmand K, Rafay H, Le J, Mohan S, Rochwerg B, Devlin JW, et al. A systematic review of risk factors for sleep disruption in critically ill adults. Crit Care Med. 2020;48(7):1066–74.
38. Kamdar BB, Knauert MP, Jones SF, Parsons EC, Parthasarathy S, Pisani MA, et al. Perceptions and practices regarding sleep in the intensive care unit. A survey of 1,223 critical care providers. Ann Am Thorac Soc. 2016;13(8):1370–7.
39. Devlin JW, Skrobik Y, Gelinas C, Needham DM, Slooter AJC, Pandharipande PP, et al. Clinical practice guidelines for the prevention and Management of Pain, agitation/sedation, delirium, immobility, and sleep disruption in adult patients in the ICU. Crit Care Med. 2018;46(9):e825–e73.
40. Bosma K, Ferreyra G, Ambrogio C, Pasero D, Mirabella L, Braghiroli A, et al. Patient-ventilator interaction and sleep in mechanically ventilated patients: pressure support versus proportional assist ventilation. Crit Care Med. 2007;35(4):1048–54.
41. Trompeo AC, Vidi Y, Locane MD, Braghiroli A, Mascia L, Bosma K, et al. Sleep disturbances in the critically ill patients: role of delirium and sedative agents. Minerva Anestesiol. 2011;77(6):604–12.
42. Roche Campo F, Drouot X, Thille AW, Galia F, Cabello B, d'Ortho MP, et al. Poor sleep quality is associated with late noninvasive ventilation failure in patients with acute hypercapnic respiratory failure. Crit Care Med. 2010;38(2):477–85.
43. Thille AW, Reynaud F, Marie D, Barrau S, Rousseau L, Rault C, et al. Impact of sleep alterations on weaning duration in mechanically ventilated patients: a prospective study. Eur Respir J 2018;51(4).
44. Parthasarathy S, Tobin MJ. Effect of ventilator mode on sleep quality in critically ill patients. Am J Respir Crit Care Med. 2002;166(11):1423–9.
45. Cooper AB, Thornley KS, Young GB, Slutsky AS, Stewart TE, Hanly PJ. Sleep in critically ill patients requiring mechanical ventilation. Chest. 2000;117(3):809–18.
46. Drouot X, Roche-Campo F, Thille AW, Cabello B, Galia F, Margarit L, et al. A new classification for sleep analysis in critically ill patients. Sleep Med. 2012;13(1):7–14.
47. Watson PL, Pandharipande P, Gehlbach BK, Thompson JL, Shintani AK, Dittus BS, et al. Atypical sleep in ventilated patients: empirical electroencephalography findings and the path toward revised ICU sleep scoring criteria. Crit Care Med. 2013;41(8):1958–67.
48. Ambrogio C, Koebnick J, Quan SF, Ranieri M, Parthasarathy S. Assessment of sleep in ventilator-supported critically III patients. Sleep. 2008;31(11):1559–68.
49. Nieuwenhuijs D, Coleman EL, Douglas NJ, Drummond GB, Dahan A. Bispectral index values and spectral edge frequency at different stages of physiologic sleep. Anesth Analg. 2002;94(1):125–9.
50. Pedrao RAA, Riella RJ, Richards K, Valderramas SR. Viability and validity of the bispectral index to measure sleep in patients in the intensive care unit. Rev Bras Ter Intensiva. 2020;32(4):535–41.

51. Reinke L, van der Hoeven JH, van Putten MJ, Dieperink W, Tulleken JE. Intensive care unit depth of sleep: proof of concept of a simple electroencephalography index in the non-sedated. Crit Care. 2014;18(2):R66.
52. Dres M, Younes M, Rittayamai N, Kendzerska T, Telias I, Grieco DL, et al. Sleep and pathological wakefulness at the time of liberation from mechanical ventilation (SLEEWE). A prospective multicenter physiological study. Am J Respir Crit Care Med. 2019;199(9):1106–15.
53. Richards KC, O'Sullivan PS, Phillips RL. Measurement of sleep in critically ill patients. J Nurs Meas. 2000;8(2):131–44.
54. Gazendam JA, Van Dongen HP, Grant DA, Freedman NS, Zwaveling JH, Schwab RJ. Altered circadian rhythmicity in patients in the ICU. Chest. 2013;144(2):483–9.
55. Knauert MP, Murphy TE, Doyle MM, Pisani MA, Redeker NS, Yaggi HK. Pilot observational study to detect diurnal variation and misalignment in heart rate among critically ill patients. Front Neurol. 2020;11:637.
56. Beyer SE, Salgado C, Garçao I, Celi LA, Vieira S. Circadian rhythm in critically ill patients: insights from the eICU database. Cardiovascular Digital Health Journal. 2021;2(2):118–25.
57. Wittenbrink N, Ananthasubramaniam B, Munch M, Koller B, Maier B, Weschke C, et al. High-accuracy determination of internal circadian time from a single blood sample. J Clin Invest. 2018;128(9):3826–39.
58. Braun R, Kath WL, Iwanaszko M, Kula-Eversole E, Abbott SM, Reid KJ, et al. Universal method for robust detection of circadian state from gene expression. Proc Natl Acad Sci U S A. 2018;115(39):E9247–E56.
59. Maas MB, Iwanaszko M, Lizza BD, Reid KJ, Braun RI, Zee PC. Circadian gene expression rhythms during critical illness. Crit Care Med. 2020;48(12):e1294–e9.
60. McKinley S, Fien M, Elliott R, Elliott D. Sleep and psychological health during early recovery from critical illness: an observational study. J Psychosom Res. 2013;75(6):539–45.
61. Chong Y, Fryer CD, Gu Q. Prescription sleep aid use among adults: United States, 2005-2010. NCHS Data Brief. 2013;127:1–8.
62. Peppard PE, Young T, Barnet JH, Palta M, Hagen EW, Hla KM. Increased prevalence of sleep-disordered breathing in adults. Am J Epidemiol. 2013;177(9):1006–14.
63. Motamedi KK, McClary AC, Amedee RG. Obstructive sleep apnea: a growing problem. Ochsner J 2009;9(3).
64. Spurr K, Morrison DL, Graven MA, Webber A, Gilbert RW. Analysis of hospital discharge data to characterize obstructive sleep apnea and its management in adult patients hospitalized. in Canada: 2006 to 2007. Can Respir J 2010;17(5).
65. Goldstein C. Management of Restless Legs Syndrome/Willis-Ekbom disease in hospitalized and perioperative patients. Sleep Med Clin 2015;10(3).
66. Rosenberg RP, Krystal AD. Diagnosing and treating insomnia in adults and older adults. J Clin Psychiatry 2021;82(6).
67. Ding Q, Redeker NS, Pisani MA, Yaggi HK, Knauert MP. Factors influencing Patients' sleep in the intensive care unit: perceptions of patients and clinical staff. Am J Crit Care. 2017;26(4):278–86.
68. Louzon PR, Heavner MS, Herod K, Wu TT, Devlin JW. Sleep-promotion bundle development, implementation, and evaluation in critically ill adults: roles for pharmacists. Ann Pharmacother. 2022;56(7):839–49.
69. Hu RF, Jiang XY, Chen J, Zeng Z, Chen XY, Li Y, et al. Non-pharmacological interventions for sleep promotion in the intensive care unit. Cochrane Database Syst Rev 2015(10):CD008808.
70. Toublanc B, Rose D, Glerant JC, Francois G, Mayeux I, Rodenstein D, et al. Assist-control ventilation vs. low levels of pressure support ventilation on sleep quality in intubated ICU patients. Intensive Care Med. 2007;33(7):1148–54.
71. Cordoba-Izquierdo A, Drouot X, Thille AW, Galia F, Roche-Campo F, Schortgen F, et al. Sleep in hypercapnic critical care patients under noninvasive ventilation: conventional versus dedicated ventilators. Crit Care Med. 2013;41(1):60–8.

72. Kahn DM, Cook TE, Carlisle CC, Nelson DL, Kramer NR, Millman RP. Identification and modification of environmental noise in an ICU setting. Chest J. 1998;114(2):535–40.

73. van de Pol I, van Iterson M, Maaskant J. Effect of nocturnal sound reduction on the incidence of delirium in intensive care unit patients: an interrupted time series analysis. Intensive Crit Care Nurs. 2017;41:18–25.

74. Olson DM, Borel CO, Laskowitz DT, Moore DT, McConnell ES. Quiet time: a nursing intervention to promote sleep in neurocritical care units. Am J Crit Care. 2001;10(2):74–8.

75. Knauert MP, Pisani M, Redeker N, Murphy T, Araujo K, Jeon S, et al. Pilot study: an intensive care unit sleep promotion protocol. BMJ Open Respir Res. 2019;6(1):e000411.

76. Darbyshire JL, Müller-Trapet M, Cheer J, Fazi FM, Young JD. Mapping sources of noise in an intensive care unit. Anaesthesia 2019;74(8).

77. Darbyshire JL, Young JD. An investigation of sound levels on intensive care units with reference to the WHO guidelines. Crit Care. 2013;17(5):R187.

78. Knauert MP, Pisani M, Redeker N, Murphy T, Araujo K, Jeon S, et al. Pilot study: an intensive care unit sleep promotion protocol. BMJ Open Respiratory Res [Internet]. 2019;6(1):e000411.

79. Knauert M, Jeon S, Murphy TE, Yaggi HK, Pisani MA, Redeker NS. Comparing average levels and peak occurrence of overnight sound in the medical intensive care unit on A-weighted and C-weighted decibel scales. J Crit Care. 2016;36:1–7.

80. Gabor JY, Cooper AB, Hanly PJ. Sleep disruption in the intensive care unit. Curr Opin Crit Care. 2001;7(1):21–7.

81. Freedman NS, Gazendam J, Levan L, Pack AI, Schwab RJ. Abnormal sleep/wake cycles and the effect of environmental noise on sleep disruption in the intensive care unit. Am J Respir Crit Care Med. 2001;163(2):451–7.

82. Elbaz M, Leger D, Sauvet F, Champigneulle B, Rio S, Strauss M, et al. Sound level intensity severely disrupts sleep in ventilated ICU patients throughout a 24-h period: a preliminary 24-h study of sleep stages and associated sound levels. Ann Intensive Care. 2017;7(1):25.

83. Fan EP, Abbott SM, Reid KJ, Zee PC, Maas MB. Abnormal environmental light exposure in the intensive care environment. J Crit Care. 2017;40:11–4.

84. Lusczek ER, Knauert MP. Light levels in ICU patient rooms: dimming of daytime light in occupied rooms. J Patient Exp. 2021;8:23743735211033104.

85. Gao CA, Knauert MP. Circadian biology and its importance to intensive care unit care and outcomes. Semin Respir Crit Care Med. 2019;40(5):629–37.

86. Tamburri LM, DiBrienza R, Zozula R, Redeker NS. Nocturnal care interactions with patients in critical care units. Am J Crit Care. 2004;13(2):102–13.

87. Le A, Friese RS, Hsu CH, Wynne JL, Rhee P, O'Keeffe T. Sleep disruptions and nocturnal nursing interactions in the intensive care unit. J Surg Res. 2012;177(2):310–4.

88. Hu RF, Jiang X, Chen J, Zeng Z, Chen X, Li Y, et al. Non-pharmacological interventions for sleep promotion in the intensive care unit. Cochrane Database Syst Rev 2018.

89. Ewing R. The rest project: how penn medicine is helping patients sleep better in the hospital. https://www.pennmedicine.org/news/news-blog/2018/april/the-rest-project-how-penn-medicine-is-helping-patients-sleep-better-in-the-hospital https://www.pennmedicine.org/news/news-blog/2018/april/the-rest-project-how-penn-medicine-is-helping-patients-sleep-better-in-the-hospital: Penn Medicine News; 2018.

90. Richardson S. Effects of relaxation and imagery on the sleep of critically ill adults. Dimens Crit Care Nurs. 2003;22(4):182–90.

91. Wang YLWY. Effect of foot massage combined with the use of a Chinese herbal sleep pillow on sleep in coronary care unit patients. Journal of Qilu Nursing. 2012;18(1):38–9.

92. Chen JH, Chao YH, Lu SF, Shiung TF, Chao YF. The effectiveness of valerian acupressure on the sleep of ICU patients: a randomized clinical trial. Int J Nurs Stud. 2012;49(8):913–20.

93. Umbrello M, Sorrenti T, Mistraletti G, Formenti P, Chiumello D, Terzoni S. Music therapy reduces stress and anxiety in critically ill patients: a systematic review of randomized clinical trials. Minerva Anestesiol. 2019;85(8):886–98.

94. Su CP, Lai HL, Chang ET, Yiin LM, Perng SJ, Chen PW. A randomized controlled trial of the effects of listening to non-commercial music on quality of nocturnal sleep and relaxation indices in patients in medical intensive care unit. J Adv Nurs. 2013;69(6):1377–89.
95. Jaber S, Bahloul H, Guetin S, Chanques G, Sebbane M, Eledjam JJ. Effects of music therapy in intensive care unit without sedation in weaning patients versus non-ventilated patients. Ann Fr Anesth Reanim. 2007;26(1):30–8.
96. Meza S, Mendez M, Ostrowski M, Younes M. Susceptibility to periodic breathing with assisted ventilation during sleep in normal subjects. J Appl Physiol. 1998;85(5):1929–40.
97. Vaporidi K, Akoumianaki E, Telias I, Goligher EC, Brochard L, Georgopoulos D. Respiratory drive in critically ill patients. Pathophysiology and clinical implications. Am J Respiratory Crit Care Med. 2020;201(1):20–32.
98. Thille AW, Cabello B, Galia F, Lyazidi A, Brochard L. Reduction of patient-ventilator asynchrony by reducing tidal volume during pressure-support ventilation. Intensive Care Med. 2008;34(8):1477–86.
99. Delisle S, Ouellet P, Bellemare P, Tetrault JP, Arsenault P. Sleep quality in mechanically ventilated patients: comparison between NAVA and PSV modes. Ann Intensive Care. 2011;1(1):42.
100. Kamdar BB, King LM, Collop NA, Sakamuri S, Colantuoni E, Neufeld KJ, et al. The effect of a quality improvement intervention on perceived sleep quality and cognition in a medical ICU. Crit Care Med. 2013;41(3):800–9.
101. Tonna JE, Dalton A, Presson AP, Zhang C, Colantuoni E, Lander K, et al. The effect of a quality improvement intervention on sleep and delirium in critically ill patients in a surgical ICU. Chest 2021.
102. Knauert MP, Redeker NS, Yaggi HK, Bennick M, Pisani MA. Creating naptime: an overnight, nonpharmacologic intensive care unit sleep promotion protocol. J Patient Exp. 2018;5(3):180–7.
103. McNett M, O'Mathuna D, Tucker S, Roberts H, Mion LC, Balas MC. A scoping review of implementation science in adult critical care settings. Crit Care Explor. 2020;2(12):e0301.
104. Brown T, Brainard G, Cajochen C, Czeisler C, Hanifin J, Lockley S, et al. Recommendations for healthy daytime, evening, and night-time indoor light exposure. Preprints 2020. 2020.
105. Vetter C, Pattison PM, Houser K, Herf M, Phillips AJK, Wright KP, et al. A review of human physiological responses to light: implications for the development of integrative lighting solutions. Leukos 2021.
106. Engwall M, Fridh I, Johansson L, Bergbom I, Lindahl B. Lighting, sleep and circadian rhythm: an intervention study in the intensive care unit. Intensive Crit Care Nurs. 2015;31(6):325–35.
107. Taguchi T, Yano M, Kido Y. Influence of bright light therapy on postoperative patients: a pilot study. Intensive Crit Care Nurs. 2007;23(5):289–97.
108. Ono H, Taguchi T, Kido Y, Fujino Y, Doki Y. The usefulness of bright light therapy for patients after oesophagectomy. Intensive Crit Care Nurs. 2011;27(3):158–66.
109. Taguchi T. Bright light treatment for prevention of perioperative delirium in elderly patients. J Nurs Educ Pract. 2013;3:10–8.
110. Simons KS, Laheij RJ, van den Boogaard M, Moviat MA, Paling AJ, Polderman FN, et al. Dynamic light application therapy to reduce the incidence and duration of delirium in intensive-care patients: a randomised controlled trial. Lancet Respir Med. 2016;4(3):194–202.
111. Zhang KS, Pelleg T, Hussain S, Kollipara V, Loschner A, Foroozesh MB, et al. Prospective randomized controlled pilot study of high-intensity Lightbox phototherapy to prevent ICU-acquired delirium incidence. Cureus. 2021;13(4):e14246.
112. Hamidi A, Roberts RJ, Weinhouse GL, Szumita PM, Degrado JR, Dube KM, et al. Characterization of nocturnal neuroactive medication use and related sleep documentation in critically ill adults. Crit Care Explor. 2021;3(3):e0367.
113. Gandolfi JV, Di Bernardo APA, Chanes DAV, Martin DF, Joles VB, Amendola CP, et al. The effects of melatonin supplementation on sleep quality and assessment of the serum melatonin in ICU patients: a randomized controlled trial. Crit Care Med. 2020;48(12):e1286–e93.

114. Nishikimi M, Numaguchi A, Takahashi K, Miyagawa Y, Matsui K, Higashi M, et al. Effect of Administration of Ramelteon, a melatonin receptor agonist, on the duration of stay in the ICU: a single-center randomized placebo-controlled trial. Crit Care Med. 2018;46(7):1099–105.

115. Skrobik Y, Duprey MS, Hill NS, Devlin JW. Low-dose nocturnal Dexmedetomidine prevents ICU delirium. A randomized, placebo-controlled trial. Am J Respir Crit Care Med. 2018;197(9):1147–56.

116. Masuyama T, Sanui M, Yoshida N, Iizuka Y, Ogi K, Yagihashi S, et al. Suvorexant is associated with a low incidence of delirium in critically ill patients: a retrospective cohort study. Psychogeriatrics. 2018;18(3):209–15.

117. Society for Critical Care Medicine: ICU Liberation Bundle (A-F) [January 4, 2022]. Available from: https://www.sccm.org/Clinical-Resources/ICULiberation-Home/ABCDEF-Bundles.

118. Garcia-Perdomo HA, Zapata-Copete J, Rojas-Ceron CA. Sleep duration and risk of all-cause mortality: a systematic review and meta-analysis. Epidemiol Psychiatr Sci. 2019;28(5):578–88.

119. Stone CR, Haig TR, Fiest KM, McNeil J, Brenner DR, Friedenreich CM. The association between sleep duration and cancer-specific mortality: a systematic review and meta-analysis. Cancer Causes Control. 2019;30(5):501–25.

120. Grandner MA, Sands-Lincoln MR, Pak VM, Garland SN. Sleep duration, cardiovascular disease, and proinflammatory biomarkers. Nat Sci Sleep 2013;5.

121. Knauert MP, Gilmore EJ, Murphy TE, Yaggi HK, Van Ness PH, Han L, et al. Association between death and loss of stage N2 sleep features among critically ill patients with delirium. J Crit Care. 2018;48:124–9.

122. Flannery AH, Oyler DR, Weinhouse GL. The impact of interventions to improve sleep on delirium in the ICU: a systematic review and research framework. Crit Care Med. 2016;44(12):2231–40.

123. Sveinsson IS. Postoperative psychosis after heart surgery. J Thorac Cardiovasc Surg 1975;70(4).

124. Harrell RG, Othmer E. Postcardiotomy confusion and sleep loss. J Clin Psychiatry. 1987;48(11):445–6.

125. Thille AW, Muller G, Gacouin A, Coudroy R, Demoule A, Sonneville R, et al. High-flow nasal cannula oxygen therapy alone or with non-invasive ventilation during the weaning period after extubation in ICU: the prospective randomised controlled HIGH-WEAN protocol. BMJ Open. 2018;8(9):e023772.

126. Blackwell T, Kriesel DR, Vittinghoff E, O'Brien CS, Sullivan JP, Viyaran NC, et al. Design and recruitment of the randomized order safety trial evaluating resident-physician schedules (ROSTERS) study. Contemp Clin Trials. 2019;80:22–33.

127. Leproult R, Holmback U, Van Cauter E. Circadian misalignment augments markers of insulin resistance and inflammation, independently of sleep loss. Diabetes. 2014;63(6):1860–9.

128. Slomko J, Zawadka-Kunikowska M, Kozakiewicz M, Klawe JJ, Tafil-Klawe M, Newton JL, et al. Hemodynamic, autonomic, and vascular function changes after sleep deprivation for 24, 28, and 32 hours in healthy men. Yonsei Med J. 2018;59(9):1138–42.

129. Dengler V, Westphalen K, Koeppen M. Disruption of circadian rhythms and sleep in critical illness and its impact on innate immunity. Curr Pharm Des. 2015;21(24):3469–76.

130. Haspel JA, Anafi R, Brown MK, Cermakian N, Depner C, Desplats P, et al. Perfect timing: circadian rhythms, sleep, and immunity—an NIH workshop summary. Jci Insight 2020;5(1).

131. Altman MT, Knauert MP, Pisani MA. Sleep disturbances after hospitalization and critical illness: a systematic review. Annals of ATS. 2017; https://doi.org/10.1513/AnnalsATS.201702-148SR.

132. Inoue S, Hatakeyama J, Kondo Y, Hifumi T, Sakuramoto H, Kawasaki T, et al. Post-intensive care syndrome: its pathophysiology, prevention, and future directions. Acute Med Surg. 2019;6(3):233–46.

133. Prokopidis K, Dionyssiotis Y. Effects of sleep deprivation on sarcopenia and obesity: a narrative review of randomized controlled and crossover trials. J Frailty Sarcopenia Falls. 2021;6(2):50–6.
134. Luetz A, Grunow JJ, Morgeli R, Rosenthal M, Weber-Carstens S, Weiss B, et al. Innovative ICU solutions to prevent and reduce delirium and post-intensive care unit syndrome. Semin Respir Crit Care Med. 2019;40(5):673–86.
135. Knauert MP, Ayas N, Bosma K, Drouot X, Heavner MS, Owens RL, et al. ATS research statement: causes, consequences, and treatments of sleep and circadian disruption in the ICU. Am J Respir Crit Care Med. 2022 (under review).
136. Tactics to address research goals in sleep and circadian biology. NHLBI (accessed July 19, 2022). https://www.nhlbi.nih.gov/sleep-research-plan/research-tactics#:~:text=Promote%20 inclusion%20of%20more%20diverse%20patient%20populations%20with,Reduction%20 and%20Treatment%20of%20Sleep%20and%20Circadian%20Disorders.

Index

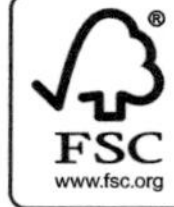